Herbal Prescriptions after 50

"Medical statistics clearly show that Americans are the most heavily medicated people in the world. In spite of this (or possibly because of this), we rank far below many other first world countries in life expectancy, cancer rates, levels of obesity, and many other chronic degenerative diseases. As our population ages many more people are realizing that in order to stay healthy into old age we need to become proactive, improving our diets and lifestyle choices, reducing stress, and becoming more knowledgeable about our health and medicine. One way we can help to prevent disease and enhance wellness is the intelligent use of herbs. Because few Americans grew up using plants as medicine, educating oneself as to their safe and rational use is essential. With so many books, Web sites, and magazines publishing information on herbs and natural health, how does one discern accurate information from the fraudulent? One answer is David Hoffmann's new book *Herbal Prescriptions after 50*. The author is one of the Western world's most respected clinical herbalists, and he offers the reader safe, effective, and relevant treatments for many of the ills that come with increasing age. If you are in your 50s, 60s, or 70s and want to prevent senior moments, menopausal symptoms, prostatic enlargement, and circulatory problems, some of the answers you are seeking can be found within these pages."

DAVID WINSTON, RH (AHG), AUTHOR OF
ADAPTOGENS: HERBS FOR STRENGTH, STAMINA, AND STRESS RELIEF

"This book of herbal recipes and restoratives will fascinate you. . . . Attractive and clearly written."

AMERICAN BOOKSELLER

"Herbal medicine can be as simple as brewing a pot of tea. However, knowing which herbs to use and how to use them requires experience, which Hoffmann amply provides. *Herbal Prescriptions after 50* gives authoritative answers to most of the commonly asked questions about when and how to use herbs medicinally."

NATURAL HEALTH

"Unlike most herbals, which summarize information, *Herbal Prescriptions after 50* takes the space to clearly explain what goes on in the body for each condition and how each suggested herb acts, deepening the reader's understanding of how to use and combine herbs medicinally."

BECCA HARBER, *THE VILLAGE HERBALIST*

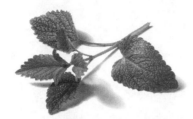

Herbal Prescriptions after 50

Everything You Need to Know to Maintain Vibrant Health

David Hoffmann, FNIMH, AHG

Healing Arts Press
Rochester, Vermont

Healing Arts Press
One Park Street
Rochester, Vermont 05767
www.HealingArtsPress.com

Healing Arts Press is a division of Inner Traditions International

Originally published in 1993 by Healing Arts Press under the title *An Elders' Herbal*
Revised and expanded second edition published in 2007 under the title *Herbal Prescriptions after 50*

Note to the reader: *This book is intended as an informational guide. The remedies, approaches, and techniques described herein are meant to supplement, and not to be a substitute for, professional medical care or treatment. They should not be used to treat a serious ailment without prior consultation with a qualified healthcare professional.*

Library of Congress Cataloging-in-Publication Data
Hoffmann, David, 1951–
  Herbal prescriptions after 50 : everything you need to know to maintain vibrant health / David Hoffmann. — Rev. and expanded 2nd ed.
      p. cm.
  Rev. ed. of: An elders' herbal. 1993.
  Summary: "A guide to herbal remedies that promote longevity and address the health concerns of the baby boom generation"—Provided by publisher.
  Includes bibliographical references and index.
  ISBN-13: 978-1-59477-180-4
  ISBN-10: 1-59477-180-4
  1. Herbs—Therapeutic use. 2. Older people—Diseases. 3. Older people—Health and hygiene. I. Hoffmann, David, 1951–. Elders' herbal. II. Title.
  RM666.H33H62 2007
  615'.321—dc22
                                                                          2007001882

Printed and bound in Canada by Transcontinental Printing
10 9 8 7 6 5 4 3 2 1

Text design by Rachel Goldenberg
This book was typeset in Sabon with OPTIPoster Bodoni as the display typeface

To send correspondence to the author of this book, mail a first-class letter to the author c/o Inner Traditions • Bear & Company, One Park Street, Rochester, VT 05767, and we will forward the communication.

For Dolores and Chris from their brother,
who will never grow up and get a real job!

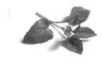

"Oh, well, a touch of grey
Kind of suits you anyway."

Robert Hunter and Jerry Garcia

My deepest thanks go to all the people who made this possible, but especially to Alan for stopping me on Main Street and seeding the idea in the first place; to Joel, Cherie, and Dylan for being such soul friends; and to Barry and Sue for so much support and help.

This country has yet to truly discover the profound wisdom and humanity of its herbalists that through some divine blessing I have encountered! Bless you all. For help and insights that are imbedded in my ramblings like gems in mud, special thanks to Rob McCaleb, Brigitte Mars, Kathi Keville, Jim Green, Jeannie Rose, Rosemary Gladstar, David Winston, Christopher Hobbs, Roy Upton, Mary Moss, Michael Tierra, and Autumn Summers.

Remember that none of this would have been possible without the Photosynthesis Angels.

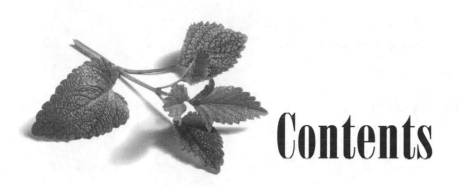

Contents

Foreword by Cheri Quincy, D.O.   xi

Introduction   1

Why Now   1

Holistic Medicine: The Healing Context   3

What Herbal Medicine Can Contribute   7

But Do Herbs Really Work?   10

The "Illness" of Health Care   20

Preventive Care   21

1. The Digestive System   22

The Healthy Digestive System   23

The Aging Digestive System   23

Herbal Actions   24

Keeping the Digestive System Healthy   26

Gastrointestinal Problem—Common and Serious   27

The Aging Colon and Its Problems   40

The Aging Liver and Its Problems   51

The Aging Gallbladder and Its Problems   53

2. The Cardiovascular System   56

Herbal Actions   56

Keeping the Cardiovascular System Healthy   60

Factors Contributing to Heart Disease   60

Cardiovascular Problems   64

3. The Pulmonary System   79

Herbal Actions   81

Pulmonary Problems   84

4. The Upper Respiratory System   96

Upper Respiratory Problems   96

5. The Nervous System   104

Herbal Actions   105

Stress and Its Impact on the Nervous System   110

Managing Stress   112

Nervous System Problems   121

6. The Urinary System   143

Signs of Kidney Disease   144

Herbal Actions   144

Keeping the Kidneys Healthy   145

Urinary Problems   146

7. The Reproductive System   156

The Female Reproductive System/Female Sexuality   157

Herbal Actions for the Female Reproductive System   157

Problems Specific to Women   160

The Male Reproductive System/Male Sexuality   166

Herbal Actions for the Male Reproductive System   168

Problems Specific to Men   169

8. The Musculoskeletal System — 172

Herbal Actions — 173

Musculoskeletal Problems — 182

9. The Skin and Hair — 197

The Skin and Its Functions — 197

The Aging Skin — 198

Herbal Actions — 199

Skin Problems — 200

Herbal "First Aid" for the Skin — 208

The Hair — 212

10. The Immune System — 213

Herbal Actions — 215

Immunological Actions — 219

Immune System Problems — 220

11. The Endocrine System — 229

The Adrenal Glands — 229

The Pancreas — 231

The Thyroid Gland — 233

12. Herbal Medicine Making — 237

Herbal Tea — 238

Tincture — 240

Dry Herb Preparations — 241

Formulations for the Skin — 242

13. Materia Medica   253

Useful Internet Addresses   317

Bibliography   321

Index   323

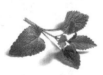

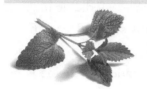

Foreword

Read this timely and delightful book for a comprehensive look at herbal health and take away a deepened understanding of a natural approach to more healthful aging. You will also get an appreciation for the personal power that results from an integrated relationship with the growing things of the earth. As an internist and geriatrician, I have been and am profoundly moved by the failures of preventive health care and the resulting helplessness of our aging population to manage their own symptoms. Though I began practicing in both hospital and outpatient settings in 1978, it was only after ten years of practice that I began to recognize the helpful role of phytotherapeutics in preventing, supporting, and toning aging metabolic systems. And it was another five years after that before I more directly experienced the remarkable help provided by herbal preparations (used in a complementary role) in acute or severe chronic conditions. David Hoffmann's encyclopedic knowledge and enthusiastic passion for his subject have provided much of the database supporting my observations of this realm of medical information.

Hoffmann's chapter on the nervous system is particularly of interest to a generation frequently living in fear of decreasing mental abilities, although only a minority will actually develop the pathological dementias of aging (Alzheimer's disease, multi-infarct dementia). Despite the demographic realities, many people suffer from fear of diminished capacities or will be profoundly affected by anxiety, loss of role in the family, situational depressions, or loneliness. Hoffmann recognizes the importance of control in the management of anxieties and stress and offers useful, self-controlled strategies for the development of adaptive responses to changing life situations, without falling into the traps of overgeneralization or oversimplification.

The chapter on herbal medicine making should appeal to all the frustrated chemists and cooks among us. The satisfaction that comes from preparing one's own concoctions, tinctures, ointments, and topicals is immense. Medicine making connects me with many earlier generations of wise herbalists, and I can, however briefly, assume that mantle of earthly healing knowledge. The independence engendered and the love transmitted by the gift of "home-made" medicine is no minor aspect of the path.

Herbal, holistic approaches also offer the family a chance to rediscover their herbal heritage and to begin building family lore and support for disorders and difficulties faced by all. Whenever the healing process can be a cooperative activity of an empowered, informed family, the potential for growth and increased richness of relationship may emerge along with recovery.

I invite you into this world of green, growing friends with enthusiasm. May you acquire many new helpers in the plant world and begin to feel a part of the garden into which you were born.

CHERI QUINCY, D.O.
INTERNAL MEDICINE AND GERIATRICS
SANTA ROSA MEDICAL GROUP
SANTA ROSA, CALIFORNIA

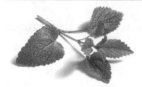# Introduction

You have in your hand a guide to using herbal medicines in addressing the health care needs of people over fifty. It emphasizes practical information that can be taken by anyone who wishes to use safe and effective herbs to promote wellness, prevent illness, and treat disease when necessary. It is not meant to replace professional medical help, and as a practical herbal, it makes no claim to be a comprehensive medical guide, stuffed with references and citations. The focus is the potential herbal contribution to ensuring a healthy aging process.

Why Now?

The Relevance of Herbal Medicine

- *It works!* This comes as a surprise to many people after years of being conditioned, by the medical and pharmaceutical establishment, to the idea that life was hell before the advent of steroids and antibiotics. Of course, there are limits to what herbalism can do, but within these limits herbalism is very effective.
- *It can be used in conjunction with other modalities.* There is no need to choose between therapies, as medicinal plants can be a part of any treatment plan.
- *It is environmentally clean.* Green issues and environmental awareness are finally becoming part of our culture's worldview, and more people recognize that green medicine is healthy for the individual and for the environment.

- *It possesses* viriditas. This Latin term (literally "the greening power") was coined by the medieval abbess and herbalist Hildegard of Bingen to describe the profoundly spiritual aspect of herbal remedies. The use of herbs allows us to experience the embrace of nature and, through it, the miraculous touch of the divine.
- *You can make friends with your medicine.* Herbalism offers the unique opportunity of developing a relationship with your medicine. People can grow their own herbs and get to know them.
- *We are undergoing an herbal renaissance.* A reawakening to the natural world is happening throughout our culture. One aspect is that herbalism is no longer considered to be weird or on the fringe of respectable knowledge, but is increasingly recognized as a valuable healing modality.

The Potential for Personal Transformation

- *Self-help and empowerment.* A sense of control over one's life and the experience of personal empowerment in taking responsibility for one's own health are vital. The simple skills of the herbalist offer such empowerment.
- *Relevance for aging hippies!* The generation that grew up thinking it could end the Vietnam war by 1969, banish world hunger by 1972, and heal the environment by 1990 can't even keep its cholesterol levels down! Many baby boomers are attracted to the natural world, but this tendency is being compromised more and more as they age and become greater medical consumers. The vision that was once so meaningful to so many can become more practically relevant through green medicine.

Societal Changes

- *A demographic shift in age.* The demographics of our culture point to an ever-increasing proportion of people over fifty. This is in marked contrast to what is arrogantly called the "Third World," which is characterized demographically by an increasingly *younger* population.
- *Rising health care costs.* The health care crisis facing society has created a situation in which few can afford insurance. Even when they can, it is often inadequate.

The Constraints of the Current Health System

- *Iatrogenic illness.* The United States is entering an ever-deeper health care crisis and paying the price for its infatuation with high-tech solutions. At a time when degenerative disease is reaching epidemic proportions, little or no attention is given to preventive approaches. Indeed, a new branch of medicine, called "iatrogenic medicine," now focuses on illness resulting from an action or attitude of a physician.
- **Orthodox Medical Treatment.** Orthodox medical treatment has been called "battlefield medicine" for good reason: it excels in emergencies and acute life threatening situations. Thank God that it does! However, this approach is inadequate to deal with the increasing challenge of chronic and degenerative illness. By contrast, herbalism offers the possibility of sustaining optimal health, in part due to its preventive capabilities.

Holistic Medicine: The Healing Context

The new understanding of health that has emerged over the past decades in both attitude and approach, often referred to as holistic medicine, promises to contribute many valuable insights to health care. What is "health" from this perspective? The World Health Organization has provided a definition that wonderfully sums up the perspective of holistic medicine: "Health is more than simply the absence of illness. It is the active state of physical, emotional, mental, and social well-being."

Holism assumes that health is a positive, active state and an inherent characteristic of whole and integrated human beings. From a holistic standpoint, a person is not a patient with a "disease syndrome," but a whole being. Thus the holistic therapist must appreciate not only the physical but also the mental, emotional, spiritual, social, and environmental aspects of his or her patients' lives. A holistic practitioner—of whatever specific therapy—has a deep respect for the individual's inherent capacity for self-healing. This respect in turn makes possible a relationship of active partnership in the healing process, rather than one of expert on one side and passive recipient on the other.

The therapeutic tradition of relating to the whole person is, of course, not new. Indeed, it is a part of the healer's heritage: ever since the teachings of Hippocrates every doctor, every herbalist, every nurse has been guided toward the deeply caring support of the patient. The reemphasis of this direction in holistic medicine today is simply an attempt to correct the tendency in modern medicine to equate health care with the treatment of a "disease entity." Holism does not predefine any medical technique or theory. It is a context in which the whole person is considered, his or her physical health as well as mental/emotional state, relationships, and life in the world. A medical doctor can be just as holistic as a medical herbalist or osteopath. The framework of holism embraces a wide range of therapeutic modalities, whether they are labeled "orthodox" or "alternative." All may be used in a relevant and coherent way while treating the whole of a person, not simply a set of symptoms or a syndrome picture.

Holistic medicine highlights the very personal nature of the healing process. An idea common to all holistically orientated therapists is that a human being is a self-healing individual; at best the medical practitioner merely facilitates this profound inner process. Addressing a pathological condition is a relatively straightforward matter, but as the World Health Organization's definition reminds us, health is much more than the absence of disease, it is an active state of well-being. Self-healing is the birthright of all, for at the core of our humanness is a spark of the divine that moves us toward wholeness and fulfillment. This approach does not negate the importance of medicine and the healing arts but provides a broad context within which to view them.

The self-healing individual is intrinsically part of what might be called a therapeutic ecology, whose various components are in relationship with each other and the wider world. The person is at the core of this therapeutic ecology, which in turn embraces four groups or branches of therapies.

The first branch comprises those techniques that involve taking some "medicine" for healing purposes. Approaches included here are medical herbalism, homeopathy, naturopathy, and drug-based allopathic medicine. All have in common the use of some physical medicine that is taken into the body to achieve a therapeutic goal. The specifics vary, of course, but all such medicines can be seen as fruits of the earth. Whether herb or synthesized drug, they share a common origin in the physical world.

Second is "bodywork," comprising those approaches that do something actively with or to the physical body. Structural factors are focused on as either causation of or contribution to illness. This area includes the manipulative therapies ranging from osteopathy and chiropractic to the many varieties of massage, as well as surgery.

The third therapeutic approach utilizes psychological techniques to identify and treat emotional and mental factors in health and disease. All the branches of psychotherapy are involved here, but especially the more holistically orientated approaches of humanistic and transpersonal psychology.

Finally, spiritual factors in human healing are increasingly recognized today even by materialistic Western medicine. This branch of therapy includes meditative and prayer-based techniques whereby the person aligns his or her being with higher spirit, and those whereby a practitioner works with the "energy body" of a patient.

Holism tells us to focus on an individual's unique situation and not simply treat a diagnosed disease syndrome. In the context of this therapeutic ecology it may be, for example, that one person diagnosed as having colitis will best respond to a treatment combining dietary advice, herbs, and osteopathic manipulation, while a second person will need drugs, psychoanalysis, and surgery.

Practitioners will have their firmly held opinions of the pros and cons concerning one approach or another, but the patient is always more important than any one doctor's belief system.

Such therapeutic interrelationships, based on a structure of mutual support, can compensate for any weaknesses inherent within a particular therapy. Homeopathic remedies will not put a fractured arm into a splint; neither do antibiotics. From a more positive perspective, cooperation can lead to synergistic support, with the whole of any treatment program being more than the sum of its parts. A geodesic relationship develops whereby extraordinary potential and strength can flow from cooperation between the therapies. Rather than giving rise to acrimonious debate and conflict, their differences can lead to a celebration of the richness of therapeutic diversity. The only fundamental obstacles to such a vision becoming a reality in our clinics are the egos of practitioners, professional organizations, and—most fundamentally—the profit motive of the medical power elite and drug companies.

This array of therapies simply represents different modalities within the broad "church" of medicine. With the healing professions changing rapidly, it would be a mistake to talk of medical herbalism as a form of alternative medicine. Is it an alternative to acupuncture, osteopathy, or psychiatry? Of course not; they complement each other, creating a complex of relationships in which the whole is much more than the sum of the parts. In light of the unique strengths and weaknesses offered by each approach, mutual support and cooperation is the way toward a truly holistic health service. All medical modalities are complementary within the perspective of the patient's needs.

Language often blocks communication and shared endeavor in medicine. Apparent disparities in vocabulary may mask fundamental agreements of ideas and approach. On the other hand, lack of clarity obscures important differences in both guiding principles and technique. All too many people have a dogmatic attachment to words and specific formulations of belief, opinion, and theory, assuming that if the "correct" words or phrases are not used, the speaker must be wrong!

Entrenched confrontation between dedicated allopathic practitioners and dedicated holistic practitioners becomes irrelevant when seen in the context of therapeutic ecology. Open-mindedness and tolerance should be characteristics common to all involved in health care, whether as practitioners, researchers, or patients. Medical modalities that have their foundations outside the biomedical model should not be ignored or discounted simply because they exemplify a different belief system or challenge the status quo. They should be respected as an enrichment of possibilities.

Everyone involved in health care provision can benefit by such a mutually supportive environment. Health service administrators will appreciate the economic savings gleaned from a drop in dependence upon costly medical technology. A proportion of procedures and treatments that currently utilize expensive drugs or surgery can be replaced by more appropriate techniques from another healing modality. For example, most run-of-the-mill gallbladder removals can be avoided by using herbs or homeopathic remedies, certain costly orthopedic techniques could be replaced with skilled osteopathy.

What is the contribution of medical herbalism to this healing framework? An enduring strength of herbalism lies in the fact that it is deeply rooted in traditional healing on the one hand and relates fully to modern science and medicine on the other. Paradoxically, herbalism is both a wonderfully simple and staggeringly complex therapy. Its simplicity is reflected in the ease of picking cleavers from a hedgerow or chewing on a stem of chickweed; its complexity is seen in research that attempts to grasp the processes that underlie the multitude of biochemical interactions between a plant's chemical constituents and the metabolic basis of human physiology. The degree and depth of interaction are breathtaking.

Practitioners of medical herbalism have the unique possibility of introducing their patients to their medicine! A bridge can be built between person and herb, empowering patients to be present and responsible in the healing process. They can be given packets of herb seeds, thus receiving a direct experience of the life of the plant. This experience of herbal vitality will be translated into a deeper rapport with the otherwise impersonal "medicine" they take. Patients will receive not only the medical benefit from the herb but also the enlivening experience of growing and preparing their own healing. If there is no garden, part of the treatment might involve a window box.

What Herbal Medicine Can Contribute

Herbalism offers such an array of health care benefits, I should start by pointing out what it does *not* offer. This is a book about using herbs to augment wellness and treat illness—not about magic bullets and "miracle herbs." Its goal is to contribute to a meaningful and fulfilling improvement in the quality of an individual's life rather than to a cumulative year count.

The more extreme proponents of what has been called the longevity movement suggest that aging is simply the consequence of bad nutrition and cramped vision, and herbs are touted as part of their approach to "life extension." An entire industry of expensive products has rapidly emerged to address the delusions of the consumer obsessed with living a long life. I must acknowledge my personal bias on these issues because of the very high cost of these products, and because of the tendency in these circles to see illness as something a person creates or attracts into his or her own life. On some level this may well be true, as illness can be a profound gift or a learning opportunity, but this insight has been distorted into a potent tool for intimidation and profit as well as a source of guilt and judgment.

Appropriate nutrition can do much to improve the quality of life and health in general and relieve specific illnesses. Vision and spirituality have a similarly important role in human life. I deeply respect this role but recall that the Bible says "Without vision the people die," *not* that with vision the people live forever. The fundamental importance of vision and spirituality is qualitative, not quantitative, and by bringing such qualities into our lives we heal and transform ourselves and the world around us. Living for a longer chronological span is beside the point.

The search for so-called longevity herbs (often expensive imported herbs) is not unlike hunting the rhinoceros to near-extinction for its horn. This small example of humanity's environmental rampage is fueled by a worldwide market for the supposedly aphrodisiac horn. One view of this is of men who, seeking to regain their lost youth, cause rhinos to be killed—could this be death by testosterone poisoning? There are many herbal parallels. The Brazilian suma plant *(Pfaffia paniculata)* has recently become popular as an "immunostimulant." Quite apart from the question of its efficacy is the fact that this vine is collected from gullies and water runoff in the Brazilian rain forest—gullies that are highly sensitive to erosion and disturbance. Isn't it ironic that in their search for increased health and longer life, longevity herbalists may be contributing to rain forest destruction, the greenhouse effect, and thus a potentially dramatic reduction in the life span of their children and grandchildren?

Although many of these "longevity herbs" are often therapeutically useful, the concept of longevity is unreal. As discussed earlier, health is an aspect of the whole system, and humanity does not live in a vacuum but within its many cultures and the planetary environment. The nurture of health in any meaningful way goes beyond high-tech intensive care devices or "longevity herbs" to take into account the health of family, society, and environment. Our culture's lunge for more-faster-easier convenience is killing us and our world, and no new "miracle" herbs will stop that. We ourselves must stop it.

Many herbalists and supplement manufacturers have jumped on the bandwagon, generating pages and pages of "information" that are fit only for the tabloid newspapers. Fortunately there are some important, noteworthy exceptions. Consider these ideas from Rob McCaleb, director of the Herb Research Foundation:

> Life extension is not so mysterious as finding secret longevity pills. By and large, it involves identifying the major predictable causes of death, and, reducing the risk that you will fall prey to them. In America, our major causes of death are heart disease and cancer. The third leading cause of death—excluding accidents—is pneumonia and influenza, but this is often a euphemism for "dying of old age." People who survive to an advanced age frequently die of pneumonia developing as a complication during bouts with influenza or cold viruses, which leave their defenses weakened. Liver disease is fourth, followed by diabetes. Herbs and other dietary supplements can help us avoid succumbing to these diseases, or at least lessen or delay them. The strategy is simple: identify the risks and minimize them.
>
> - *Protect your heart and arteries.* Beneficial effects of herbs include lowering blood fat levels, including cholesterol; improving the ratio of high density to low density cholesterol; "thinning" the blood to resist clots, heart attack, and stroke; and cardiac tonification, strengthening and slowing the heartbeat.

- *Reduce cancer risk.* Many herbs are anticarcinogens or stimulate the immune system, increasing your body's ability to detect and destroy aberrant cells.
- Protect yourself against damage from pollutants and radiation; contaminants in food, water, and air; and self-inflicted pollutants like alcohol.
- *Take advantage of the general protective effects of antioxidants and "free-radical scavengers."* These eliminate highly reactive ions in our cells that can cause liver damage and cell mutations.
- *Reduce your stress and improve sleep.*
- *Increase your resistance to infectious disease,* including colds and flu.

I could not agree with Mr. McCaleb more when he locates the herbal contribution of remedies that reduce the identifiable risks. As will become clear in the book, this can be achieved with safe, effective, and relatively inexpensive herbal remedies. He goes on to identify some important remedies that can contribute to achieving this goal. (All of them will be discussed again later in this book.)

- *Astragalus:* A nonspecific stimulant to the immune system that promotes healthy activity of all its diverse functions.
- *Echinacea:* One of the best-known herbal antimicrobials, it effectively increases resistance to infections.
- *Garlic:* Garlic is a wonderful remedy with a range of useful actions. As an antimicrobial herb it helps the immune system resist and deal with infections. It lowers blood cholesterol levels and elevated blood pressure. There is increasing evidence that it possesses some antitumor activity.
- *Ginkgo:* This ancient plant stimulates peripheral and cerebral circulation and increases oxygen availability to the brain. It also has antioxidant properties.
- *Ginseng and Siberian ginseng:* These contain effective adaptogens that help the body cope with stress.
- *Hawthorn:* The safest of the herbal heart remedies, it dilates the coronary arteries, lowers blood pressure and cholesterol levels, and generally strengthens heart tone.
- *Milk thistle:* Possibly the most important herb for treating or preventing liver damage due to toxins or liver disease.
- *Valerian:* An example of a group of herbs that help ensure a deep and revivifying sleep.

But Do Herbs Really Work?

In light of cultural amnesia and modern medical disdain for natural therapics, no one will be blamed for asking whether herbs actually work! In fact, plants can play an important part in health care, but this does not mean that herbs are always the preferable therapy of choice. Herbalism is *not* the best technique when one is troubled with a broken arm or with a life-threatening infection such as meningitis. The diversity of health care techniques available is something to celebrate, not a cause for conflict and exclusivity. All can work together and support each other. The strengths of one technique can support the weaknesses of another with much mutual benefit when cooperation rather than dogmatic conflict is the keynote. The needs of the patient are always more important than the beliefs of the practitioner!

Herbs can play a unique role in all healing work. Any health problem that is medically treatable will benefit from herbal therapy, but it is especially relevant in preventive medicine and the treatment of chronic illness. For most common acute medical problems it will also be useful, but the herbs may not act fast enough or be sufficiently specific in their mode of action. This is especially the case with acute infections. Yet, with degenerative diseases of all kinds reaching epidemic proportions throughout the Western world, herbal therapeutics may now be coming into their own. Diseases that reflect a degenerative breakdown within the body, such as osteoarthritis, respond badly to orthodox treatments but may do well with appropriate herbal therapy.

How do these remedies work? Usually there is no answer to this question because academic research to find a mechanism to explain the clinical findings has not been undertaken. This may be because no researcher has been interested or funded, or because the factors involved are so complex that coherent analysis is almost impossible.

Demonstrating or "proving" herbal efficacy is not always straightforward. The first step is to ascertain what form the "proof" needs to be in for the person concerned! Some need only have the subjective experience of personal benefit gained from using herbal medicine, or the similarly subjective observation of another's experience. For the medical establishment, and for the many who perceive the world from this perspective, however, such subjective experiences are invalid. There must be some objective, quantifiable, and reproducible data—laboratory or clinical findings that are then put through statistical analysis—so that evidence and proof become a dispassionate mathematical process rather than a messy human one. Thus, the striving for scientific objectivity has obscured the reality of working with human beings with all their diversity and idiosyncrasies.

A book like this one is not the place to explore the strengths and weaknesses of the scientific method. However, some clear problems arise for the medical herbalist in a world where the arbiters of medical veracity still consider statistical methodology to be the only valid measurement of truth.

On the most basic experiential level, it is often easy to show that herbs "work"—in other words, that there are a range of remedies with a demonstrable impact upon human physiology. One of the most widely used plants in the world is senna, a laxative that works within twelve hours of ingestion through its biochemical triggering of peristalsis, the muscular contractions along the colon that lead to an emptying of the bowels. This effect does not involve belief, placebo effect, or even knowledge that the herb has been ingested. Similarly, the leaves of the common dandelion have a strong diuretic effect. The plant's French name *pissenlit* hints at this function. Not an herb to take last thing at night!

The medical herbalists of the world have abundant evidence that their remedies work, as does the person using senna for constipation. However, the professional journals of medicine and science also provide a wealth of evidence. Anyone who considers herbalism quackery, or herbs placebo medicine at best, is simply demonstrating ignorance.

Choosing Herbs for Health

The therapeutic possibilities of herbal medicine in the hands of skilled professionals become most exciting when herbs are used to augment and nurture that which is "well." The deep toning, nutritional, and functional support that herbs often provide can particularly help the body in times of formidable change. A challenge for the medical herbalist is to transcend our conditioned perception of herbs as medicines suited for symptomatic relief only.

The alleviation of distress and suffering through treatment of symptoms such as pain or inflammation is certainly a vital role for the practitioner. Yet healing is not simply a matter of easing symptoms but a deeper process that must address pathology, psychology, and even spirituality. In the hands of a practitioner with the personal integrity and insight to embrace the holistic perspective, herbal remedies can bring about profound physical transformations, supporting the body's innate striving to heal itself and move toward greater well-being.

Unfortunately, much modern herbalism remains mired in the allopathic mold that has affected medical practice for the past sixty years. Perhaps the problem with herbal medicine is that it *does* work! Too often the practitioner uses herbs to treat a surface manifestation while avoiding the challenges of the holistic approach. The patient experiences the removal of symptomatic discomfort and even the "curing" of the disease, but the profound healing that is the goal of holistic medicine does not occur. Using the earth's wealth of herbal medicines in a broad context opens possibilities for practitioners of all therapeutic modalities to work with the body and its metabolism in a safe yet profoundly transforming way.

Nothing inherent in a plant defines the way it should be used. Such a wealth of herbs is provided by the earth that some coherent selection criteria are essential to guide herbalists in their healing work. Well over half a million plant species are thought to be sharing the planet with us. A British medical herbalist routinely uses 250 species, whereas a Chinese herbal practitioner has about 2,000 readily available in community pharmacies. Some set of guidelines is obviously being applied to whittle down 500,000 to a more manageable figure, but what is it? There are a number of useful ways to group the relevant criteria, but three categories are most helpful in Western herbalism:

- Assessment of each herb's impact upon the body and mind
- Use of herbs within the context of a system of some kind
- Nontherapeutic criteria such as aesthetics, economics, and ecology

Applying these three sets of criteria facilitates the formulation of treatments that can be wholly specific for an individual's unique needs and at the same time environmentally sensitive and economically reasonable. We will review each of them in more detail below.

Assessment of the Herb's Impact

The herbal remedies of the world vary in strength from potential poisons (if taken at the wrong dosage) to gentle remedies that might be considered foods. The herbalist works with the underlying idea that the body is self-healing and the therapist simply supports this innate healing process. *Thus, the tonic herbs are of paramount importance, as this is exactly what they do.* Tonics are gentle remedies, having a mild yet profound effect upon the body. Not *all* herbal remedies are tonics, of course. Many have such a powerful impact upon human physiology that they must be used with the greatest respect, being reserved for those illnesses that necessitate strong medicine.

By identifying the intensity of an herb's impact upon the individual, a useful selection criteria is found. The remedies may be categorized as either normalizers or effectors.

NORMALIZERS

Normalizers are remedies that nurture the body in ways that support inherent processes of growth, health, and renewal. These are the tonic herbs mentioned above, which are often seen as "herbal foods." The value of tonic herbs lies first in their normalizing, nurturing effects, yet these invaluable remedies usually have some associated action that further indicates their *best* use. An excellent example is the cardiovascular tonic hawthorn, which tones the whole system while specifically dilating blood vessels and lowering blood pressure. Whenever possible, the herbalist focuses on the use of such remedies; stronger effectors are used only when absolutely necessary. The chemically based effectors—the foundation of modern allopathic medicine—are rarely used at all.

Tonics and gentle normalizer remedies not only avoid most side-effect complications but offer possibilities for the maintenance of wellness and the prevention of many problems associated with aging. Indeed, the tonics can play a specific role in ensuring that an individual maintains a personal peak of health and vitality. This state of well-being will vary from person to person, but any individual should sense an improvement in his or her general experience of life. Tonics may also be used specifically to ward off a known health problem or a family weakness by addressing a specific system of the body. Examples of remedies that act as tonics for the various systems of the body are listed below.

- *Cardiovascular:* Hawthorn, ginkgo, and garlic.
- *Digestive:* No one herb is an all-around tonic, as the digestive system is so varied in its form and functions. The bitter tonics are often helpful: examples are gentian, agrimony, and dandelion root. Chamomile and meadowsweet are so generally useful to the digestive process that they may also be considered as general tonics here.

- *Infection:* Garlic, echinacea, and system-specific antimicrobials such as bearberry for the urinary system.
- *Liver:* Bitter tonics, hepatics, and especially milk thistle.
- *Musculoskeletal:* Celery seed, bogbean, and nettle will help prevent any systemic problems manifest as disease in this system. Horsetail can help strengthen bones and connective tissue.
- *Nervous:* Oats, skullcap, St. John's wort, vervain, and mugwort are all excellent tonic remedies.
- *Reproductive:* For women, consider raspberry leaves, false unicorn root, and other uterine tonics; for men, use saw palmetto, and possibly sarsaparilla.
- *Respiratory:* Mullein, elecampane, and coltsfoot.
- *Skin:* Cleavers, nettle, red clover, and most of the alterative remedies (see pages 198–99) will help.
- *Urinary:* Bearberry and corn silk.

EFFECTORS

Effectors are remedies that have an observable impact upon the body. Used in the treatment of the whole range of human illnesses, they can be divided into the two following groups depending upon how they work.

- *Whole plant actions.* Here the effects are those of the whole plant upon the human body. An example would be the antimicrobial remedy echinacea or the anti-inflammatory herb meadowsweet.
- *Specific active chemicals.* In such cases a specific impact is so overpowering that whole plant effects are not usually seen. Such intense chemicals are potentially poisonous if taken in the wrong dosage or in the wrong way. The cardioactive herb foxglove and the opium poppy are examples.

Using Herbs in a Holistic Context

The medical herbalist formulates prescriptions based on a model that addresses the needs of the whole person. The herbal component must be used in a context of nonherbal factors such as diet, lifestyle, and emotional, mental, and spiritual factors—all within a specific socioeconomic context. Such a model enables the practitioner to identify and address a whole range of issues, from symptoms and disease pathology to constitution and whole-body toning.

This model is not new; little is truly new in such an ancient field as herbalism! Rather, it is a formulation of well-established and proven approaches described in holistic terms. Choosing specific remedies from the vast range that nature offers can be a daunting task. The herbalist/prescriber must first have a basic grasp of human physiology and the disease process and then take into account the following five factors: herbal actions; system affinity; specific remedies for the illness in question; herbal biochemistry; and intuition.

HERBAL ACTIONS

Herbal actions are the ways by which the specific remedy or remedies affects human physiology. Since plants have a direct impact on physiological activity, by knowing what body process you want to help or heal, the appropriate action can be selected. Obviously the selection of actions that are suitable for a specific person will depend on accurate diagnosis.

Much pharmaceutical research has gone into analyzing the active constituents of herbs to find out how and why they work. A much older, and far more relevant, approach is to categorize herbs according to the kinds of problems they help to treat. In some cases the action is due to a specific chemical in the herb (as with the antiasthmatic effects of ma huang); in others, it is due to a complex synergistic interaction between various constituents of the plant (as with the sedative valerian). However, it is best to view the actions as attributes of the whole herb, and any understanding of the chemistry as simply an aid in prescription. Actions are the basis for remedy selection used throughout this book, and they are as follows:

Adaptogen: These herbs increase resistance and resilience to stress, enabling the body to avert various problems and avoid collapse by adapting to external pressures. Adaptogens work through support of the adrenal glands. Examples include Siberian ginseng and panax ginseng.

Alterative: These herbs gradually restore proper functioning of the body, increasing health and vitality. Some alteratives support natural waste elimination via the kidneys, liver, lungs, or skin. Others stimulate digestive function or are antimicrobial, while others "just work." Examples include burdock and cleavers.

Anticatarrhal: Anticatarrhals help the body remove excess mucus, whether in the sinus area or elsewhere in the body. Catarrh is not of itself a problem, but when too much mucus is produced it is usually in response to an infection or serves as a way to remove excess carbohydrate from the body. Examples include goldenrod and eyebright.

Anti-inflammatory: These plants soothe inflammations or directly reduce the inflammatory condition of the tissue. They work in a number of different ways but will rarely inhibit the inflammatory reaction as such; rather, they support and encourage the body's natural processes. Examples include chamomile, meadowsweet, and wild yam.

Antimicrobial: Antimicrobials help the body to destroy or resist pathogenic microorganisms. They help the body strengthen its own resistance to infective organisms and throw off illness. While some contain antiseptic chemicals or act as specific poisons to certain organisms, in general they boost the body's natural immunity. Examples include echinacea and garlic.

Antispasmodic: Antispasmodics ease muscle cramps, alleviate muscular tension, and, as many are also nervines, can ease psychological tension as well. Some antispasmodics reduce muscle spasm throughout the body; others work on specific organs or systems. Examples include cramp bark and valerian.

Astringent: Astringents have a binding action on mucous membranes, skin, and other tissue, due to chemicals called tannins (after their use in the tanning industry). Such herbs have the effect of precipitating protein molecules and thus reducing irritation and inflammation by creating a barrier against infection (especially helpful in wounds and burns). Examples include agrimony and oak bark.

Bitter: Herbs with a bitter taste have a special role in preventive medicine. The taste triggers a sensory response in the central nervous system, releasing digestive hormones that in turn lead to a range of effects including stimulation of appetite; general stimulation of the flow of digestive juices; increased bile flow, an aid in the liver's detoxification work; and stimulation of the gut's self-repair mechanisms. Examples include agrimony and gentian.

Cardiac remedies: This is a general term for herbal remedies with a beneficial action on the heart. Some of the remedies in this group are powerful cardioactive agents such as foxglove, whereas others are gentler, safer herbs such as hawthorn and motherwort.

Carminative: Plants that are rich in aromatic volatile oils stimulate the digestive system to work properly. They soothe the gut wall, reduce any inflammation present, ease griping pains, and help to remove gas from the digestive tract. Examples include lemon balm and peppermint.

Demulcent: Herbs rich in mucilage soothe and protect irritated or inflamed tissue. They reduce irritation down the whole length of the bowel; reduce sensitivity to potentially corrosive gastric acids; help to prevent diarrhea and reduce the muscle spasms that cause colic; ease coughing by soothing bronchial tension; and relax painful spasm in the bladder. Examples include marshmallow and slippery elm.

Diaphoretic: These herbs promote perspiration, the process of elimination of waste through the skin; thus they help to ensure a clean and harmonious inner environment. Some produce observable sweat, while others aid normal perspiration. Diaphoretics often promote dilation of surface capillaries and thus help to improve poor circulation. They support the work of the kidney by increasing cleansing through the skin. Examples include boneset and ginger.

Diuretic: Diuretics increase the production and elimination of urine. In herbal medicine, with its ancient traditions, the term is also often applied to herbs that have a beneficial action on the urinary system. They help the body eliminate waste and support the whole process of inner cleansing. Examples include dandelion and bearberry.

Emmenagogue: Emmenagogues stimulate menstrual flow and activity. In most herbals, however, the term is used in the wider sense of a remedy that normalizes and tones the female reproductive system. Examples include false unicorn root and pennyroyal.

Expectorant: Strictly speaking, these herbs stimulate removal of mucus from the lungs, but the term is often used to refer to any tonic for the respiratory system. Stimulating expectorants "irritate" the bronchioles, thereby causing expulsion of material. Relaxing expectorants soothe bronchial spasm and loosen mucous secretions, helping in cases of dry, irritating cough. Examples include mullein and horehound.

Hepatic: Hepatics aid the liver. They tone, strengthen, and in some cases increase the flow of bile. In a broad holistic approach to health they are of great importance because of the fundamental role of the liver in the working of the body. Examples include dandelion root and gentian.

Hypotensive: These plant remedies lower abnormally elevated blood pressure. Examples include hawthorn and linden blossom.

Laxative: Laxatives stimulate bowel movements. However, stimulating laxatives should never be used long term. If this appears to be necessary, then diet, general health, and stress should all be closely considered. Examples include senna and yellow dock.

Nervine: Nervines help the nervous system and can be meaningfully subdivided into three groups. Nervine *tonics* strengthen and restore the nervous system. Nervine *relaxants* ease anxiety and tension by soothing both body and mind. Nervine *stimulants* directly stimulate nerve activity. Examples of relaxing nervines include skullcap and valerian.

Rubefacient: Herbs in this category generate a localized increase in blood flow when applied to the skin and thereby promote healing, cleansing, and nourishment. They are often used to ease the pain and swelling of arthritic joints. Examples include mustard and ginger.

Tonic: The tonic herbs are gentle remedies that nurture and enliven. See the description and examples on pages 13–14.

Vulnerary: These remedies promote wound healing. The term is mainly used to refer to herbs for skin lesions, yet the action is just as relevant for wounds such as stomach ulcers. Examples include comfrey and calendula.

TONIC AFFINITY

Some herbs show a tonic *affinity* for certain organs, body systems, or even specific types of tissue. They work as specific tonics or nutrients for the areas involved. Many herbs can be used freely and safely as part of one's lifestyle without thinking of them as "medicines." They are at their best when used to nurture health and vitality. During illness the system affinity herbs will enhance the general health of the organ or system concerned when combined with remedies selected for their specific actions. They are especially useful where a tendency toward illness is recognized but no overt disease is present. In this way herbs may help to overcome a weakness that could lead to disease later in life.

SPECIFIC REMEDIES

The wealth of herbal knowledge that has been garnered over many generations is rich in plants that are traditionally *specific* in the treatment of certain diseases or symptoms. While holistic healing aims at going beyond symptomatic therapy, knowledge of specific remedies can add much to a prescription based on appropriate herbal action and system support.

HERBAL BIOCHEMISTRY

Increasing attention is being given to the *biochemistry* of herbal active constituents. This has led to the development of many lifesaving drugs but is limited as an approach to using whole plants. In the hands of an experienced herbalist, knowledge of plant pharmacology can add to the healing possibilities, but not as much as is often thought.

INTUITION

There is a flowering of *intuitive* rapport between herbalists and their plants. Intuition has a special role to play in healing, and the unique relationship between plant and person augments it well. Rarely can such insightful intuition be made to flow, but it should be embraced when it does. Intuitive knowledge should always be verified if at all possible. For example, if a practitioner is not clear on the difference between bearberry, barberry, and bilberry, it might lead to an unfortunate misunderstanding!

Nontherapeutic Criteria

In addition to the therapeutic criteria used to select a herbal remedy or remedies, further help in selecting an herbal remedy may be obtained by considering a number of *nontherapeutic* factors.

AESTHETIC CRITERIA

There is no reason for herbal medicines to always taste unpleasant! When the choice arises, do take into account taste, aroma, and visual appeal. Such factors are a matter of personal taste, and it is fine to select herbs from among those indicated by a combination of therapeutic criteria and personal aesthetic preference. Bitter herbs make the only general exception here: if bitterness is indicated, then the bitterness must be actually tasted; otherwise the healing value is lost.

An example is a cough remedy widely used in France, composed of the flowers of herbs that ease the cough reflex and help remove phlegm from the lungs. It is straightforward enough to make an herbal cough mixture that works well, but such effective combinations are often composed of acrid or unpleasant-tasting plants. In this case, the same therapeutic results are achieved, but in addition there is a wonderful aroma, a delicate taste, and beautiful color.

ECONOMIC CRITERIA

Ideally, herbs should be free of charge. Nature does not impose a financial levy on herbs, as they grow wild and free. There may be environmental costs incurred from the impact of picking, but that is another matter. When the choice arises, use common and inexpensive herbs. Expensive, rare, or imported plants may not be any more effective in a particular case than common (and not very glamorous) nettle or cleavers. Naturally, the fast-developing herb industry has a financial stake in the promotion of expensive "new wonder herbs" from exotic parts of the world—but just remember that Fresno and Hoboken are exotic locales to most of the world!

ENVIRONMENTAL CRITERIA

Seeing ecological relationships as having a bearing on the healing arts can lead to some important conclusions. The choice of most relevant therapy should be based on individual needs; however, Donne's insight that "no man is an island" is crucial. In a world where human impact has become life threatening, the broader implications of health practices must be taken into account. In addition to the range of criteria already described, environmental impact can be used as one way to identify appropriate or inappropriate treatments.

The "Illness" of Health Care

Far too many illnesses occurring in the years after fifty are directly due to previous medical treatment. The impact of years of medication (including the various side effects involved) combined with subjection to medical procedures of all kinds eventually takes its toll in the increased incidence of iatrogenic disease, that is, illness caused in some way by previous medical treatment.

Obviously, if symptoms are recognized as being produced by some commonly prescribed medication, the best treatment in such a case is abstinence from that pharmaceutical agent. It may not be appropriate, however, and may even be dangerous to simply stop taking a prescribed medication. In consultation with the doctor involved, a useful strategy of elimination of one medication at a time, with close observation, can often be negotiated. (In fact, the usefulness of occasional "drug holidays" is widely recognized.)

Preventive Care

Except where some specific pathogen or causal factor is involved, prevention of illness is an outcome of promoting health. Health is more than the absence of illness, and the active experience of wellness can be achieved, not merely accepted when (or if) it occurs. Balance and harmony in all areas are the keys to successful preventive medicine:

- *Nutrition* must be of a quality that nurtures the body in a way that ensures health and wholeness.
- *Structural factors* must be addressed, by skilled practitioners if this is indicated, but also through appropriate exercise, dance, or any enjoyable expression of the body. The structure of general alignment of the skeleton has a profound effect upon all aspects of human life, and, of course, herbs can't move the bones around.
- A conscious and free-flowing *emotional life* is fundamental to achieving any inner harmony. This does not mean that everyone must get involved in psychotherapy, but that attention must be given in the appropriate form to each individual's emotional needs. (Not that everyone should be smiling all the time. What's "appropriate" in this case might mean facing one's anger or grief.)
- *Mental factors* are crucial as we are what we think! Without a personal vision, life becomes a slow process of degeneration and decay. Attention must be given to self-image, personal purpose, and so forth.
- Some openness to *spirituality* is vital. This may take the form of experiencing the upliftment of a sunset, being touched by poetry or art, religious faith, or a dogma-free joy in being alive.

1 The Digestive System

Herbs are an unequaled form of medicine for treatment of the digestive system. Many beneficial effects are due to the metabolism and absorption of the whole range of plant constituents; others are brought about by a direct action upon the tissue through contact. Furthermore, much digestive illness in our society is simply due to abuse. Today's average diet is marked by a high proportion of overly processed foods, chemical additives, and irritants such as alcohol and carbonated drinks. Even tobacco is a gastric irritant; swallowed tars are linked with ulcers. In this context it is easy to see why herbal remedies are so helpful in the various inflammations and reactions that plague so many. The direct soothing of demulcents, the healing effect of astringents, and the general toning of bitters can do much to reverse this damage.

However, as with all true healing, any potential "cure" ultimately lies beyond the range of medicines, whether they be herbal or drug in nature. The healing process must involve a change of whatever dietary indiscretions are occurring as well as attention being given to lifestyle changes that may be called for to reduce stress. Herbal medicine can bring about dramatic improvements in even profound digestive problems, but the long-term maintenance of benefit lies in the hands of the person seeking treatment.

This chapter contains a discussion of how herbs can beneficially impact disorders of the digestive system, including disorders of the liver and gallbladder.

The Healthy Digestive System

The digestive system is basically a long tube, measuring about forty feet long from the mouth to the anus. In simplified terms, a healthy digestive process would work as follows:

1. As the food is chewed saliva mixes with it, initiating the digestion of starches.

2. Once swallowed, the food moves down the esophagus, a tube that leads from the base of the tongue to the stomach.

3. In the stomach the food is physically broken down further by the stomach's churning action and chemically digested to produce a thick liquid mixture called chyme.

4. The chyme passes into the duodenum, the upper portion of the small intestine. As the chyme is moved through the intestine by muscle contractions (peristalsis), intestinal juices, pancreatic juices, and bile complete the enzyme-facilitated breakdown of the food. The nutrients released by this process are absorbed through the walls of the small intestine and enter the bloodstream to be distributed around the body.

5. Undigested material moves into the large intestine, or colon, where the water is absorbed back into the body.

6. The remaining material passes into the rectum, where it is eliminated.

If problems develop in any of these steps, they may be attributable to changes that occur quite normally in the aging process rather than being signs of a disease process.

The Aging Digestive System

Throughout the human body the aging process is reflected in changes in both functioning and structure. These in turn lead to certain repercussions that scientists consider normal. The degree of change, or the response of the rest of the body to these changes, varies from person to person. Again the question arises: what is a normal person? Age-related changes will affect digestive juices, strength of the abdominal muscles, and general control and integration of functions. Thus, as a person ages:

1. Smaller amounts of digestive juices are produced.
   - The salivary glands produce less saliva with a lower concentration of digestive enzymes.
   - In the stomach, production of gastric juices declines from age twenty on. In the middle years, there is an increased incidence of chronic inflammation of the stomach with associated degeneration of the mucous lining. Such changes can prevent an older body from absorbing as much iron and vitamin B_{12} as a younger one can absorb.
   - One intestinal age-related change that does bother some people is increased *intolerance of milk products,* as over time the enzyme that breaks down milk sugar (lactose) disappears from the intestinal tract.
   - The liver experiences age-related changes, including reduction of enzyme concentrations.
   - The pancreas also shows age-related changes in the making and secretion of digestive enzymes.

2. The muscles of the whole system grow weaker, the lining of the intestines grows thinner, and the intestines themselves grow less resilient and elastic. Because of this, small pouches called diverticula may balloon out from the colon wall. In some people, the pouches become inflamed and infected.

3. The movements of the bowels grow weaker, and the functioning of the colon becomes less efficient.
   - Food takes longer to make its way down the esophagus because of a decrease in the wavelike motion that pushes the food toward the stomach.
   - Food may take longer to travel through the small intestines.
   - There is more opportunity for water to be absorbed from the feces, increasing the chance of constipation.

Herbal Actions

The use of herbs to aid digestion has long been part of the tradition of modern Europe and North America. Whether culinary herbs such as rosemary or "medicinal" alcohols such as vermouth, therapeutic remedies are used in large quantities. The very name "vermouth" comes from that of the bitter remedy wormwood. Even today, herbs maintain their foothold in the official pharmacopoeias as the major therapeutic agents in the categories of digestive bitters, carminatives, and laxatives.

A number of herbal actions (listed in order of importance) are of direct value for the digestive system.

Demulcent: These mucilage-rich herbs soothe and protect irritated or inflamed tissue; reduce irritation down the whole length of the bowel; reduce sensitivity to potentially corrosive gastric acids; help to prevent diarrhea; and reduce the muscle spasms that cause colic. Herbs to consider include comfrey root, marshmallow root, slippery elm, licorice, and Irish moss.

Bitter: Herbs with a bitter taste have a special role in preventive medicine. The taste triggers a sensory response in the central nervous system. A message goes to the gut, releasing digestive hormones and ultimately giving rise to stimulation of appetite; general stimulation of the flow of digestive juices; increased bile flow, an aid to the liver's detoxification work, and stimulation of gut self-repair mechanisms. (All this from a nasty taste in the mouth!) Herbs to consider include yarrow, gentian, agrimony, goldenseal, and wormwood.

Astringent: The astringents, with their binding action on mucous membranes, denature proteins, thereby reducing irritation and inflammation, creating a barrier against infection and reducing fluid loss. Herbs to consider include agrimony, oak bark, cranesbill, and meadowsweet.

Carminative: Plants rich in aromatic oils that stimulate the digestive system to work properly and with ease, soothing the gut wall, reducing any inflammation that might be present, easing griping pains, and helping the removal of gas from the digestive tract. Herbs to consider include fennel, ginger, caraway, peppermint, chamomile, and lavender.

Anti-inflammatory: These soothe inflammation of the tissue directly. They work in a number of different ways but rarely inhibit the natural inflammatory reaction as such; rather they support and encourage the body's natural processes. Herbs to consider include chamomile, lemon balm, and meadowsweet.

Antispasmodic: Antispasmodics ease muscular cramping. They alleviate muscular tension and, as many are also nervines, ease psychological tension as well. There are antispasmodics that reduce muscle spasming throughout the body, and also those that work on specific organs or systems. Herbs to consider include chamomile, valerian, cramp bark, and wild yam.

Laxative: Laxatives stimulate bowel movements. Stimulating laxatives should not be used long term. If this appears to be necessary then diet, general health, and stress should all be closely considered. Herbs to consider include psyllium seed, yellow dock, dandelion root, and senna.

Hepatics: Hepatics aid the liver. They tone, strengthen, and in some cases increase the flow of bile. In a broad holistic approach to health, they are of great importance because of the fundamental role of the liver in the working of the body. Herbs to consider include dandelion, bitters, milk thistle, goldenseal, and balmony.

Nervine: Nervines help the nervous system and can be meaningfully subdivided into three groups. Nervine tonics strengthen and restore the nervous system. Nervine relaxants ease anxiety and tension by soothing both body and mind. Nervine stimulants directly stimulate nerve activity. Herbs to consider include the relaxing nervines chamomile, lavender, valerian, rosemary, and mugwort.

Keeping the Digestive System Healthy

Even more important than treating disease is the maintenance of vitality and health. This may sound like an unattainable ideal, but in practice some basic guidelines will help prevent illness. To nurture the digestive system's inherent "wellness," follow these basic guidelines:

- *Eat a high-fiber diet.* Sufficient bulk in the colon keeps the system working smoothly. Lack of dietary fiber is linked to many bowel problems, including constipation and diverticulosis. High-fiber foods include bran, whole-grain breads and cereals, fresh fruits, and vegetables.
- *Eliminate foods that cause digestive distress.* This will, of course, vary from person to person. It may be problems with gas-producing vegetables such as broccoli, cauliflower, and cabbage. Others may find milk products less and less digestible. If cramps, gas, diarrhea, or constipation occur, the key may be what was eaten in the previous forty-eight hours.
- *Overeating can cause stomach bloat, heartburn, and bowel distress.* High-calorie diets have been linked to gallstones.
- *Make mealtime an enjoyable and relaxing experience.* Meals should never be rushed. Such simple advice can be the key to avoiding indigestion, heartburn, and even ulcers.
- *Reduce or eliminate the use of alcohol, caffeine, and nicotine.* These commonly used drugs are irritants that may cause heartburn and indigestion

as well as aggravate an existent condition such as ulcers or irritable bowel syndrome.

- *Some medications are not kind to the digestive tract.* Aspirin, antihistamines, diuretics, antihypertensives, sedatives, and other substances can cause distress. Ask your doctor, pharmacist, or herbalist about the potential side effects of any medications you are taking.
- *Ideally avoid—but at least don't overuse—laxatives or antacids.* At best they relieve symptoms. At worst they encourage the digestive tract to become dependent on them.
- *Develop ways of coping with stress.* Burying tension and internalizing anger are two good ways to wreak havoc on the digestive system.
- *Exercise regularly.* It helps to control weight, reduce stress, and promote normal bowel functioning.

Gastrointestinal Problems—Common and Serious

It has been estimated that gastrointestinal distress in one form or another affects some two hundred thousand Americans daily severely and enough to keep them from work. This highlights the importance of knowing the difference between an innocuous upset and a serious one. Here are types of digestive discomfort that are likely to be innocuous:

- *Drug reactions.* Many drugs interact with gastric acid, sometimes causing cramps, severe diarrhea, heartburn, or indigestion. Antibiotics and anti-inflammatory drugs are the commonest causes. Aspirin can cause heartburn, indigestion, stomach irritation, ulcers, and internal bleeding.
- *Gas.* The commonest cause of discomfort is excess stomach gas. Such gas can cause feelings of bloating, discomfort, mild pain, and social embarrassment.
- *Indigestion* is a very vague term used to describe almost any stomach discomfort. Symptoms include gas, belching and flatulence, a feeling of distention in the stomach, and minor pain.
- *Irritable bowel syndrome.* Symptoms include "butterflies" in the stomach, diarrhea or constipation, cramps, nausea, indigestion, and gas.
- *Lactose intolerance* is caused by a deficiency of lactase, an enzyme that digests lactose, a dietary sugar. If a milk product is consumed, the undigested lactose causes distention, gas, nausea, diarrhea, and cramps.

- *Reflux* or *heartburn* caused by eating or drinking too much or eating any foods that "disagree" with the person. A common symptom is severe heartburn pain in the center of the chest that might be mistaken for a heart attack.
- *Stomach flu,* one of the major causes of lost work days. Symptoms include nausea, vomiting, diarrhea, and cramps.

If these generally benign signs occur two to four times a month, if there is no obvious cause, or if they are extremely painful or distressing, a more serious condition may be present. Discomfort in the abdomen may be caused by any of several conditions discussed later in this chapter. They include:

Appendicitis. Symptoms include dull pain that begins around the belly button, moves to the lower right side of the abdomen, and becomes more severe as time passes. This may be accompanied by nausea, vomiting, and fever.

Cancer of the colon, pancreas, stomach, or esophagus. Unfortunately, cancers in the gastrointestinal tract are difficult to diagnose until they are far advanced.

Diverticulitis. Symptoms include fever and a dull, steady pain on the lower left side of the stomach that worsens when you move around.

Gallstones. The first symptom is often a tightening just below your ribs. Extreme pain usually occurs in waves on the right side of your upper abdomen, extending all the way around to the middle of the back and possibly up to the right shoulder blade.

Inflamed pancreas. Symptoms include severe stomach pain, often radiating to the back. It starts as slight pain but gets steadily worse within hours and then stays severe. Sitting up or bending forward often gives temporary relief. Similar symptoms may also be caused by disorders of the spleen, appendix, or liver.

Intestinal blockage will prevent materials from passing through. There will be vomiting, nausea, and intense pain. Vomiting of material that looks like coffee grounds indicates stomach bleeding.

Kidney problems, such as kidney stones, can cause excruciating waves of pain in the middle of the back on either side, at the point where the ribs join the spine.

Peptic ulcers. A gnawing, burning pain that may feel like hunger pangs but that generally comes one to two hours after eating or when the stomach is empty can signal an ulcer.

How can a "serious" symptom be identified? The following are signs and symptoms that warrant skilled professional diagnosis:

- Blood in the vomit or bowel movement.
- Symptoms last several hours, recur two or more times in a month, and are accompanied by chills.
- Pain is very severe.
- The skin or eyes develop a yellowish tinge or the urine appears brownish.
- The stomach bloats and doesn't go back to normal in a day or two.
- Mucus is present in the bowel movements.
- A swelling or a hard lump can be felt in the area where the pain is experienced.
- The frequency or appearance of bowel movements changes.

If You Experience:	Cut Back on These Common Offenders:*
Constipation	White bread, pastries, and other highly processed, refined foods; antidepressants, antihistamines, and diuretics
Gas, bloating, bowel distress, diarrhea	Milk and milk products, saccharin-sweetened products, coffee, tea, peanuts, broccoli, cabbage, beans, and garlic
Heartburn	Coffee, chocolate, alcohol, onions, and peppermint
Stomach pain	Coffee and caffeine drinks, alcohol, nicotine, aspirin, arthritis medications, asthma medications, antihypertensives, and antibiotics*

*Always consult your physician before cutting back on any prescribed medications.

Next we will review specific problems associated with the digestive tract, beginning with problems in the mouth.

Canker Sores

These painful ulcers can be single or clustered almost anywhere in the mouth. They usually go away within seven to twenty-one days but can be a recurrent problem in some people. Their cause is unclear but is often associated with a lowered immune response, either locally or as a sign of a systemic problem. Stress is a strongly implicated cause, as are food sensitivities and nutritional deficiencies.

The best remedy for symptomatic relief is red sage, which is an effective anti-inflammatory that reduces the localized reaction in the mouth and a mild antimicrobial that will inhibit any development of infection. Red sage is a variety of ordinary culinary sage but has a stronger volatile oil. Rarely used in cooking, it makes a perfect herb to use as a mouthwash in canker sores and other inflammatory conditions of the mouth. If it is not available, the culinary variety will help.

For a more deep-seated treatment that addresses general health, herbs that support immunity and act as tonics are helpful. Echinacea, cleavers, and nettle are often best. If stress is an aggravating factor, consider the relaxing remedies known as nervines. Of the many possible nervines, I suggest vervain, as it is also helpful for the liver.

Mouthwash

- red sage
- chamomile

Equal parts of dried herbs.
An infusion of 2 tsp (10 ml) of the mixture to a cup of water can be gargled often.

Internal Remedy

- echinacea
- cleavers
- vervain

Equal parts of tinctures.
Take $1/2$ tsp (2.5 ml three times a day).

Iron, vitamin C, vitamin B complex, and zinc supplements can be very helpful, in some cases even enough to clear the problem. Dental attention may be important, as a tooth abscess or gum disease may be the focus of the underlying problem. Similarly, a history of stomach ulceration or other gastric problems point to the need to herbally focus on these conditions. The diet must exclude irritants of all kinds, whether physical irritants (e.g., very hot or coarse food) or chemical irritants (acidic food, alcohol, tobacco, and very spicy food).

Dental and Periodontal Disease and Gingivitis

During the aging process a number of normal changes occur in the teeth and gums that in themselves are not signs of disease.

- Teeth darken as dark, dense dentin takes the place of pulp inside the tooth. The enamel coating thins, allowing the darker layer underneath to show through.
- Teeth discolor from accumulated food, beverages, and tobacco stains.
- Teeth wear away. It is estimated that the normal rate of wear in teeth is so small they could serve us through three lifespans. However, years of incorrect brushing, teeth grinding, high-acid diets, or chronic vomiting can wear them away far more quickly.
- Gums damage more easily and heal more slowly as the body's circulatory and immune systems slow down.
- Plaque tends to accumulate faster with age and cause gum inflammation.
- Teeth may become loose and unstable in their sockets as a result of gum disease or loss of jawbone density caused by osteoporosis.
- Because of plaque buildup and gum sensitivity, gum disease may take hold, resulting in anything from minor gum bleeding to major tooth loss.

Pyorrhea, or periodontal disease, commonly begins as gingivitis but may occasionally be the initial sign of a more serious disease. Ordinarily the major factor is poor dental hygiene. As gingivitis is also common during puberty and pregnancy, a hormonal role has been suggested as well.

Herbs can help these problems in a number of ways but can never replace professional dental attention. They will, however, augment the efficacy of such work. Antimicrobial plants are fundamental in reducing bacterial populations that contribute to the decay process. Myrrh is considered a specific medication in cases in which its antimicrobial effects can be utilized topically. Red sage mouthwashes and echinacea taken internally are also helpful. Anti-inflammatory and astringent plants will lessen bleeding and ease irritation. An astringent herb from Peru, *Krameria triandra* (rhatany), is often effective for such gum diseases, and though rarely available in herb stores, it is often a constituent in herbal gum preparations.

Gum Application

- myrrh
- echinacea
- rhatany (replace with oak bark if unavailable)

Equal parts of tinctures.
Mix and apply to the gums three times a day, using a very fine brush.
Red sage or chamomile infusions may be used as a gargle. Do not swallow.

Internal Remedy

- echinacea
- cleavers
- prickly ash

Equal parts of tinctures.
Take 1 tsp (5 ml) three times a day.

Some proprietary herbal toothpastes can aid the treatment by supplying the indicated herbs in this form as well. The following supplements may prove helpful in the long-term treatment of periodontal disease:

vitamin C: 3–5 g daily
vitamin E: 400–800 IU daily
vitamin A: 20,000 IU daily
selenium: 400 mcg daily
zinc picolinate: 30 mg daily
folic acid: 2 mg daily

Esophagitis and Gastroesophageal Reflux Disease (GERD)

Stomach acid rising into the throat will cause a burning sensation, uncontrollable coughing, or, if some slips down the windpipe into the lungs, even difficulty in breathing. It is often associated with an abnormal relaxation of the esophageal sphincter, the ring of muscle at the end of the esophagus that controls the flow of food into the stomach. Relaxation of this muscle allows gastric juices to flow back up into the lower end of the esophagus, causing heartburn (pain behind the breastbone). As a person ages, this muscular valve becomes weaker. The result is that it occasionally fails, causing reflux. Reflux often becomes a chronic problem among those over age forty because of hiatal hernia, a condition in which the valve becomes stretched and weakened so that it no longer is able to do its job properly. It is common in healthy people, especially following a meal.

The most important component of treatment is the identification and avoidance of suspected irritants. A number of causes of reflux are listed below with the appropriate preventive steps.

- Many foods are known to relax the esophageal sphincter, including chocolate, peppermint, spearmint, fats, fried foods, and coffee. Avoidance of them may reduce gastroesophageal reflux in those who are susceptible.
- Alcohol affects the sphincter, so avoid alcohol.
- Smoking relaxes the sphincter and has been shown to increase reflux, so stop smoking.
- Commonly used drugs that may cause gastroesophageal reflux include theophylline, meperidine (Demerol), diazepam (Valium), morphine, and oral contraceptives.
- Physical factors promoting reflux include stooping; bending; wearing tight-fitting clothing, girdles, or belts; and lying down after meals or lying flat to sleep. Raise the head of the bed or sleep with several pillows, and do not consume any food in the three hours before bedtime.
- Obesity is a common factor.

Herbal treatment will help reduce discomfort if used in conjunction with application of the guidelines listed above. Demulcent remedies will soothe and coat the tissue of the esophagus, insulating the sensitive lining from irritation by the gastric contents. Comfrey and marshmallow root are very effective. Anti-inflammatory herbs such as chamomile or calendula will reduce any localized mucosal reaction. Carminatives may be needed if there is a more general disruption of the digestive process. Bitters are best avoided, as they may aggravate the symptoms by stimulating secretion of stomach acid.

Soothing GERD Remedy

- comfrey root   2 parts
- marshmallow root   2 parts
- calendula   1 part
- chamomile   1 part

As tincture: take 1 tsp (5 ml) of this mixture three times a day.
As dried herb: infuse 2 tsp to a cup and drink three times a day.

An infusion of balm or chamomile sipped slowly throughout the day will help.

Gastritis

Gastritis, an inflammation of the stomach lining, may be acute or chronic, corrosive or noncorrosive, but from the herbal perspective these differences are not too crucial. The approach described here may be applied in all cases unless there is a specific underlying problem. Acute gastritis may be caused by severe burns, major surgery, aspirin or other anti-inflammatory drugs, steroids, drugs, food allergens, or by the presence of viral, bacterial, or chemical toxins. The symptoms—appetite loss, nausea, vomiting, and discomfort after eating—usually abate after the causative agent has been removed. Chronic gastritis is usually a sign of some underlying disease such as peptic ulcer.

Demulcent herbs (comfrey root, marshmallow root, slippery elm) will soothe the lining of the stomach. Anti-inflammatory remedies such as chamomile and lemon balm will reduce localized mucosal reaction. Commercial antacids have little to offer other than symptomatic relief. Their main drawback is that the body responds to the neutralization of stomach acid by increasing production. Meadowsweet and peppermint will act in an antacid-like way but without the associated problems. Relaxing herbs, or nervines, will help where stress is a factor.

Lifestyle is fundamental to both the cause and treatment of gastritis. Food irritants (chemicals, extreme temperature, fiber) must be avoided, as must acidic foods, alcohol, and tobacco. Underlying stress-producing factors (e.g., work conditions) must be considered. A remedy for gastritis can be found on the following page.

Gastritis Remedy

- comfrey root   2 parts
- marshmallow root   2 parts
- meadowsweet   1 part
- chamomile   1 part

As tincture: take 1 tsp (5 ml) of this mixture three times a day.

As dried herb: infuse 2 tsp to a cup and drink three times a day.

An infusion of balm, chamomile, or peppermint sipped slowly throughout the day will help.

Peptic Ulceration

Ulcerative conditions of the stomach, duodenum, and esophagus are very common in our society; hence nonprescription symptomatic relief medicines are major moneymakers for the pharmaceutical industry. Drug treatment is based primarily upon reduction of the corrosive impact of stomach acid on the mucosal lining, through antacid chemicals or other drugs that directly or indirectly reduce acid production. A range of plants are available that appear to work in a broader way to facilitate a reversal of the particular syndrome.

Peptic ulcers usually have a chronic, recurrent course, with a variable symptom picture. In fact, only about half of all ulcer patients present the characteristic picture of burning, gnawing, or aching pain, or a distress described as soreness, an empty feeling, or "hunger pains." Epigastric pain is relieved by antacids or milk.

The typical picture in duodenal ulcers is that of hunger pains, whereas pain in gastric ulcers may be brought on by eating.

The skilled application of plants with demulcent, antacid, astringent, and vulnerary actions can bring about a rapid and complete healing of any ulceration. Herbs such as comfrey, marshmallow, meadowsweet, calendula, chamomile, and goldenseal are examples of remedies that may be used.

As with the conditions already discussed, the demulcents have the most to offer in the treatment of peptic ulcers. The insulation-like coating of the stomach wall allows tissue to heal itself. When the demulcent used is also an herb that speeds wound healing, even more gratifying results are achieved. Comfrey, marshmallow, meadowsweet, calendula, and chamomile are used extensively in Europe for these problems. Their validity is highly predictable, based upon an understanding of their actions. In addition to the demulcency of comfrey and marshmallow, the anti-inflammatory flavonoid content of calendula and chamomile is thought to be very significant. Licorice root is another effective remedy now being used in allopathic medicine as a treatment for ulceration.

Successful herbal therapy in the treatment of peptic ulceration is a two-stage process.

1.   To reduce inflammation and initiate healing using demulcents and vulneraries:

- comfrey root   2 parts
- marshmallow root   1 part
- chamomile   1 part

As tincture: take 1 tsp (5 ml) of this mixture three times a day.
As dried herb: infuse 2–3 tsp to a cup and drink three times a day.

An infusion of the fresh or dried herbs may be drunk often to ease symptoms.
Balm or chamomile infusion drunk on an empty stomach will reduce inflammation and help reverse the ulcerative process.

2.   To tone and complete healing:

- comfrey root   2 parts
- chamomile   2 parts
- goldenseal   1 part

As tincture: take 1 tsp (5 ml) of this mixture three times a day.

CAUTION: If symptoms have not subsided within a week, seek skilled diagnosis.

Ulcer patients should be aware of certain commonly found consequences of the nonherbal treatment of peptic ulceration: excessive use of antacids can lead to the impaired absorption of certain nutrients from the diet.

- Excessive drinking of milk or consumption of antacids can lead to elevated levels of calcium in body tissues and urine, which can result in the formation of kidney stones.

- Eating a bland and milky diet can lead to obesity.
- Consumption of milk may aggravate problems associated with sensitivity to dairy products.
- Poor appetite associated with ulceration may lead to nutritional deficiency.

Dietary factors are fundamentally involved in both the causation and treatment of peptic ulceration. In some cases ulceration may be due to a specific food allergy, but the condition will always be aggravated by exposure to irritants. Pepper, coffee, and anything that the patient experiences as a problem should be removed from the diet. Among nondietary factors, alcohol and tobacco are especially implicated. Avoidance of aspirin and other nonsteroidal anti-inflammatories is essential. Small meals often are better than large meals. Increasing the proportion of fiber in the diet has been shown to reduce the rate of recurrence of peptic ulceration; however, a bland diet is recommended in the early stages of treatment to avoid physical irritation. Rest and reevaluation of a lifestyle that may be causing stress is important. An individually designed stress management program should be a priority.

Recommended supplements to support the herbal work include:

> **vitamin A:** 20,000 IU three times a day
> **vitamin C:** 500 mg three times a day (take with food to avoid irritation of the ulcer)
> **vitamin E:** 100 IU three times a day
> **zinc:** 20 mg daily

Hiatal Hernia

This condition is based upon a herniation in the diaphragm that then pinches the stomach, leading to a range of gastric symptoms. A hernia is a protrusion of an organ through a wall of the cavity in which it is enclosed. In the case of a hiatal hernia, a portion of the stomach protrudes through a teardrop-shaped hole in the diaphragm where the esophagus and the stomach join. The most frequent known cause of hiatal hernia is increased pressure in the abdominal cavity produced by coughing, vomiting, straining during bowel movement, or sudden physical exertion. Pregnancy, obesity, or excess fluid in the abdomen are other contributing factors.

Hiatal hernias may develop in people of all ages and both sexes, although it is considered to be a condition of middle age. In fact, the majority of otherwise normal people past the age of fifty have small hiatal hernias. The symptoms are treatable with remedies that focus on stomach symptoms but do not necessarily attack the cause directly. Comfrey, marshmallow, meadowsweet, sweet flag, and chamomile can all be helpful. Comfrey has an especially valid role because of its allantoin content (which promotes wound healing). Horsetail may help through a toning of connective tissue, but it may be too irritating to the stomach for some individuals.

The main goal is to reduce inflammation and so facilitate natural healing through the use of demulcents and vulneraries.

■ comfrey root	2 parts
■ marshmallow root	2 parts
■ calendula	1 part
■ chamomile	1 part

As tincture: take 1 tsp (5 ml) of this mixture three times a day.

As dried herb: infuse 2 tsp to a cup and drink three times a day.

An infusion of balm or chamomile sipped slowly throughout the day will help.

As in the other digestive system conditions discussed so far, all irritant foods must be avoided. Alcohol and tobacco are especially implicated. Pepper, coffee, and anything that the patient experiences as a problem should be removed from the diet. Small meals often are better than large meals. Rest and reevaluation of a lifestyle that may be causing stress are essential.

"Indigestion"

This is a vague and variable problem that is functional in nature, meaning that no organic disease (i.e., no underlying structural cause) has been found. Belching, distension, and borborygmus (intestinal rumbling) often occur, associated with abdominal or epigastric pain. A psychological component is frequently present, but it is too easy to conclude that all indigestion is psychosomatic. Dietary factors are often crucial. However, as discussed at the beginning of this section, the symptom picture may be similar to that brought about by more severe conditions ranging from heart disease to stomach ulcers and gallbladder problems. Thus any intransigent case of "indigestion" needs skilled diagnosis.

The key to correcting such functional problems lies in "tuning up" the fine control of both metabolic and physical aspects of digestion and assimilation, while easing the discomfort with appropriate remedies.

Herbs that have a bitter stimulation effect will promote an integrated and adequate secretory response to food or hunger, as well as increase the muscular tone so important for proper bowel movement. Carminatives will ease flatulence and reduce localized inflammation and the muscular spasms that lead to colic. These also act as mild antimicrobials. Antispasmodics may be indicated if the carminatives do not adequately ease abdominal cramping. Nervines can be used to help reduce stress, anxiety, and tension. They are usually also antispasmodic.

Every culture and every individual herbalist has some favorite remedy for indigestion. These are, as would be expected, often bitter carminatives or nervine carminatives. European specifics include gentian, peppermint, chamomile, lemon balm, hops, and valerian. Hence the possibilities for herbal blends can be endless, though often the traditional simple blend, or even simply tea made from a single fresh remedy, is best. This is ideally a pleasant tasting herb with an agreeable aroma. From the herbs that are most therapeutically indicated for a specific individual, choose a plant that can be readily cultivated in a garden or windowbox to provide a steady supply of fresh leaves.

- peppermint
- chamomile
- balm

This basic therapy may be augmented by a combination of tinctures that generally aids the digestive system through a bitter/carminative approach:

- chamomile
- peppermint
- gentian
- valerian

Equal parts of tinctures.
Take $1/2$ tsp (2.5 ml) of this mixture 10 minutes before eating three times a day.

Persistent or unresponsive problems with indigestion call for skilled medical diagnosis. Because of the functional nature of this problem, the therapy indicated is whatever helps the patient to be at ease with himself or herself or aids physiological activity. Attention to diet is fundamental, but therapies ranging all the way from chiropractic to Rolfing may be of help, as may counseling about stress or deeper psychological issues.

The Aging Colon and Its Problems

Many plants have a direct impact on colitis and other conditions of the colon. With astringents such as bayberry, wound-healing demulcents like comfrey root or plantain, and the colic-relieving properties of the antispasmodics wild yam and cramp bark, much can be done to facilitate the healing of these distressing problems.

Colitis, an inflammation of the colon, appears to be caused by any of a number of factors. Mucous colitis, also called irritable or spastic colon, is a functional disturbance in which the colon secretes abnormally large amounts of mucus, which appears in the stools. The most common symptom is abdominal cramping accompanied by either constipation or diarrhea, sometimes alternately.

Constipation

Constipation is not itself a "disease" but a symptom that demands skilled diagnosis. Acute constipation occurs as a definite, recognizable change for that individual. This change in bowel habits can be a sign of organic disease. Chronic constipation is characterized by an ongoing hampering of normal bowel movements. In such cases the ideal is to work through the diet to normalize and regularize movements.

The most common cause of constipation in Western cultures is lack of dietary fiber. However, a number of significant if less common causes must be borne in mind by the practitioner:

- drugs that affect bowel motility, including opiates, iron supplements, certain antidepressants, chemical antacids, antihypertensives, and muscle relaxants; drugs used to control Parkinson's disease; anesthetics; and the overuse of laxatives

- cancer
- dehydration
- depression
- diverticular disease
- endocrine conditions such as hypothyroidism and hyperparathyroidism
- food sensitivity
- irritable bowel syndrome
- lead poisoning
- long periods of immobility or prolonged bed rest
- narrowing of the colon
- obstruction of the bowel
- painful anal conditions that make the person afraid to relax the sphincter
- serious abdominal infection (e.g., appendicitis)
- stress

As in the treatment of many other functional problems of the digestive system, different herbs are used by different herbalists. It cannot be stressed enough that constipation is a symptom requiring skilled diagnosis if it is unresponsive to herbal treatment or is a longstanding condition. Laxative herbs are extremely effective and thus maintain their place in official pharmacopoeias. However, if laxatives—herbal or chemical—are used over a long period of time, the bowels become dependent on them, so that without their stimulation a bowel movement becomes exceedingly difficult. This is why laxatives are one of the commonest indirect causes of constipation.

The many plants that stimulate the bowels range from very mild and gentle aperients to the drastic cathartic plants that are best left in the Middle Ages. The safe laxative remedies can be divided into three categories depending upon how they work.

1. Bulk laxatives increase the bulk of the intestinal contents, which in turn stimulates the stretch receptors in the intestinal wall to contract and move the contents along. These fiber-rich foods and herbs are the only truly safe long-term treatments and are best gradually increased in dosage each morning and evening until a softer, bulkier stool results. Herbal examples are psyllium and flax seeds.

2. Secretory laxatives promote bowel movement through stimulation of bile production by the liver and release of bile into the intestinal tract by the gallbladder. These herbs are usually hepatics or bitters, that is, herbs with a beneficial effect on the liver. Yellow dock and dandelion root are good examples.

3. Stimulant laxatives usually contain a group of natural constituents, called anthraquinones, herbs that stimulate peristaltic movement directly by affecting the nerves in the region. They are very effective but likely to cause dependency if used for a long time. Commonly used stimulant laxatives are cascara sagrada, senna, and purging buckthorn. They are best used in conjunction with carminatives to ease the griping pain and discomfort they may cause.

Any long-term approach must include dietary fiber, to provide bulk and "retraining" of the bowel musculature. A dietary approach focusing on the rational use of fiber is also the most effective. (I stress *rational;* addiction to oat bran is, after all, an addiction like any other.) The following guidelines will be helpful:

- Identify any cause of the constipation and address it.
- Set a regular time every day for a bowel movement (ideally after breakfast or morning exercise).
- Do not delay bowel movements.
- Include a high content of fiber in the daily diet. Fiber is found in whole grains, fresh fruit, and vegetables.
- Drink plenty of fluids (6–8 glasses a day).
- Avoid chemical or stimulating herbal laxatives as much as possible.
- Exercise regularly, at least twenty minutes three times a week.

A gentle yet effective laxative that avoids dependency problems can be made as follows:

■ yellow dock	2 parts
■ dandelion	2 parts
■ aniseed	1 part

As tincture: take 1 tsp (5 ml) of this mixture three times a day.
As dried herb: decoct 2 tsp to a cup and drink three times a day.

Diarrhea

Diarrhea is a condition marked by an increase in frequency, fluid content, and volume of bowel movements. It is a symptom of many conditions, ranging from infectious gastrointestinal diseases to anxiety and drug reactions. The following abbreviated list will make it clear why skilled diagnosis is so important if the condition is not responsive to herbal treatment. Diarrhea may be related to:

- antibiotic use
- dietary factors such as lactose intolerance
- fecal impaction (hardened stools in the colon or rectum)
- food allergy or allergies
- food poisoning
- inflammatory bowel disease
- malabsorption conditions
- malnutrition
- metabolic disease
- pancreatic disease
- stress and anxiety
- viral, bacterial, and parasitic infections

Many herbs can help to alleviate the symptom of diarrhea, but the underlying cause must be addressed for any real healing to take place. The primary herbs to consider are the astringents, which act as binding agents on the mucosal lining of the colon. Meadowsweet may well be the best gentle treatment for diarrhea in general, as it seems to tone the lining of the small intestine as well as act as an astringent. Other excellent remedies include agrimony, shepherd's purse, and cranesbill. The stronger astringents such as oak bark and *Acacia catechu* should only be used as a last resort. Carminative remedies such as chamomile and lemon balm will ease any associated colic or flatulence. These gentle relaxants also help to alleviate anxiety.

Antimicrobials will be indicated if infection is suspected. Infectious diarrhea usually takes an acute form with rapid onset. Associated with debility and often with fever, it may affect many or all members of the family at once. Herbs containing the alkaloid berberine—goldenseal or barberry—may be especially helpful here.

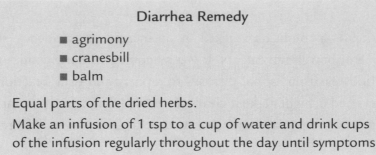

Diarrhea Remedy

- agrimony
- cranesbill
- balm

Equal parts of the dried herbs.
Make an infusion of 1 tsp to a cup of water and drink cups of the infusion regularly throughout the day until symptoms subside.

The symptoms of acute diarrhea will be gone within anywhere from a few hours to three days.

Rest until the diarrhea has stopped and drink clear liquids such as herbal teas or broth. In case of stomach cramps, use a hot water bottle or electric heating pad on the stomach to relieve pain. After the diarrhea has subsided, eat semisolid foods for two or three days, then gradually return to a normal diet. The main complication of acute diarrhea is dehydration from the loss of fluids and vital electrolytes in the body; this is why it is important to take in as much fluid as possible. Symptoms of dehydration include:

- dry mouth
- headache
- increased thirst
- irritability
- lethargy
- small amounts of dark-colored urine
- sunken eyes

Besides alleviating the diarrhea itself, electrolytes that are lost through the bowels must be replaced. This is essential; the major killer of babies around the world is electrolyte loss through diarrhea. The abysmal state of worldwide health care economics is demonstrated by the fact that a five-cent package of replacement salts would save a child's life yet is often unattainable. The standard WHO formulation has been adapted into an herbal equivalent proposed by Dr. Weiss in *Herbal Medicine* and is presented here.

> ### Herbal Electrolyte Formula
> - ■ $^1/_2$ tsp table salt
> - ■ $^1/_4$ tsp baking soda
> - ■ $^1/_4$ tsp potassium chloride
> - ■ 2 tbsp glucose
>
> Add to a cup of an infusion of equal parts peppermint and fennel seeds, 1–2 tablespoons to a liter of water.

Irritable Bowel Syndrome

In this condition, a whole panoply of symptoms can occur, including abdominal distress, erratic frequency of bowel movements, and variability in stool consistency. Unpleasant abdominal sensations are frequently associated with a whole range of generalized symptoms, from bloating and flatulence to headaches and anxiety.

The diverse and sometimes obscure causation of this condition leads some allopaths to put it down to purely psychological causes. Yet although stress, anxiety, and the like are often pivotal factors, they are still no more than components in a complex matrix. The diagnostician must also consider food intolerance to such staples as wheat, corn, dairy products, coffee, tea, and citrus fruit; intolerance to lactose; excessive bran consumption (often involved through overenthusiasm for "healthy fiber"). Occasionally infectious or parasitic organisms may be involved (e.g., giardia, threadworm, and candida), but differential diagnosis here is problematic. Sensitivity to prescription drugs, especially antibiotics, is a major cause.

Two extreme varieties of irritable bowel syndrome are seen, with a spectrum of shades in between. The *spastic colon* type is characterized by alternation between constipation and diarrhea associated with and often triggered by eating. The other extreme is a painless but "precipitous" diarrhea. *Mucous colitis* is a functional disturbance in which the colon secretes abnormally large amounts of mucus that appear in the stools. The possibilities for herbal treatment of this condition are obvious; indeed, herbal therapy often has more to offer here than other therapeutic modes.

Like indigestion, this functional problem may be relieved by many remedies. Carminatives such as chamomile and peppermint are examples of plants that have a direct impact on irritable bowel. Bitters will promote appropriate digestive secretions and often can normalize bowel function by themselves. Gentian and agrimony are often used for this purpose. Astringents such as bayberry, agrimony, and cranesbill will reverse the diarrhea and reduce pathological mucous production. The colic-relieving properties of the antispasmodics wild yam, cramp bark, and peppermint can do much to promote healing. Garlic can be most valuable, although it is difficult to say whether this is due to an antimicrobial effect or some broader impact of the garlic. Laxatives may be indicated temporarily but must never be strong as the swing back to diarrhea may be quick.

■ bayberry	2 parts
■ mugwort	1 part
■ chamomile	1 part
■ peppermint	1 part
■ wild yam	1 part
■ valerian	1 part

As tincture: take 1 tsp (5 ml) of this mixture three times a day.

An infusion of a carminative nervine such as chamomile should be drunk warm at frequent intervals.

As in the case of indigestion, just about anything that helps the patient to be at ease or promotes normal physiological activity will be indicated. Adjustment of the diet is fundamental; start with the following basic guidelines:

- Cut back on milk products. If symptoms subside, lactose is the villain.
- Eliminate common gas-producing vegetables (legumes, cabbage, etc.).
- Omit candy, pastries, and other foods loaded with refined sugars.
- Add fiber to your diet, including bran, whole grains, and fresh fruits.
- Increase fluids.
- Avoid laxatives. They will only aggravate an already irritable bowel.
- Exercise regularly to reduce tension.

Diverticulitis

Diverticula are small, pouchlike herniations of the lining of the colon through the muscular wall. They are found in 30 to 40 percent of all people over the age of fifty. Diverticulosis, which often has no symptoms, is the term for the presence of these small pouches, which are usually identified by X-ray. It is thought that a highly refined low-fiber diet is a primary cause. Differential diagnosis is required to rule out colon cancer. When the diverticula become inflamed (a condition called diverticulitis), they can break open a tear in the intestinal lining or wall. This is called perforation. Symptoms of diverticulitis include:

- chills, fever, or nausea
- diarrhea, alternating with constipation
- severe, intermittent cramping in the lower left abdomen
- tenderness in the lower left side of the abdomen

Herbs have a lot to offer in the treatment of diverticulitis, but their use does not supplant the need for medical supervision. Antispasmodics will help relieve the pain caused by abdominal cramping around the diverticula. Wild yam, a good antispasmodic and anti-inflammatory for the colon, also has a quite specific impact upon this condition. Carminatives will relieve the discomfort caused by flatulence, and nervines will ease the stress involved, which may be causal or the result of the condition. Care has to be taken not to induce constipation through overuse of astringent herbs in a diarrheal stage.

■ wild yam	2 parts
■ valerian	1 part
■ cramp bark	1 part
■ peppermint	1 part

As tincture: take 1 tsp (5 ml) of this mixture three times a day.

Infusions of balm, chamomile, or peppermint sipped slowly throughout the day will help. Garlic should be eaten raw (one clove a day) in the diet or as a supplement in capsule form.

As diverticular disease appears to be associated with a low-fiber diet, there is little doubt that most people gain some relief from their symptoms on a high-fiber diet. The underlying bowel abnormality remains but does not cause the same degree of problems. However, when symptoms are acute and severe, a low-fiber diet is called for initially to ensure that no physical irritation is caused by roughage intake, especially when the person is not accustomed to a high-fiber content. As soon as the discomfort is brought under control, the proportion of fiber can be gradually increased to that of a high-fiber diet first by adding unprocessed bran (¼ cup daily) to foods or mix into juice. Bulk additives such as psyllium may also be included in the day's regimen. The person suffering from diverticular disease needs to be aware of any changes in bowel movements and see that the condition is monitored professionally.

Ulcerative Colitis

This serious disease—a true colitis in that active inflammation is present—seems to be autoimmune in nature, posing real challenges to any therapist, herbalist, homeopath, and allopath alike. The disease usually presents as a series of attacks of bloody diarrhea varying in intensity and duration, alternating with periods of no symptoms at all.

Ulcerative colitis must be differentiated from inflammations with an infectious cause, as the symptoms of *Shigella, Salmonella,* and a range of bacteria can be very similar. (A history of recent travel or extensive antibiotic use may be a diagnostic clue.)

CAUTION: Blood in the stools is always a sign that must be investigated further by skilled diagnosticians.

Astringents help reduce the symptoms of loose bowels and blood loss. Bayberry is excellent here; agrimony and cranesbill can be added. Demulcents such as slippery elm and marshmallow root may soothe the surface irritation. Vulneraries (wound-healing plants) such as comfrey root will promote the healing of ulceration in the mucosal lining. Anti-inflammatories will help the body in its attempt to get the inappropriate inflammatory reaction under control. Carminatives may help alleviate abdominal discomfort. Chamomile will fulfill both roles. Antispasmodics will help ease muscular cramping in the bowels, which causes much of the pain. Wild yam, cramp bark, and valerian will prove effective. Nervines will aid in addressing any psychological component of this condition. Following is a colitis remedy that incorporates herbs from most of these categories to help soothe the symptoms of ulcerative colitis.

■ bayberry	2 parts
■ wild yam	2 parts
■ comfrey	2 parts
■ valerian	1 part
■ agrimony	1 part
■ chamomile	1 part

As tincture: take 1 tsp (5 ml) of this mixture three times a day.

At least one clove of raw garlic should be eaten every day, and an infusion of an appropriate carminative nervine should be drunk warm at frequent intervals.

Nutrition becomes a crucial issue in cases of colitis, as there will probably be some degree of malnutrition. A good multivitamin/mineral supplement will help. In their *Textbook of Natural Medicine,* Pizzorno and Murray recommend vitamin supplementation at least five times the RDA. Important minerals appear to be zinc, magnesium, iron (where there is loss of blood via the gut), and electrolyte replacement if there is much diarrhea.

Initially the patient should avoid high fiber to minimize irritation of the inflamed mucosa, but as symptoms are brought under control, build up gradually to a high-fiber diet. Lactobacillus-rich yogurt can be most helpful. It has been found that some people respond well to diets that limit the naturally salicylate-containing foods.

Suggested supplementation to support the work of the herbs might include the following multivitamin/mineral supplement at high dosage:

magnesium: 200 mg daily
zinc picolinate: 50 mg daily
vitamin A: 50,000 IU daily
vitamin E: 200 IU daily

Hemorrhoids

The symptoms of hemorrhoids are bleeding, protrusion, and pain. However, bleeding can never be merely assumed to be due to hemorrhoids but must be correctly diagnosed. Various herbs enjoy a reputation in one culture or another as the best remedy for this common problem. In Europe there is nothing to match the aptly named pilewort! Apart from this plant, most astringents or anti-inflammatories will help.

Cardiovascular tonics will help improve muscle tone and the general state of well-being of the veins involved. Astringents will reduce any bleeding and tighten tissues locally, but if taken internally, they must be used with care to avoid constipation. Bitters will help both digestive and eliminative processes; aperients or mild laxatives will ensure easier bowel movements. Vulnerary herbs will speed local healing of inflamed tissues, emollients will soothe if applied externally, and anti-inflammatories will soothe the inflamed tissue.

- ginkgo
- horse chestnut
- dandelion root
- goldenseal
- cranesbill

Equal parts of herbs or tinctures.

As tincture: take 1 tsp (5 ml) of this mixture three times a day.

As dried herb: infuse 1–2 tsp to a cup and drink three times a day.

A topical application is essential to alleviate symptoms and speed healing.

- horse chestnut tincture   10 ml
- distilled witch hazel   80 ml

Apply to area after every bowel movement and as needed.

Salves may also be used containing any of the many possible herbs, such as calendula, St. John's wort, chamomile, plantain, yarrow. Avoidance or elimination of constipation is often the key to the alleviation of hemorrhoids. Thus, in addition to direct herbal treatment of the hemorrhoids themselves, the following factors need to be explored:

- drugs that affect bowel motility (e.g., opiates, iron supplements, some antidepressants, antacids, laxative abuse)
- digestive conditions such as irritable bowel syndrome, diverticular disease, and food sensitivities

- long periods of immobility
- stress
- depression

For easy bowel movements, a diet with medium- to high-fiber content is necessary. Introduce fiber gradually if the patient is accustomed to low-fiber food.

The Aging Liver and Its Problems

Another organ that is highly receptive to herbal treatment in health as well as in disease is the liver. In the language of traditional herbalists, much mention is made of "detoxifying the liver." The incredible complexity of liver chemistry and its fundamental role in human physiology is so daunting that researchers often dismiss claims for the effectiveness of simple plant remedies as laughable nonsense. However, objective studies of these liver remedies, such as milk thistle, usually bear out the claims.

The liver is a vital organ that serves to metabolize carbohydrates and store them as glycogen; metabolizes lipids (including cholesterol and certain vitamins) and proteins; manufactures bile; filters impurities and toxic material from the blood; produces blood-clotting factors; and destroys old, worn-out red blood cells. The specialized Kupffer cells of the liver play a role in immunity. The liver is able to regenerate itself after being injured or diseased, but if a disease progresses beyond the tissue's capacity to regenerate new cells, the body's entire metabolism is severely affected.

From the ecological perspective offered earlier, it is to be expected that our evolutionary home—the environment in which we live—will nurture and heal many of the ills of the liver. After all, the liver and its wonderful biochemistry is part of the ecosystem as well. With remedies such as dandelion, milk thistle, licorice root, balmony, fringe tree bark, and the bitter tonic herbs mentioned earlier, a powerful materia medica is available. Herbal treatment can be useful for a wide range of conditions, from those requiring gentle stimulation all the way to profound liver disease.

Cirrhosis

Cirrhosis is the second biggest killer of Americans between the ages of forty-five and sixty-five. Most often this condition is related to chronic alcohol abuse. In the so-called third world, cirrhosis is secondary to viral hepatitis B. Many Western sufferers are largely asymptomatic until generalized weakness, anorexia, weight loss, malaise, and loss of libido become evident.

The hepato-regenerative potential of milk thistle makes this wonderful remedy an essential in any treatment of cirrhosis. Also relevant are the tonic hepatics, including dandelion root, boldo, fringe tree bark, black root, and balmony. Goldenseal may be useful, as may the vegetable artichoke.

■ milk thistle	2 parts
■ vervain	1 part
■ balmony	1 part
■ fringe tree bark	1 part

As tincture or glycerate: take $^1/_2$ tsp (2.5 ml) of this mixture three times a day, building up to 1 tsp (5 ml) three times a day.
As dried herb: infuse 1 tsp to a cup and drink three times a day.

The alcohol base of the tincture may be a problem for persons with an alcohol problem. In that case, if these remedies cannot be obtained in an alcohol-free glycerate form, the medicine must be put into a small amount of hot water. The alcohol will quickly evaporate, leaving behind the herbal component. Strict avoidance of any specific tissue irritants such as alcohol is essential. Alcohol abuse must be addressed if this is a factor. Treatment will include dietary counseling and psychological support. In their *Textbook of Natural Medicine*, Pizzorno and Murray recommend the following supplementation:

vitamin A: 25,000 IU daily
vitamin B complex: 20 times the RDA
vitamin C: 1 g twice a day
vitamin E: 400 IU daily
magnesium: 250 mg twice a day
selenium: 200 mg daily
zinc: 30 mg daily
carnitine: 500 mg twice a day
glutamine: 1 g daily
lactobacillus acidophilus: 1 tsp daily

Jaundice

Jaundice is a symptom, not a disease in itself; skilled diagnosis is needed to elucidate the cause and thus the treatment needed. However, a number of plants can have a direct effect upon the metabolism and buildup of bilirubin in the body, and these can be used to ease discomfort while focusing upon the underlying cause.

The most frequent cause of jaundice is cholestasis, a state in which the flow of bile is impaired, leading to a backup behind the blockage. Here the cause of the blockage must be sought: it may be due to inflamed tissue swelling, ducts blocked by gallstones, cancer, or even parasites.

Hepatic herbs have a positive metabolic effect upon liver metabolism and functioning. Dandelion root and vervain are the hepatics traditionally used in Europe; in America an herbalist might prescribe fringe tree bark, balmony, or goldenseal. The intense itching often experienced by jaundice patients may be alleviated to some degree by antipruritic herbs. Chickweed is one of the most effective of these, but the itching associated with jaundice will only really resolve when the condition itself resolves. The regenerative potential of milk thistle will ensure that no liver damage is caused by backed-up bile.

■ dandelion root	2 parts
■ vervain	1 part
■ milk thistle	1 part
■ fringe tree bark	1 part
■ boldo	1 part

As tincture or glycerate: take ¹/₂ tsp (2.5 ml) of this mixture three times a day, building up to 1 tsp three times a day.

An infusion of chickweed or distilled witch hazel may be applied topically to reduce itching.

The Aging Gallbladder and Its Problems

Allopathic medicine tends to downplay the roles of the gallbladder and of bile in digestion. That may be why the gallbladder is so often surgically removed when gallstones are present, and it is said that such people lead perfectly normal lives thereafter. Even though the absence of the gallbladder is tolerable, a healthy gallbladder helps to ensure efficient digestion, which, in turn, directly decreases the chances of arteriosclerosis, irritable bowel syndrome, hypertension, heart disease, stroke, and many other conditions. Next we will discuss gallbladder inflammation (cholecystitis) and gallstones.

Gallbladder Inflammation

This condition, also called cholecystitis, is characterized by severe pain that becomes localized in the upper right quadrant and radiates to the right lower scapula. Nausea is common. Cholecystitis is responsive to herbal treatment over time, but this may not be an option because of the extreme pain. Diet is pivotal, as intake of fats precipitates the pain.

What actions are most appropriate in the case of gallbladder inflammation? Hepatic tonics such as balmony, fringe tree bark, and milk thistle will support the work of the liver. Anti-inflammatories may help in reducing the severity of swelling. Antispasmodics may help ease the colic in the gallbladder or ducts but are rarely strong enough to alleviate the extreme pain involved. Nervines help ease the strain from pain and general worry. Antimicrobials are helpful as surface immune support even if there is no infection present.

CAUTION: Bitters and strong cholagogues are contraindicated because they increase the strength of muscle contraction.

■ wild yam	2 parts
■ fringe tree bark	2 parts
■ valerian	2 parts
■ dandelion root	1 part
■ black root	1 part

As tincture: take 1 tsp (5 ml) of this mixture three times a day.

An infusion of a carminative-antispasmodic-nervine should be taken on a regular basis throughout the day. Chamomile and balm are excellent examples.

Gallstones

The gallbladder contains bile, a viscous fluid made in the liver that drains via the common bile duct into the intestine. When the gallbladder becomes diseased, some of the material normally held in suspension in the bile forms stones in the gallbladder. Stones may close the narrow end of the gallbladder or the common bile duct, creating pressure that may cause acute pain on the right side of the abdomen. Common duct stones usually begin in the gallbladder and travel to the common bile duct, but they may also form spontaneously in the duct. Once they become lodged there, the resulting blockage produces pain as well as impaired functioning of the liver and gallbladder.

Many factors appear to influence the development of gallstones, from sex to ethnic origin, but its fundamental causes are not understood. Diet contributes to the major type of stones in that they are made primarily of cholesterol. Antilithics are plants with a long tradition of use in easing the pain as well as in moving or even dissolving gallstones. Hepatic tonics support the work of the liver and so have a positive metabolic effect through the makeup of the bile. Antispasmodics may help ease colic in the gallbladder or ducts. Nervines help ease strain from the pain and general worry. Alteratives/tonics will support the body as a whole in its healing work.

■ wild yam	2 parts
■ boldo	2 parts
■ valerian	2 parts
■ balmony	1 part
■ black root	1 part
■ fringe tree bark	1 part

As tincture: take 1 tsp (5 ml) of this mixture three times a day. An infusion of a carminative-antispasmodic-nervine (e.g., balm or chamomile) should be taken regularly throughout the day.

2 The Cardiovascular System

Plants still maintain a central position today in orthodox medical treatment of various heart problems. Herbs containing constituents called cardiac glycosides are used worldwide for treating heart failure and arrhythmias. These herbs help strengthen the heartbeat and normalize its rate. Yet their real value lies in the fact that the increased efficiency does not necessitate an increase of oxygen supply to the heart muscle. Heart problems are often marked by a deficiency in blood supply because of blockage in the coronary arteries. Foxglove is the source of the widely used medication digoxin, but it is not the sole herb with such valuable properties. Indeed, lily of the valley shares its therapeutic value but has fewer side effects. However, herbal remedies nurture the heart in deeper ways as well. Consider the cordial, a warming drink and a word for heartfelt friendliness. The original cordial was a medieval drink based on borage that warmed the heart and gave the recipient *heart*.

Herbal Actions

Treatment of cardiovascular conditions can be based on an understanding of herbal actions and the way in which they affect physiology. The cardiovascular tonics offer a range of remedies uniquely suited for treating problems of the heart and blood vessels. While they cannot boast the dramatic, rapid, often lifesaving effects of many of the synthetic drugs on the market today, they have a definite advantage in addressing the chronic degenerative conditions often found among

56

people as they age. In addition to tonic remedies for the heart, there are also tonics for the vessels. Vascular tonics are often rich in plant constituents called flavones (found, for example, in horse chestnut and ginkgo).

It is essential to avoid the inappropriate use of cardiac glycoside-containing herbs, as toxic levels of these chemicals are rapidly built up. If such support of heart function is needed, it is safest to use the glycosides in a standardized form to ensure correct dosage. This is almost impossible for the herbalist to calculate in the case of the very variable leaf of foxglove, which points to the value of pharmaceutical preparations of the digitalis glycosides. Such potent treatment is not always necessary and not the only option. The cardiotonic remedy hawthorn, arguably the most valuable tonic for the cardiovascular system, contains no cardiac glycosides. The plant kingdom offers many cardioactive remedies in addition to foxglove, such as lily of the valley, oleander, autumn squill, and Scots broom. Great care must be taken with these remedies, which are best left to the trained and experienced practitioner.

Circulatory stimulants such as cayenne, ginger, and prickly ash help warm the periphery of the body by increasing blood flow; they will also support oxygenation of tissue and the elimination of waste, which makes them important in circulatory problems as well as conditions such as rheumatism. Peripheral vasodilators such as prickly ash and ginkgo yield similar results but work by dilation of the small blood vessels. They are especially relevant where arteriosclerosis is present.

Hypotensives are plants that lower high blood pressure. Many such plants exist; the most widely used in the west are hawthorn, linden blossom, European mistletoe, and garlic. Conversely, hypertensives are plants that raise the blood pressure. Scots broom and ma huang are two examples; hence these herbs are strongly contraindicated in the treatment of hypertension.

Diuretics often help, as water retention is widely seen in those whose hearts are not pumping efficiently. (Less blood goes through the kidneys and so less water is filtered.) Of the many plant diuretics, dandelion and yarrow are especially helpful in cardiovascular disease.

Nervine remedies have an effect upon the nervous system in some way, and some have a specific effect upon the neurological control of the heart and blood vessels. Motherwort, linden blossom, and valerian are especially helpful. Antispasmodic plants have a more focused impact upon muscle tone; these are useful in situations where relaxation is appropriate but general sedation is not. Cramp bark is a noteworthy example.

A number of remarkable cardiac tonics are available to us. Each of the herbal traditions of the world has its own excellent plants, but the following are most often used in Western therapy:

garlic   hawthorn   yarrow
ginkgo   linden flowers

Garlic and ginkgo are discussed elsewhere in the book (see pages 62–63 and 125–28), but here we shall consider hawthorn.

Hawthorn

This wonderful gift of nature is the most valuable tonic remedy for the cardiovascular system found in the plant kingdom. There are stronger herbs, but none that provide the nourishing regeneration that hawthorn does. The renowned turn-of-the-century American medical herbalist, Dr. Finley Ellingwood, said of hawthorn that "it is superior to any of the well-known and tried remedies at present in use for the treatment of heart disease, because it seems to cure while other remedies are only palliative at best." (This was at a time when hawthorn was new to North American medicine and was viewed as the wonder herb of its time, much like ginkgo is viewed today!)

Hawthorn offers a way to strengthen the heart with a medicine that is remarkably free of side effects, effective in its actions, and dramatically cheaper than equivalent synthetic preparations. Its chemical constituents make clear the importance of flavones and flavonoids in treatment of the cardiovascular system. This invaluable heart remedy does *not* contain cardiac glycosides.

Hawthorn is a relevant remedy in most cases of cardiovascular disease. A tonic in the true sense, its therapeutic benefits are gained only when a whole-plant preparation is used. When the isolated constituents were tested separately in the laboratory, their individual effects were found to be insignificant, whereas the whole plant has unique and valuable properties. Herbal synergy again! A double-blind clinical trial done in 1981 demonstrated marked improvement of heart function in patients with reduced cardiac output following treatment with hawthorn. Following a four-year study commissioned by the German Federal Ministry of Health, hawthorn has gained full recognition as a heart remedy in Europe.* The monograph reporting this study concludes that the herb has three properties:

---

*H. P. Ammon and M. Handel, "Crataegus, Toxicology and Pharmacy, Part I; Toxicity" [author's translation], *Planta Medica* 43/2 (Oct. 1981): 105–20.

1. It increases the strength of contraction of the heart muscle.

2. It normalizes irregular heartbeat.

3. It increases coronary circulation through dilation of the coronary arteries.

The Ministry of Health concluded that hawthorn's main clinical applications are in the long-term treatment of "loss of cardiac function," any case involving subjective feelings of congestion and "oppression" in the heart region, mild arrhythmias, and especially for conditions of the aging heart that do not warrant the use of foxglove. Most significant is the finding that no contraindications or side effects were noted at all.

How does the herb achieve such results? The research suggests that many of its observable effects are linked to its improvement of coronary circulation. By dilating the coronary arteries, hawthorn relieves cardiac hypoxemia, thus relieving symptoms of angina and reducing the likelihood of anginal attacks. The herb thus directly affects the cells of the heart muscle, enhancing both activity and cell nutrition. It is quite different in activity from the cardiac-glycoside-containing remedies. These impact the contractile fibers, whereas hawthorn promotes the availability and utilization of energy, resulting in a gentle but long-term, sustained affect on degenerative, age-related changes in the myocardium. It does not produce rapid results, but they are persistent once achieved.

In modern herbal therapy the indications for hawthorn are numerous. Any degenerative condition of the cardiovascular system will benefit from its use. Specific examples are myocardial problems and coronary artery disease and its associated conditions. Angina pectoris and similar symptoms will be eased and prevented. Where no disease state exists but a gradual loss of function is experienced due to the aging process, hawthorn is a specific. Because it is nontoxic, does not build up, and is not habit-forming, it may be used over long periods of time to attain therapeutic goals safely. It speeds recovery from heart attacks and lowers hypertension. Used in conjunction with other hypotensives, hawthorn will help keep the heart healthy, preventing the development of coronary disease. It will guard against heart weakness following infectious disease such as pneumonia or diptheria. For arteriosclerosis and its complications, hawthorn is often combined with linden flowers or garlic. Cramp bark, linden, and skullcap complement it well in cases of hypertension.

As hawthorn is one of the better-tasting herbal remedies, a very pleasant tea can be made from one to two teaspoonfuls of the dried herb infused in hot water and drunk daily. Using the tincture is a convenient and effective way to gain the therapeutic benefits from this special remedy; for optimal results, take thirty to forty drops three times daily, then morning and evening for as long as is needed, as a maintenance dose once the desired lower blood pressure has been achieved.

Keeping the Cardiovascular System Healthy

Half of all annual deaths in the Western world are ascribed to heart and blood vessel disease led by atherosclerosis, the most common lethal disease. Any contribution that herbal medicine can make to its treatment is to be welcomed. Heart disease is often the result of an inappropriate lifestyle comprised of features such as stress, poor diet, a destructive belief system, and alcohol abuse. Preventive measures are by far the best way to keep the cardiovascular system healthy. But are people willing to change? This raises questions that herbal medicine cannot answer!

Unfortunately, the causes underlying heart disease are complex and can be confusing. Some of the factors involved are well known and suggest guidelines for possible prevention: for example, the death rate from heart disease in North America is 300 percent higher in smokers than in nonsmokers; and while occasional modest intake of alcohol may actually be beneficial to the circulatory system, there is no doubt that alcohol abuse is a major contributing factor in heart disease. On the other hand, simplistic statements about saturated fats or jogging can be misleading. The following discussion is an overview of factors that contribute to heart disease.

Factors Contributing to Heart Disease

Diet

Whole forests have been turned into pulp to provide paper for articles about cholesterol, polyunsaturated fats, and heart disease. Anyone who attempts to read them all may be inviting a hypertensive crisis! Still, from the wealth of research done, it is clear that heart disease has definite links with dietary fat, raised blood cholesterol, raised blood pressure, smoking, obesity, short stature, and underactivity. The precise role of these factors is unclear, but enough is known to formulate general guidelines about a preventive diet.

The involvement of fats is one well-studied factor. While the saturated fats may be the "worst," it seems that an overpreponderance of *all* fat in the diet is at fault. Stress, a well-recognized factor in cardiovascular aetiology, is known to interact with fat metabolism: A stressful lifestyle leads to the sustained production of adrenaline and noradrenaline, hormones that act to mobilize fatty acids from the body's fat store, which in turn provide a rapid source of energy. However, in the absence of exercise to use this energy, the fatty acids are believed to accumulate and interact with other fatty substances to form yet another fatty substance called atheroma, which is deposited in plaques on the walls of blood vessels. This deposition does the most damage in the blood vessels close to the heart and in the brain and kidneys, because it causes a narrowing of the vessels and so limits the amount of blood available to these organs.

Cholesterol

The name *cholesterol* has come to carry fearful connotations to many people, yet it plays an important and natural role in human metabolism. Cholesterol is found in all cells of the body, mainly as a component of cell membranes, but it has other vital important functions as well. Stored in the adrenals, testes, and ovaries, it is converted into various hormones.

In the liver, cholesterol is the precursor of the bile acids, which are secreted into the intestine to aid in the digestion of food, especially fats. There can be no doubt, however, that high cholesterol levels represent a major factor in the development of many cardiovascular diseases.

Diets rich in saturated fats, cholesterol, and calories appear to be chiefly responsible for high blood cholesterol; such diets are therefore believed to promote the fatty deposits known as plaques, which are symptomatic of atherosclerosis (which we will further discuss in a moment). The atherogenic (plaque-forming) tendency of cholesterol is, however, influenced by the type of lipoproteins that transport it in the blood. The low-density lipoproteins (LDL) are clearly atherogenic, but the high-density lipoproteins (HDL) appear to prevent accumulation of cholesterol in the tissues. The blood levels of these lipoproteins are partially governed by dietary factors, especially the type of vegetable lipids (phytosterols) eaten. The processes involved are complex, but simply stated, plants provide a way to balance cholesterol absorption in a way that has evolved as our bodies evolved, affecting fat metabolism and blood chemistry in an integrated manner. As medical research has focused on this issue, a number of common dietary components have been shown to be active in lowering cholesterol levels in the blood.

Cayenne pepper and other plants that contain the phenolic compound capsaicin lower blood cholesterol levels, as does the spice fenugreek. Caraway is another aromatic spice with demonstrable cholesterol-lowering properties. Finally, garlic and onion have an international reputation as remedies for lowering blood pressure and generally improving the health of the cardiovascular system, and recent research supports this traditional lore. A study was conducted on two groups who were fed garlic for six months, one consisting of twenty healthy volunteers and the other of sixty-two patients with coronary heart disease and raised serum cholesterol. Beneficial changes were found in all involved and reached a peak at the end of eight months. The improvement in cholesterol levels persisted throughout the two months of clinical follow-up. The clinicians concluded that the essential oil of garlic possessed a distinct hypolipidemic, or fat-reducing, action in both healthy people and patients with coronary heart disease. When garlic oil is fed to animals maintained on high fat-high cholesterol diets, cholesterol levels are significantly reduced, often nearing those seen in untreated control animals. This suggests that garlic oil enhances the breakdown of dietary cholesterol and fatty acids.

Great attention has been given by Indian research workers to the value of such findings in humans. In one study, a group of volunteers were given a fat-rich diet for seven days; on the eighth day the fasting blood was analyzed for cholesterol and other fats. They were then given a fat-rich diet with garlic for seven days and on the fifteenth day the fasting blood was analyzed again. On the fat-rich diet the cholesterol levels were significantly increased as compared to normal diet. When garlic was added to the fat-rich diet for seven days, it significantly reduced serum cholesterol levels.

Garlic also reduces the tendency for unnecessary clotting to occur within the blood vessels. It appears to work on the "stickiness" of blood platelets, reducing aggregation and inhibiting the release of clotting factors in the blood. This is thought to be a property of allicin, a unique chemical in garlic well known for its strong antibiotic and antifungal properties. Garlic can work selectively, inhibiting the synthesis of enzymes involved in plaque formation while sparing the vascular synthesis of important prostaglandins. This would make it a safe and effective antithrombotic agent. Following studies on the effect of raw garlic on normal blood cholesterol level in men, research scientists advocated its daily use to lower one's blood cholesterol. Traditional use of onion as well as garlic in the treatment of hypertension is now being supported by research. Onion oil was recently found to contain a blood pressure–lowering prostaglandin. An interesting note is that the blood pressure-normalizing and cholesterol-lowering actions of garlic are not lost in cooking, unlike its antimicrobial effects.

Stress and Personality

An association between a particular type of personality and heart disease has been suggested for many years. As early as 1959, researchers showed that there was a difference in the risk of developing heart disease between people with two types of behavior, called type A and type B.

Type A behavior is characterized by a chronic sense of urgency, aggressiveness (which may be repressed), and striving for achievement. Such people will drive themselves to meet deadlines, many of which are self-imposed. They have feelings of being under pressure, both of time and responsibility, and often do two or three things at once. They are likely to react with hostility to anything that seems to get in their way and are temperamentally incapable of letting up. They are liable to think of themselves as indispensable. All of these factors add up to a state of constant stress!

Type B behavior is characterized by the opposite traits. Type B people are less preoccupied with achievement, less rushed, and generally more easygoing. They don't allow their lives to be governed by a sense of deadlines. They are less prone to anger and do not feel constantly impatient or rushed. They are also better at separating work from play, and they know how to relax.

Studies done over a period of eighteen months to two years with a group of type A and type B people showed that type A people had a 31 percent increased risk of developing heart disease. Physical differences have been identified in people who exhibit one or the other of these two types of behavior. For example, there appear to be more plaque deposits in the coronary arteries of people who fit into the type A category. Type A behavior also was closely associated with other medical risk factors, such as smoking, shortened blood-clotting time, higher than normal blood fat levels, and increased daily secretion of adrenaline (which in turn increases the oxygen requirement of the heart muscles and releases fatty acids from the body fat).

In considering such studies, we need to bear in mind that each person is an individual; while it may be useful for the purpose of a specific study to sort people into categories, these categories are ultimately artificial and cannot stamp any individual once and for all.

Cardiovascular Problems

Angina Pectoris

This relatively common condition occurs when the work of the heart and thus myocardial oxygen demand exceeds the coronary arteries' ability to supply oxygenated blood. The characteristic pain is caused by the resultant lack of oxygen. The intermittent chest pain is usually precipitated by exercise, emotional stress, or other factors such as exposure to cold. Anginal pains are evidence of coronary insufficiency, since the coronary arteries are so narrowed by deposits or clots that the heart cannot receive sufficient blood to support its functions during periods of greater demand.

The phytotherapeutic approach to angina pectoris is similar to that for arteriosclerosis and hypertension. (See pages 65 and 71–75.)

■ hawthorn	3 parts
■ motherwort	2 parts
■ linden blossom	1 part
■ cramp bark	1 part
■ ginkgo	1 part

As tincture: take I tsp (5 ml) of this mixture three times a day.

As dried herb: infuse 2 tsp to a cup and drink three times a day.

One teaspoon of hawthorn tincture can be taken at the first sign of an attack. This should not replace the use of prescription medication. Garlic should be a regular part of the diet.

Arteriosclerosis

The term *arteriosclerosis* refers to several diseases that involve arteries of different sizes as well as different layers of the walls of the arteries. Taken from the Greek for "hardening of the arteries," the term originally signified the tendency of arteries to become hard and brittle through the depositing of calcium in their walls. This is not, however, an important characteristic of the most familiar form of arteriosclerosis, called *atherosclerosis*.

Atherosclerosis, as we noted earlier, is a disease characterized by fatty deposits on the inner lining of the arteries. The presence of these fatty deposits or plaques, leads to a loss of elasticity and a narrowing of the artery. This constriction to smooth blood flow can ultimately deprive vital organs of their blood supply. Clots may lodge in arteries supplying the heart, causing heart attacks, or in the brain, causing stroke. A number of risk factors have been identified that increase the chances of developing arteriosclerosis, including:

- *Hypertension.* High blood pressure is critical in the atherosclerotic process, which does not normally occur in the low-pressure pulmonary arteries and veins, despite their being bathed by the same blood concentration of lipids.
- *Elevated serum lipid levels.* The plaque-forming tendency of cholesterol is influenced by the presence of certain lipoproteins, four types of which transport cholesterol in the blood. The low-density lipoproteins are clearly atherogenic, but the high-density lipoproteins appear to prevent accumulation of cholesterol in the tissues.
- *Obesity* promotes all the risk factors.
- *Cigarette smoking* increases the chances of developing this disease as well as many others.
- *Diets* rich in saturated fats, cholesterol, and calories appear to be chiefly responsible for high blood cholesterol; such diets are therefore believed to promote atherosclerosis.
- A *family history* of premature atherosclerotic disease appears to indicate either a propensity to higher levels of the risk factors for atherosclerosis or an increased susceptibility to them. Inborn errors in lipid metabolisms also increase susceptibility.
- *Diabetes mellitus* is one disease that may lead to arteriosclerosis.
- *Sex.* Between the ages of thirty-five to forty-four the death rate from coronary heart disease among white men is 6.1 times that among white women. This is thought to be due to hormonal influences. Overt manifestations are rare in either sex before the age of forty because more than a 75 percent narrowing of the arteries must occur before blood flow is seriously impeded.
- *Aging* brings about degenerative arterial changes such as dilatation, tortuosity, thickening, and loss of elasticity.

- *Physical inactivity* increases the chances of complications developing, but the disease affects both the active and the sedentary.
- *Personality type* appears to predispose individuals to a range of cardiovascular problems.
- *Lifestyle* considerations may contribute (diet, stress level, etc.).

Herbal tonics that help the heart and blood vessels will support the tissue of the cardiovascular system, possibly maintaining flexibility and tone in affected vessels. Hawthorn berries and garlic are especially important. Herbs that produce a dilation of the small vessels have an obvious value due to their potential for lessening the impact of vessel blockage. Ginkgo is a good example. The hypotensive herbs described in the section on raised blood pressure (page 71) are often indicated. Relaxing remedies such as linden blossom, motherwort, and cramp bark will be indicated if stress is an issue (and when is it not?).

■ hawthorn	2 parts
■ linden blossom	1 part
■ yarrow	1 part
■ cramp bark	1 part
■ ginkgo	1 part

As tincture: take 1 tsp (5 ml) of this mixture three times a day.
As dried herb: infuse 2 tsp to a cup and drink three times a day.

Garlic should be used as a dietary supplement.

Cold Hands and Feet

This common problem in cold climates has many possible causes and presents a challenge to the therapist, as success will result only from careful diagnosis. Herbs will immediately alleviate the symptoms, but unless they also address the underlying cause(s), there will be no long-term change. Factors that can influence vasodilation/constriction include:

- the autonomic nervous system
- the endocrine system
- basal metabolic rate

- locally produced hormones (prostaglandins)
- allergy
- diet
- state of mind

Each one of these factors is in itself multifactorial; thus clear diagnosis is problematic and all too often sidestepped for "convenience." For example, a case of cold hands might have as its cause a prior whiplash injury to the neck, which led to "pinching" of the nerves that control the vascular muscles in the arms. Here, warming herbs will help but not undo the damage of the injury.

Circulatory stimulants will promote better circulation of blood from the trunk of the body to the periphery, and so warm the tissue. Peripheral vasodilators will also increase the warming efficiency of the bloodstream by allowing more blood through. Antispasmodics will ease the tightness of voluntary muscles in the limbs that may be constricting the blood vessels passing through them. Spicy herbs such as ginger, cayenne, mustard, and horseradish are the traditional symptomatic remedies. Prickly ash also has much to offer.

■ hawthorn	2 parts
■ ginkgo	2 parts
■ prickly ash	2 parts
■ cramp bark	1 part
■ ginger	1 part

As tincture: take 1 tsp (5 ml) of this mixture three times a day.
As dried herb: mix 2 tsp to a cup and drink three times a day.

Structural factors must be assessed by a competent practitioner. Exercise is important to ensure that metabolic rate is raised to a healthy level. Nutritional supplements can be very helpful.

vitamin B$_3$ (nicotinic acid): 50 mg three times a day
vitamin C: 1 g daily
vitamin E: 600 IU daily
evening primrose oil: 500 mg daily
magnesium: 200–400 mg daily

Congestive Heart Failure

In cases of congestive heart failure, the heart is not pumping efficiently enough. This leads to a range of problems, with most symptoms resulting from congestion that develops in the lungs or from backup pressure of blood in the veins of the body. Breathlessness and water retention result. Such conditions occur either because the heart itself is diseased or as a result of lung disease, which makes the heart work harder to pump blood to the lungs. In spite of its name, heart failure does not mean that the heart stops pumping. In general, heart failure is not an immediate threat to life; the outcome will depend on the cause and the severity of the problem.

In any type of heart failure, if the heart cannot pump out a normal volume of blood, blood backs up in the veins leading to the heart. Most types of heart disease initially affect the left side of the heart, and clinicians divide associated heart failure into left-sided heart failure and right-sided heart failure. Peripheral edema (water retention) occurs in connection with right-sided heart failure and breathlessness in connection with left-sided heart failure.

Orthodox medicine's approach to heart failure is based upon the successful use of plants that contain cardiac glycosides, such as foxglove. As dramatically effective as these medications are, the key to safe and successful use is skilled diagnosis and interpretation, without which such plants are potentially highly poisonous. The noncardioactive approach described here will prove effective in two particular situations: to support the work of the medication a patient may be on, but not to replace it; and for patients with mild heart failure that does not warrant the use of stronger medication. (This is often the case in older people who have chronic congestive heart failure.)

Cardioactive remedies will be the core treatment for such problems but should be used only under the supervision of skilled diagnosticians who can follow the changes brought about in the heart and its functioning. Cardiac tonics are herbs that safely aid the heart and support the work of the more active drugs. (Hawthorn and garlic are excellent examples.) Safe herbal hypotensives will be indicated if there is associated hypertension. Diuretics can ease water retention problems; dandelion leaf is an herbal diuretic that replaces all the potassium that the diuresis flushes out. Nervines will ease the stress component, whether it is seen as causal or a result of the heart disease.

As the primary cardioactives are often out of the range of what can be safely used by the herbalist, lily of the valley and its equivalents are not included in the following prescription. Our aim is to either strengthen the heart muscle or to support the work of allopathically prescribed cardiac glycosides. Hawthorn, linden blossom, and garlic are essential.

■ hawthorn	3 parts
■ ginkgo	1 part
■ linden blossom	1 part
■ dandelion leaf	1 part
■ motherwort	1 part
■ cramp bark	1 part

As tincture: take 1 tsp (5 ml) of this mixture three times a day.

As dried herb: infuse 2 tsp to a cup and drink three times a day.

Garlic should be used as a dietary supplement.

The dietary and lifestyle issues already discussed all apply in cases of congestive heart failure. (See pages 60–66.)

Heart Attack (Recovery From)

A heart attack occurs when the blood supply to some part of the heart muscle stops abruptly, often because of clotting in a coronary blood vessel. Blood supplying the heart muscle comes entirely from two coronary arteries, both lying along the outside surface of the heart. If one of these arteries or any part of one suddenly becomes blocked, the area of the heart being supplied by the artery dies. The death of a portion of the heart muscle is a myocardial infarct, a heart attack, and the amount of the heart affected by the sudden occlusion will determine the severity of the attack. If the heart continues to function, the dead portion is eventually walled off as new vascular tissue supplies the needed blood to adjacent areas.

As is so often the case, stress can be a contributing factor here, too. The details of this relationship are not entirely clear, but it may be that stress increases the stickiness of blood and makes it more likely to clot. Anxiety, fear, and stress may bring on an attack, as increased adrenaline and noradrenaline are released at such times, and in turn stimulate the heart to beat faster. The pain experienced creates further stress, and the fear of having an attack actually increases the likelihood of one occurring.

As in the case of heart failure, the cardiac tonic remedies will aid in the renewal of tissue and the regaining of as much cardiac function as possible. Hawthorn is the most appropriate remedy. Peripheral vasodilators (e.g., hawthorn and ginkgo) help in the process of reoxygenation of oxygen-starved tissue as well as helping to prevent another attack. Relaxing nervine herbs as well as adaptogens will help the person to cope with the stress component, which may be either causal or a result of experiencing cardiac trauma.

■	hawthorn	3 parts
■	ginkgo	2 parts
■	linden blossom	1 part
■	Siberian ginseng	1 part

As tincture: take 1 tsp (5 ml) of this mixture three times a day.

As dried herb: infuse 2 tsp to a cup and drink three times a day.

Garlic should be used as a dietary supplement.

Hypertension

A differentiation must be made between elevated blood pressure with no obvious medical cause (primary or essential hypertension) and that due to an underlying pathology such as kidney, hormonal, or cerebral disease (secondary hypertension). The following section is concerned with essential hypertension.

There are more than thirty-five million hypertensives in the United States. Twice as many African Americans as Caucasians are afflicted, but the reasons for this are not understood. A common problem in our culture, hypertension is rare in cultures that are relatively untouched by the Western lifestyle. Lifestyle plays a major role in causing and maintaining hypertension. Dietary, psychological, and social factors must all be addressed for any real change to occur.

Hypertension is typically free of symptoms until complications arise. The symptoms associated with the condition can be caused by other problems as well and include dizziness, flushed face, headache, fatigue, nosebleed, and nervousness. Observable changes in retinal blood vessels are diagnostic indicators of the degree of damage caused to the body by hypertension. Diagnosis includes finding that both systolic and diastolic blood pressure are usually, but not always, higher than normal; other causes must be excluded. Hypertension is considered to be shown by a blood pressure reading of greater than 140/90, but "normal" must be considered as a range rather than as one specific figure for the whole population.

Temporary increase in blood pressure is a common and normal response to the ups and downs of life. Sustained hypertension is caused by increased peripheral vascular resistance. This is initiated by increased arteriolar tone and leads to the damaging structural changes of arteriosclerosis.

A number of herbs have a reputation as being specific for hypertension, usually because of their impact on one or another of the processes involved in the condition's development. The hypotensives, remedies that have been found by generations of herbalists to reduce elevated blood pressure, fit this description. The most important such plant remedy known to Western medicine is hawthorn, but there are many more. Included here is a partial list:

black cohosh	hawthorn berries	passionflower
black haw	linden	Siberian ginseng
blue cohosh	mistletoe	skullcap
buckwheat	motherwort	valerian
cramp bark	nettle	vervain
fenugreek	onion	yarrow (European)
garlic	parsley	

Each of these hypotensives has other effects that are known as secondary actions; thus the herbalist can select remedies that address the individual's range of needs, not merely the hypertension. Following is a selection of safe and effective hypotensives grouped by their other actions.

- *Adaptogen:* Siberian ginseng
- *Anti-inflammatory:* black cohosh, blue cohosh, buckwheat, valerian
- *Antispasmodic:* black cohosh, cramp bark, linden, motherwort, passionflower, skullcap, valerian
- *Bitter:* yarrow

- *Carminative:* parsley, valerian
- *Demulcent:* fenugreek
- *Diaphoretic:* garlic, linden, onion, vervain, yarrow
- *Diuretic:* linden, nettle, parsley, yarrow
- *Expectorant:* fenugreek, garlic, onion, parsley
- *Hepatic:* onion, vervain
- *Nervine:* black cohosh, cramp bark, linden, motherwort, passionflower, skullcap, valerian, vervain

Where hypertension is associated with water retention, more emphasis will be placed upon the diuretic herbs listed above; where stress is a major factor, consider the adaptogens and nervines, and so forth. Here is a safe and effective sample combination that will gradually normalize the blood pressure:

■ hawthorn	2 parts
■ linden blossom	1 part
■ yarrow	1 part
■ cramp bark	1 part
■ valerian	1 part

As tincture: take 1 tsp (5 ml) of this mixture three times a day.
As dried herb: infuse 2 tsp to a cup and drink three times a day.

Garlic should be used as a dietary supplement.

The ingredients in this mixture are all hypotensives but also offer a well-rounded range of relevant secondary actions. Hawthorn is also an excellent cardiac tonic and thus plays a fundamental role in strengthening and toning the whole cardiovascular system. Diuretics such as yarrow help remove any excessive buildup of water in the body and overcome any decrease in renal blood flow that may accompany the hypertension. Peripheral vasodilators will lessen high resistance within the peripheral blood vessels, thus increasing the total volume of the system and so lowering the pressure within it. The nervines valerian, linden, and cramp bark address any tension and anxiety present. Antispasmodics will ease peripheral resistance to blood flow by gently relaxing both the muscles that the vessels pass through and the muscular coat of the vessels themselves. Cramp bark is probably the most effective and safe of these herbs; valerian is a second.

Other plants might be added as well, depending upon the individual's specific symptom picture. For example, if palpitations are present, add motherwort. If stress is a factor, increase the nervine content and possibly include an adaptogen. An alternative prescription for hypertension with stress as a major factor might be the following:

■ hawthorn	2 parts
■ linden blossom	1 part
■ yarrow	1 part
■ Siberian ginseng	1 part
■ skullcap	1 part
■ cramp bark	1 part
■ valerian	1 part

As tincture: take 1 tsp (5 ml) of this mixture three times a day.

As dried herb: infuse 2 tsp to a cup and drink three times a day.

Garlic should be used as a dietary supplement

Another example might take into account heart palpitations (tachycardia). If the cause of the palpitations is not heart disease as such, a prescription for hypertension with palpitations might be the following:

■ hawthorn	2 parts
■ motherwort	2 parts
■ linden blossom	1 part
■ yarrow	1 part
■ cramp bark	1 part
■ valerian	1 part

As tincture: take I tsp (5 ml) of this mixture three times a day.

As dried herb: infuse 2 tsp to a cup and drink three times a day.

Garlic should be used as a dietary supplement.

A wide array of factors have been identified as important in the cause and treatment of essential hypertension. However, it must be remembered that causation is *always* multifactorial and any general statements (e.g., about alcohol or calcium) are often too simplistic. For example, one study failed to show any association between heavy coffee consumption and long-term hypertension. Since many coffee drinkers tend to be heavy smokers as well, this may mean a lower body weight and thus a lower blood pressure—but such people will nevertheless be subject to an increased risk of heart attack!

Many dietary factors must be taken into account, including the following:

- *Alcohol.* There appears to be a link between alcohol and hypertension, but not a simple one. Statistics show that people who drink moderately tend to have lower blood pressure than either teetotalers or heavy drinkers. Alcohol withdrawal causes an initial, temporary increase in blood pressure before there is a fall. All in all, it is safe to say that any individuals with a tendency to hypertension should avoid alcohol.
- *Caffeine.* Tea, coffee, and cola drinks will aggravate hypertension because of the stimulating effect of caffeine and other alkaloids they contain. This is also true for the herbal stimulants on the market, such as ephedra, guarana, and cola.
- *Calcium and magnesium.* Supplementation with these minerals can have a marked hypotensive effect.
- The *Contraceptive Pill* (used in hormone replacement therapy). Controversy still rages over its side effects. One area of debate concerns its possible hypertensive effects.
- *Dietary salt.* The average Western salt intake is about fifteen times that needed by the body. A low salt diet is strongly indicated.
- *Drugs.* A number of medications raise blood pressure as an unwanted side effect. Check the labels of all prescription drugs being used, and note that even over-the-counter nonsteroidal anti-inflammatories may cause mild water retention that can elevate blood pressure.
- *Obesity.* It has long been recognized that obesity is linked to hypertension, as well as to risk of heart attack, diabetes, gallstones, osteoarthritis, and kidney disease. Weight reduction is essential and will often lower blood pressure more effectively than drug treatment.
- *Potassium.* The relative balance between sodium and potassium is crucial for many cardiovascular factors. In addition to restricting salt intake, elevate potassium levels in the diet by eating potassium-rich foods. Such

natural sources of potassium include fruit, legumes, meat, fish, green leafy vegetables, whole grains, and especially apricots, avocados, bananas, blackstrap molasses, brewer's yeast, dates, and figs.

- *Saturated fats.* Apart from the impact upon blood cholesterol and other lipids, there appears to be an association between overly high levels of saturated fats and hypertension. Here, as in other cardiovascular conditions, increasing the ratio of polyunsaturated fats to saturated fats will assist the healing process.
- *Sugar.* In some individuals heavy sugar intake may raise blood pressure, possibly by causing sodium retention or by a direct effect upon the stress response hormone system.
- *Tobacco.* Experts disagree about the connection between tobacco and hypertension, but as there is no doubt about the impact of smoking upon the heart, it should be avoided.
- *Vegetarian diets.* A diet free of animal products definitely lowers blood pressure and is strongly advised for hypertensive patients. At the very least, there should be an avoidance of red meat.

Lifestyle can often be the key in reversing this condition. Exercise, massage, and other approaches to the body are important, as are relaxation techniques and meditation. The nature of the individual's work, relationships, worldview, self-image, and so on may all contribute to hypertension, creating a challenging job for the herbalist!

Intermittent Claudication

Peripheral vascular diseases such as intermittent claudication are caused by narrowing of the arteries in the legs, which restricts the flow of blood to muscles in the calves, thighs, and buttocks. Although such conditions are usually symptom free in the early stages, the restricted availability of oxygen eventually causes major problems. The most striking symptom occurs upon exertion, such as walking. The increase in oxygen required cannot be provided by the limited blood supply, resulting in a buildup of lactic acid and other products of enforced anaerobic metabolism in the muscles. These metabolites cause pain and cramps and bring any attempts at walking to a halt. On resting, the pain and discomfort stops, enabling the walking to be resumed. There is a close association between this problem and the aetiology of arteriosclerosis.

Cardiovascular tonics are indicated because the pathology that is manifesting in the legs is suggestive of disease processes almost certainly affecting the whole of the cardiovascular system. Peripheral vasodilators facilitate the flow of blood through the extremities, and antispasmodics may ease muscular spasm.

- hawthorn
- horse chestnut
- ginkgo
- prickly ash
- cramp bark

Equal parts of herbs or tinctures.

As tincture: take 1 tsp (5 ml) of this mixture three times a day.

As dried herb: infuse 2 tsp to a cup and drink three times a day.

Garlic should be used as a dietary supplement.

Varicose Veins

This common problem affects between 10 and 20 percent of the population, incidence increases with age and is most common in those individuals who are fifty years of age and older. It is four times more common in women than men. The core problem is that some degree of reversal of blood flow in the veins of the legs occurs due to valve incompetency. This causes dilation of the veins and loss of tissue tone. The abnormal swelling of veins in the legs is a symptom of a generally poor circulatory system, with a loss of elasticity in the walls of the veins and particularly in their valves. When they are functioning normally, these valves prevent blood from flowing back away from the heart, but if their efficiency decreases some blood may stagnate in the vein, which then becomes swollen and twisted, causing aching and abnormal fatigue of the legs. A number of factors can be identified as contributory to two aspects of varicosity:

1. Lack of support of the vein walls:
   - *Heredity.* About 40 percent of cases have a family history of varicosity.
   - *Obesity.* The fatty tissue that builds up in the legs provides inadequate support and leads to loss of tone.

- *Age.* The aging process leads to degenerative changes in the supporting connective tissue, compounded by decreased muscular activity.
- *Posture.* Occupations that involve prolonged standing or sitting increase the chances for this problem to develop. This is due to a combination of the pull of gravity and not enough muscular activity in the thighs.

2. Increased resistance to free flow of blood back into the trunk:
   - *Pregnancy.* The growing baby will act as an obstacle to venous return.
   - *Thrombosis.* Any tendency to blockage of the blood vessels increases resistance to the free flow of blood.
   - *Tumors.* For example, uterine fibroids or ovarian cysts can become obstructive.
   - *External pressure.* Constriction caused by tight clothing will weaken the tissue.

Flavonoid-rich plants have a major role to play in toning up these vessels. In Europe, horse chestnut has traditionally been considered an effective specific.

Internal Remedy

- hawthorn
- prickly ash
- ginkgo
- yarrow
- horse chestnut

Equal parts of herbs or tinctures.
As tincture: take 1 tsp (5 ml) of this mixture three times a day.
As dried herb: infuse 2 tsp to a cup and drink three times a day.

A Lotion for External Use

- distilled witch hazel   80 ml
- horse chestnut tincture   10 ml
- comfrey tincture   10 ml

Apply liberally as needed to ease irritation and discomfort.
Rose water may be added to the lotion for cosmetic reasons.

Lifestyle factors are very important in the long-term treatment of this sometimes intransigent condition. Diet is as important here as for the rest of the cardiovascular system. The main insight is the avoidance of postures or situations that aggravate the resistance to easy venous return from the legs. Anything that counters the effects of gravity will be helpful.

Resting with the legs higher than the head for at least ten minutes every day will help in the long run and also decrease any immediate discomfort. This may be achieved through the inverted postures of yoga, use of a slanted board, or simply lying on the floor with the legs and feet supported by a chair. The foot of the bed can be elevated between six and twelve inches, thus facilitating drainage at night. Gentle exercise is helpful. Walking and gentle stretching exercises are suitable, but jogging, skipping, aerobics, or other exercises that involve repeated impact can do more harm than good. (However, such exercise would be so uncomfortable for anybody with varicose veins that she or he would be unlikely to try it for more than a very short time.)

Aromatherapy can help improve the general tone of the veins when used in a broad holistic context. Cypress oil has a good reputation for strengthening the veins in the legs. It can be used as a bath oil and applied very gently over the area of the affected veins. Massage can be used above the affected area of the vein but must never be used below the varicosity, as this will increase the pressure in the vein. Cypress oil should be blended in a carrier oil such as almond oil (see pages 242–49).

3 The Pulmonary System

Much of the disease commonly associated with both the upper and lower respiratory systems is preventable. Air quality is the key. If everyone could avoid particulate air pollution and chemical irritants such as sulphur dioxide, many of the disabling conditions of the lungs that are seen today would not develop. Thus smoking—both active and passive—as well as urban and industrial pollution are important issues for "therapist" and "patient" alike.

Keeping lungs healthy in an industrialized nation, where air pollution and cigarette smoking are significant hazards, is no easy task. A city dweller may feel helpless against the emission from buses and automobiles, yet organized civic action has succeeded in reducing these pollutants. Far worse, from the viewpoint of health, are the fumes smokers willingly suck into their lungs with every puff of a cigarette.

The best thing to do for the lungs is to avoid cigarettes. The numbers are persuasive. The Surgeon General's office estimates that tobacco kills as many as 340,000 Americans each year. In a twenty-five-state study conducted by the American Cancer Society, the following findings about smoking and longevity emerged:

- A 30-year-old nonsmoking man can expect to live, on average, another 43.9 years.
- A 30-year-old man who smokes from one to nine cigarettes daily can expect to lose, on average, 4.6 years of his life; if he smokes ten to nineteen

cigarettes daily, he can expect to lose 5.5 years; if he smokes twenty to thirty-nine cigarettes daily, he can expect to lose 6.1 years; if he smokes forty or more cigarettes daily, he can expect to lose 8.1 years.

On the positive side, stopping the habit *at any age* can dramatically reduce the risk of contracting heart disease, lung cancer, or emphysema. Damaged cilia within the lungs will regrow in about six months after all smoking has stopped. Studies have shown improvement in pulmonary function as early as three weeks after the last cigarette has been smoked.

Furthermore, the physiological benefits are many. No longer will nicotine cause the heart to beat faster and your blood pressure to rise, and no longer will nicotine affect the automatic nervous system in other dangerous ways. No longer will the ex-smoker have to deal with a fuzzy mouth, lowered taste sensations, and yellow teeth stains. Finally, the ex-smoker suffers less from coughs and colds, laryngitis, and sinusitis.

Some people are able to stop smoking on their own, others need group support. Many groups exist to help smokers quit the habit. Contact the local chapter of the American Cancer Society or the American Lung Association, which has a free program entitled "Freedom From Smoking," available to visitors of their website (www.lungusa.org), or call your state's Quit Line for a free or low-cost kit. Breathing exercises are advised for both ex-smokers and nonsmokers to relieve tension and also to maintain healthy lungs throughout life. The American Lung Association recommends the following four-step deep-breathing exercises to be done twice a day:

1. Lie flat on your back with your mouth closed, hands folded on your stomach, and your knees flexed. Let your shoulders relax and inhale as deeply as you can—to the count of eight. Push your stomach out as you inhale.

2. Hold your breath to the count of four.

3. Exhale slowly to the count of eight.

4. Repeat this inhale-hold-exhale cycle five times.

Herbal Actions

When the lungs are affected, several herbal actions are of direct value as explained in the following list.

Anticatarrhal: Anticatarrhals help the body remove excess catarrh, whether in the sinus area or other parts of the body. Catarrh is not of itself a problem, but when too much is produced it is usually in response to an infection or as a way to remove excess carbohydrates from the body. Many herbs can help here (these are discussed in more depth elsewhere); consider goldenrod, hyssop, and coltsfoot.

Antimicrobial: These help the body to destroy or resist pathogenic microorganisms. More important, they help the body strengthen its own resistance to infective organisms and throw off the illness. While some contain chemicals that are antiseptic or specific poisons to certain organisms, in general they aid the body's natural immunity. Of the many herbs that are antimicrobial in the respiratory system, consider garlic, echinacea, eucalyptus, thyme, and osha.

Antispasmodic: Antispasmodics ease muscle cramps in general, but some will reduce muscle spasm in specific organs or systems. For the respiratory system, they will be helpful in conditions such as asthma. Consider gumweed, lobelia, wild cherry bark, and wild lettuce.

Cardiac Tonics: This term refers to herbal remedies that have a beneficial action on the heart without having the powerful cardioactive effect of agents such as foxglove. Hawthorn, motherwort, and linden blossoms are excellent examples of safe yet effective herbs for supporting the heart.

Demulcent: Rich in mucilage to soothe and protect irritated or inflamed tissue, the demulcents are usually considered primarily useful for the digestive system, but they will ease coughing by soothing bronchial tension. Herbs that are especially useful for the lungs include plantain, lungwort, Iceland moss, and pleurisy root.

Expectorant: Strictly speaking, these herbs stimulate removal of mucus from the lungs, but often they provide a tonic for the respiratory system as a whole. Stimulating expectorants "irritate" the bronchioles, causing expulsion of material. Relaxing expectorants soothe bronchial spasm and loosen mucous secretions, helping in dry, irritating coughs. The differences are discussed in more depth in the next section. Stimulating expectorants include elecampane, horehound, and bloodroot; relaxing expectorants include coltsfoot, lobelia, and mullein.

Nervines: Nervines generally help the nervous system and form three groups. Nervine tonics strengthen and restore the nervous system. Nervine relaxants ease anxiety and tension by soothing both body and mind. Nervine stimulants directly stimulate nerve activity. They often help in respiratory problems where there is associated tension and anxiety. Examples most relevant to this system include hyssop, motherwort, lobelia, and wild lettuce.

Pulmonary Tonic: Tonics specifically nurture and enliven the lungs and thus the whole process of breathing. They may be safely used whenever such tonic work is needed. The most important ones also have other beneficial properties as well. Elecampane has associated stimulating expectorant properties and is helpful in clearing the lungs of phlegm. Mullein has a more soothing expectorant effect.

Herbal Expectorants

Expectorants are herbs that help in the removal of excess mucus from the lungs. However, the same term is often used to loosely mean a remedy that "does something" for the respiratory system. To be more precise, the various remedies called "expectorants" can be subdivided as follows:

Stimulating expectorants can act in any of various ways to produce the same effect, and it is not always clear how a specific remedy is working, but current ideas suggest the following processes:

- The irritation of the bronchioles stimulates the expulsion of any material present.
- The viscous sputum is made thinner so that it can be cleared by coughing. The sputum is moved upward from the lungs by the fine hairs of the cells lining the bronchiole tubes; reducing viscosity through expectorants facilitates this transport.

Most stimulating expectorants contain alkaloids, saponins, or volatile oils. However, not all chemicals in these groups, or plants with these constituents, act in this same way.

Relaxing expectorants would seem to act also by reflex, but here it is to soothe bronchial spasm and loosen secretions; thus they are especially useful in treating dry, irritating coughs.

Pharmacopeias abound in plant remedies, and most of the herbs still in the official lists are expectorants, antitussives, or decongestants. However, the allopathic focus on "effect" has led to elimination of the tonic remedies such as the pulmonaries. They provide phytotherapy with the possibility of strengthening both tissue and function, in addition to addressing the symptoms of respiratory disease.

Tonics for the Lower Respiratory System

Pulmonary herbs have a beneficial effect upon both the tissue of the lungs and their functioning and are a valuable addition to any treatment of a lung-related problem. They often mark the difference between simple removal of symptoms and a more fundamental healing. Important remedies include elecampane, mullein, and coltsfoot.

The differential indications will be found in the Materia Medica section of this book for each of the remedies, but in general elecampane can be said to have stimulating expectorant effects, whereas mullein is generally a relaxing expectorant. Coltsfoot is the best of the three for the very frail.

Several remedies are appropriate for respiratory problems, each having its distinct area of application. The criteria for their inclusion in this list are that they are both safe and effective.

aniseed	hyssop	pleurisy root
coltsfoot	Irish moss	thyme
elecampane	lungwort	wild cherry bark
garlic	motherwort	
horehound	mullein	

The following stronger effectors may be found useful in more intransigent conditions but should be reserved for cases where the gentler herbs have not produced the results desired:

bloodroot	ipecacuanha	senega
gumweed	lobelia	

Pulmonary Problems

Asthma

This is a noncontagious condition in which the small airways of the lungs temporarily constrict so that it is difficult to exhale. This leads to breathlessness and the characteristic wheezing sound associated with an asthma attack. Such difficulty is caused by muscle spasm in the bronchi of the lungs. Because the passages are narrowed and air flow reduced, mucus also builds up in the lungs, making breathing even more difficult. The mucus is also a breeding ground for bacteria, so bronchitis may arise as a complication of the asthma.

Many asthma attacks are triggered by allergens such as dust, mold spores, animal hair, or feathers, but the onset may also be caused by cold air or may be preceded by a respiratory infection. Stress and specifically acute anxiety are known to trigger many attacks, and this can sometimes give rise to a vicious circle in which asthma generates anxiety about the asthma, which in turn provokes further attacks.

The symptoms of people with asthma differ greatly in frequency and degree. Some have occasional episodes that are mild and brief, otherwise they are symptom free. Others have mild coughing and wheezing much of the time, punctuated by severe exacerbations of symptoms following exposure to known allergens, viral infections, exercise, or nonspecific irritants. A series of stages have been characterized for describing the severity of an acute asthma attack:

1. *Mild:* mild breathlessness

2. *Moderate:* respiratory distress and wheezing at rest

3. *Severe:* marked respiratory distress

4. *Respiratory failure:* severe respiratory distress (life threatening)

Herbalism has much to offer in the treatment, control, and even cure of asthmatic problems but will not replace emergency allopathic support in stages 3 and 4. Most successful are the antispasmodic and bronchodilator plants, but they will do little for short-term relief of attacks. When used over a period of time, however, especially in conjunction with pulmonary tonics that strengthen the lungs, they can reduce both the frequency and severity of attacks. Expectorant remedies will be essential to ensure minimum buildup of sputum in the lungs. However, as stimulant expectorants can potentially aggravate breathing difficulties, only the relaxing expectorants are used. Antimicrobial support will guard against secondary infection. Anticatarrhals will help the body to deal with any overproduction of sputum in the lungs or sinuses, and cardiotonic herbs will support the heart in the face of lung congestion or strain. Nervines can help either where stress is a primary trigger or where the asthma itself becomes a source of stress that in turn triggers attacks.

Ma huang, the original source of the widely used alkaloid l-ephedrine, is exceptionally useful as a bronchodilator. This natural form has advantages over the synthesized version, as it is better tolerated and in particular causes fewer heart symptoms. Ephedrine stimulates the sympathetic nervous system, relieving the bronchial spasm that underlies the asthmatic state, as well as other conditions with a bronchospasm component such as emphysema. Besides ma huang, other plants prominent in Western herbal therapy for their marked antispasmodic and bronchodilating effects are gumweed, sundew, and wild cherry bark.

Asthma Mixture (Chronic Asthma)

■ gumweed	5 parts
■ wild cherry bark	2 parts
■ lobelia	1 part
■ licorice	1 part
■ motherwort	1 part
■ ma huang	1 part

As tincture: take 1 tsp (5 ml) of this mixture three times a day.

A good deal can be done by the asthmatic to prevent attacks. Every effort should be made to stay in good physical condition, to avoid colds and respiratory infections, and to seek prompt and adequate treatment if a cold threatens. Extremes of heat, cold, and dampness should be avoided; if it is necessary to go out in inclement weather, dress warmly. On the other hand, air that is too dry, as is the case in many homes in winter, may be harmful. A relative humidity of 40 to 50 percent is desirable.

Infected teeth and sinuses should be treated. The diet should be as balanced and nutritious as possible, with foods selected to compensate for any omitted allergenic foods. Food sensitivities must also be identified. It may be wise to exclude eggs, wheat, gluten (found in wheat, oats, barley, and rye), or dairy products for a time. Another source of concern is alcohol (wine and beer) and dried fruit, which often contain sulphur dioxide. Many asthmatics react to preservatives in amounts as small as five parts of sulphur dioxide per million. Asthmatics should keep away from drafts, paint fumes, chemicals, and dust; smoking must be avoided entirely. In persistent or severe asthma, exercise should be moderate. Getting enough rest is particularly important.

The asthmatic's emotional life may also need regulating, for our lungs are connected to our emotions in an obvious way (think about laughing or crying). If a person with asthma has difficulty in expressing his or her feelings, it is worth exploring why this should be. The Bach Flower Remedies can help here. Deep breathing can strengthen our connection to our feelings and can help improve asthma if practiced regularly. Other regular exercise, such as walking, swimming, yoga, t'ai chi, or other relaxation classes, can also help to deepen and relax breathing and provide emotional balance.

The whole thoracic area—back and chest—should be regularly massaged with aromatic oil, with particular emphasis on strokes that open out the chest and shoulders. The choice of an essential oil will depend on many factors, such as whether or not there is infection present, whether the asthma is known to be an allergic response, or whether emotional factors are involved. During an actual crisis, inhaling an antispasmodic oil is the only practical herbal help, and direct sniffing from the oil bottle, or from drops put on a tissue, will be safer than a steam inhalation, as the heat of the latter will increase any inflammation of the mucus membranes and make the congestion even worse. Useful oils include hyssop, aniseed, lavender, pine, and rosemary.

The *Textbook of Natural Medicine* by Pizzorno and Murray recommends the following nutritional supplements:

> **vitamin B$_6$:** 25 mg twice a day
> **vitamin B$_{12}$:** 1,000 mcg daily
> **vitamin C:** 1–2 g daily
> **vitamin E:** 400 IU daily
> **selenium:** 250 mcg daily

Bronchitis (Acute)

Bronchitis is an acute or chronic inflammation of the mucous lining of the bronchial tubes, the main passageways carrying air from the trachea to the lungs. Acute bronchitis is often a feverish condition, usually lasting a few days, with a harsh and painful cough. The development of acute bronchitis is often preceded by symptoms of upper respiratory infections such as those that characterize the common cold: chilliness, slight fever, back and muscle pain, and sore throat. At first the cough is very dry, but as the lungs produce additional mucus in response to the infection, the cough becomes easier and less painful as the mucus lubricates the bronchi. Persistent fever suggests a complicating condition such as pneumonia.

The form of acute bronchitis may be severe in debilitated people and those with chronic lung or heart disease.

Pulmonary tonics are crucial when treating acute bronchitis, as toning will speed recuperation and lessen the chances of a secondary infection. The type of expectorant indicated—stimulating or relaxing—depends upon the individual case. Antimicrobials are essential to deal with any infection or to help the body protect itself against the development of secondary infection. Cardiotonic herbs are essential if there is any history or suspicion of cardiovascular problems. Antispasmodic herbs may be of help if coughing proves too troublesome.

The world's many herbal traditions provide a wealth of possible remedies for bronchitis. For example, osha *(Ligusticum porterii),* a plant from the American Southwest, is excellent in cases of tracheobronchitis. Below is a partial listing of herbs commonly used in Europe and parts of North America. They may be appropriate for different individuals at different times, the range covering stimulant and demulcent expectorants, antimicrobials, antispasmodics, and so on. Thus no one herb is guaranteed to work in all cases.

aniseed	horehound	mullein
balm of Gilead	hyssop	osha
bloodroot	Iceland moss	plantain
coltsfoot	ipecacuanha	pleurisy root
comfrey	Irish moss	skunk cabbage
elecampane	licorice	thyme
fenugreek	lobelia	vervain
garlic	lungwort	
goldenseal	marshmallow	

The use of soothing, relaxing expectorants, with their distinctive demulcency, in conjunction with antimicrobials is often the key to successful treatment. The following combination of relaxing expectorants may be especially helpful:

- mullein
- coltsfoot
- marshmallow
- aniseed

Equal parts of dried herbs.
Infuse 2 tsp to a cup of boiling water for 10 minutes. Drink hot several times a day. (It is in the form of an infusion partly for the benefit of increasing fluid intake.)

Another approach is to add stimulating expectorants; the resultant mixture is more appropriate for those stages of bronchitis that are characterized by excessive sputum production. An example of a mixture to promote expectoration and combat infection in acute bronchitis is the following:

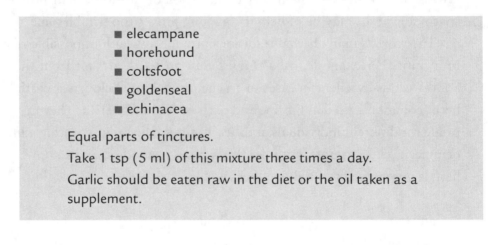

- elecampane
- horehound
- coltsfoot
- goldenseal
- echinacea

Equal parts of tinctures.
Take 1 tsp (5 ml) of this mixture three times a day.
Garlic should be eaten raw in the diet or the oil taken as a supplement.

STEAM INHALATIONS

Volatile oil-rich plants are often used for steam inhalations, a form of treatment that can often abort the development of a cold or even flu. When the problem is already established, using inhalations will loosen a cough and clear the sinuses. Many different combinations can be utilized; often the final choice is one of personal preference concerning aroma. For a simple and safe preparation, place a handful of chamomile flowers in a bowl and pour boiling water over them. The vapor is inhaled with a towel draped over the head and bowl to create a "tent" that keeps the vapor trapped in. Thyme and eucalyptus are often used as well, or try the following mixture:

> - chamomile flowers
> - thyme
> - marjoram
>
> Equal parts of dried herbs.
> Infuse 1 tbsp of the mixture to a pint of boiling water.

Alternately, pure volatile oils may be used for steam inhalations. Traditionally, the oil of dwarf pine needles *(Pinus pumilio)* has been the main oil used, but with growing interest in aromatherapy, many volatile oils are now recognized as valuable remedies for inhalation. Aromatherapy treatment aims to combat the infection, reduce fever, ease cough, and expel mucus. In the first stages, when the cough is dry and painful, steam inhalation with any of the following oils may give a great deal of relief. Bergamot and eucalyptus oils are also effective in lowering fever, and all the oils listed here will help to reinforce immune response to the infection.

Asian mint	eucalyptus	pine, dwarf or white
benzoin	lavender	sandalwood
bergamot	peppermint	thyme

Oil of an Asian mint, *Mentha arvensis* var. *piperascens,* is a constituent of many Chinese and Japanese oils and is especially rich in menthol. Menthol is anti-inflammatory, especially on the mucous membranes of the upper respiratory tract. It is also antimicrobial, a stimulant to mucosal secretions, and mildly anesthetic. Like many other oils, it is best used at the initial onset of symptoms. Place three to five drops of the oil in a bowl and add boiling water. Inhale for five to ten minutes. Keep the eyes closed, as the vapor can be irritating.

Massaging or applying the oils to the chest, neck, or back allows absorption through the skin (percutaneous absorption). Oils absorbed this way are often eliminated from the body via the lungs, thus enabling effective treatment of lung infections or inflammations. A good technique is to apply the oil and then place a dry pack or dressing over the oils to ensure that they are absorbed and don't evaporate.

The cough may persist for some time after the fever has subsided, but inhalations, baths, and local massage to the chest and throat with the appropriate oils will shorten the time needed for full recovery. The patient needs to be kept warm and rested. It is important to avoid anything that can aggravate the cough, such as smoke or very dry air. Most adults will recover from an attack of bronchitis fairly quickly and without complications, but the very elderly and frail, as well as people with heart conditions or a history of lung infections, are at much greater risk.

POST-BRONCHITIS RECOVERY

A period of debility often follows an acute attack of bronchitis. Appropriate herbs will not only speed recovery but help the body use this time of convalescence to revivify and recuperate. Emphasis should be given to respiratory tonics such as the bitter tonics of coltsfoot, horehound, and mullein.

Horehound is especially useful, for it is not only an excellent lung remedy but also has valuable bitter properties (see page 286). If antibiotics have been used, please follow the guidelines for herbal therapy support in the section on the immune system (see page 224).

Bronchitis (Chronic)

Chronic bronchitis is a long-term condition without fever, affecting over 5 percent of the American population. It is characterized by the presence of a mucous-producing cough most days of the month, three months of a year for two successive years, without indication of some other underlying disease that would explain the cough. Healthy lungs normally produce a small amount of mucus all the time, and this is constantly swept up the bronchi by the cilia. This process goes on continually without our noticing it as the amount of mucus is very small and is swallowed imperceptibly along with our saliva. However, when irritation of the bronchi through infection, air pollution, smoking, or some other external irritant provokes the production of abnormally large amounts of mucus, this literally swamps the minute cilia so they can no longer propel it upward. Then the body can only get rid of the mucus by coughing. Once the bronchial tubes have been irritated over a long period of time, excessive mucus is produced constantly, the lining of the bronchial tubes becomes thickened, an irritating cough develops, and air flow may be hampered. The bronchial tubes then make an ideal breeding place for infection.

Chronic bronchitis is often a preventable condition, as the main causal factors are pollutants. Climate and air pollution are serious problems associated with bronchitis, especially when they combine to produce fog, but in fact the two most important contributing factors are poor nutrition and smoking. Workers with certain jobs, especially those involving high concentrations of dust and irritating fumes, are at high risk of developing this disease, but no matter what their occupation or lifestyle, people who smoke cigarettes are those most likely to develop chronic bronchitis.

Chronic bronchitis is often neglected until it is in an advanced state, because people mistakenly believe that the disease is not life threatening. By the time a patient goes to his or her doctor the lungs have frequently been seriously injured. Then the patient may be in danger of developing serious respiratory problems or heart failure. Chronic obstructive pulmonary disease (chronic bronchitis and/or emphysema) increased by 87.5 percent in the United States between 1970 and 1987!

In this chronic and debilitating condition, tonic support is vitally important. The inherent strength of herbal medicine can reveal itself here, for plants may be selected that not only address the symptom picture but also serve as appropriate tonics. Expectorant remedies are the core of successful treatment. Stimulants will be important in the more productive cases, and whereas relaxing remedies will not be as important in cases of chronic bronchitis as for acute bronchitis, they often provide good support for more active remedies. Cardiotonic herbs are essential for supporting cardiac function in anyone with a weak heart.

Antispasmodics may be helpful in severe coughing or breathlessness. Antimicrobials will support the body's attempts to rid itself of any accompanying infection. Examples of combinations to address specific symptom pictures are:

For Chronic Recurrent Bronchitis Associated with Debility

- elecampane
- Irish moss
- coltsfoot
- mullein

Equal parts of herbs or tinctures.

As tincture: take 1 tsp (5 ml) of this mixture three times a day.

As dried herb: infuse 1–2 tsp to a cup and drink three times a day.

This combination is formulated for the patient who is becoming debilitated and weakened by the chronic problem. Thus there is a blending of stimulating and relaxing pulmonary tonics. Irish moss has long been used in Britain (the world's capital of chronic bronchitis) as a nutritive support in such cases. To this may be added whatever else is appropriate for the individual concerned: hawthorn for the heart, or Siberian ginseng for associated stress.

For Chronic Recurrent Bronchitis Associated with Infection

- elecampane
- echinacea
- horehound
- mullein

Equal parts of herbs or tinctures.
As tincture: take 1 tsp (5 ml) of this mixture three times a day.
As dried herb: infuse 2 tsp to a cup and drink three times a day.

Garlic should be eaten raw in the diet or the oil taken as a supplement.

For Chronic Recurrent Bronchitis Associated with Excessive Congestion

- elecampane
- bloodroot
- horehound
- mullein

Equal parts of tinctures.
Take 1 tsp (5 ml) of this mixture three times a day.

Garlic should be eaten raw in the diet or the oil taken as a supplement.

Much of the information listed above for acute bronchitis is relevant for chronic bronchitis as well. Smokers are more likely to die from chronic bronchitis than from lung cancer, and to give up smoking is the first and most important preventive measure. The other is to improve the level of nutrition, and particularly to eliminate or greatly reduce the intake of foods that encourage the production of mucus. For most people, these are dairy products and refined starches (white flour and all products made from it). Of the two, dairy products seem to be the worse culprits, and cutting them totally from the diet for a time—maybe several weeks, or even months if the bronchitis is of long standing—will often bring about improvement. Thereafter, cheese, milk, yogurt, and so on may be cautiously reintroduced but in very small amounts only. Some people may need to omit them from the diet permanently.

Goat's milk is often found to be less mucous forming than cow's milk. Starches also provoke excessive mucous production, and refined starches are far worse than unrefined grains. Additives such as chemical flavorings, colorings, and preservatives often trigger mucous excess as well and should be avoided. The best and simplest rule is to eat foods in a state as near as possible to that in which they were grown—in other words, not processed, dried, frozen, packaged, or precooked, but as often as possible raw or very lightly cooked.

Cough

Should one soothe, stimulate, or suppress a cough? It is always preferable to focus on the underlying cause of the cough, as removing the cause will, of course, alleviate it. In the sections that follow, a number of cough remedies are discussed. Always select the approach appropriate to the individual's unique case. The key is finding the balance between the various stimulating, demulcent, antimicrobial, or cough-suppressing herbs available. Treat the person and his or her experience, not the cough.

Acute inflammatory conditions of the respiratory system are primarily treated with mucilage-rich demulcents that act to soothe the inflamed tissue. It would be inappropriate to use the stimulating, saponin-containing expectorants in all cases, as they are best for subacute or chronic bronchitis, where active expectoration is required. Any increased irritation in chronic bronchitis will indicate the need for increased demulcancy. The therapist's sensitivity to the differentiated stages of cough therapy can rapidly address the symptoms and shorten the duration of respiratory illness.

Coughing is a reflex response to whatever is blocking the airways—usually an excess of mucus secreted by the membranes lining the respiratory tract. Normally such mucous secretions help to protect the respiratory tract from irritants and trap and flush out smoke particles, bacteria, and viruses. Any cough that lasts more than a few days, does not respond to treatment, or produces blood should be investigated further, as it may be a sign of serious organic disease.

A simple cough remedy may be made by slicing a large onion into rings and putting them into a deep bowl. Cover the onion slices with organic honey and let it stand overnight. In the morning, strain off the mixture of honey and onion juice to obtain a simple cough elixir. Honey itself, which is often included in cough mixtures, has antimicrobial properties and is also an expectorant. Take a dessert spoon of this mixture four or five times a day. A basic herbal cough tea is as follows:

Herbal Cough Tea

■ coltsfoot	2 parts
■ marshmallow	2 parts
■ hyssop	2 parts
■ licorice	1 part
■ aniseed	1 part

As dried herb: infuse 2 tsp of the mixture to a cup and drink as often as needed until symptoms subside.

Emphysema

Emphysema, which often accompanies chronic bronchitis, is characterized by overinflation and destructive changes of the alveolar walls, resulting in a loss of lung elasticity and decreased gas exchange. Such changes are caused by constant coughing to try to dislodge the bacteria and mucus blocking the swollen bronchi. Normally, the cilia—microscopic hairs that line the airways—act as a respiratory "escalator" to push out particles of dust, soot, and bacteria. In chronic bronchitis the cilia become paralyzed due to the constant secretion of viscid mucus.

Emphysema is not curable but can be treated, and those who develop it can be helped to live with it. It is a destructive disease for hundreds of thousands of Americans and their families, third among the diseases for which Social Security gives disability benefits. A high percentage of those with emphysema have been heavy smokers for many years and often live in areas with high levels of air pollution.

The issues to be addressed herbally are similar to those facing asthma patients. Treatment is long-term and palliative; herbal medicine will not cure this condition. Pulmonary tonics are important to strengthen the lungs over time. Expectorant remedies will be essential to ensure that there is minimum buildup of sputum in the lungs. Stimulant expectorants such as elecampane or bloodroot are usually necessary because of the lessening of tone in the alveoli walls. Antispasmodic plants will ease the spasm response in the muscles of the lungs. Antimicrobial support is called for if there is potential for secondary infection, which is to be guarded against at all costs. Cardiotonic herbs such as hawthorn will support the heart in the presence of lung congestion or strain.

To Ease Emphysema

- "Asthma Mixture" (see page 85)
- bloodroot
- hawthorn
- elecampane

Equal parts of the four tinctures.
Take 1 tsp (5 ml) of this mixture three times a day.

Great care must be taken with general health and well-being, as any health problem will aggravate this condition. Keeping fit not only helps prevent emphysema and other diseases but also speeds recovery from illness. Avoid polluted air to whatever extent possible, and do not expose yourself unnecessarily to dust or fumes of any kind. Continued smoking definitely makes emphysema worse.

4 The Upper Respiratory System

Prevention is largely a matter of avoiding pollutants and taking care with certain dietary factors. Air pollution will aggravate or even cause a whole spectrum of problems. This includes both particulate matter and irritant gases, so stop smoking and move out of Los Angeles!

Nature is abundant in herbs that have an anticatarrhal effect upon the upper respiratory system. These plants, which directly affect the production of catarrh, include goldenrod, elder flower, hyssop, coltsfoot, goldenseal, and the volatile oils. Antimicrobials will often clear the sinus congestion that is a response to infection by some pathogen. Important examples are garlic, echinacea, eucalyptus, thyme, wild indigo, and osha.

Upper Respiratory Problems

Many of the common chronic catarrhal states are a response by the body to a diet that is too rich in mucous-forming foods. Thus, for a patient with such problems, a low-mucous diet is essential. This is discussed below.

The Common Cold

The common cold is a viral infection of the upper respiratory tract. Many different strains of virus can cause cold symptoms, and these are constantly mutating. While the mucous membranes of the nose and throat are inflamed as a result of the infection, they are far more vulnerable to attack by bacteria, and this can give rise to secondary infections (such as sinusitis, ear infections, and bronchitis) that are more serious than the original cold. Thus, antibiotic drugs are often prescribed by allopathic therapists to ward off secondary infection. As they destroy bacteria, however, they cannot touch a cold virus.

Unfortunately, there is no universally miraculous herbal cold cure! However, herbal medicine can do more than most therapies in treating and preventing this all too common problem. Herbs can be selected to fit the individual's unique needs, while at the same time immune support, diet, and lifestyle are addressed.

Regional and traditional herbs favored for the common cold include:

cayenne	horseradish	peppermint
echinacea	linden	thyme
elder flower	mustard	yarrow
eucalyptus	onion and garlic	

A very popular and traditional tea used throughout Europe consists of the following herbs.

> ■ elder flower
> ■ peppermint
> ■ yarrow
>
> Equal parts of herbs.
> Infuse 1–2 tsp to a cup and drink hot often until symptoms pass.

A number of essential oils can help to diminish the discomfort of a cold as well as to reduce the risk of secondary infections; these are antimicrobial and also stimulate the immune response. For the immediate relief of congestion, a steam inhalation with essential oil is often effective. Very hot steam—as hot as can be tolerated without actually burning the nose and throat—is in itself a hostile environment for viruses, and the addition of an antiviral oil increases the effectiveness of the steam. Together they not only ease the congestion but also help to combat the infection that has caused it. For catarrh caused by pollen and other irritants, lavender and chamomile are probably the best choices. The steam inhalation described in the section on bronchitis (pages 88–90) will prove helpful. Other plant oils that may prove beneficial include:

Asian mint	marjoram	sandalwood
basil	myrrh	thyme
bergamot	peppermint	tea tree
eucalyptus	pine, white or dwarf	
lavender	rosemary	

A steam inhalation with one of these essential oils combines several beneficial effects. It clears the congested nasal passages and soothes the inflamed mucous membrane, while at the same time the essential oil will kill many bacteria. Some of the oils, especially eucalyptus and tea tree, have an inhibiting effect on the cold virus. Use either of these two oils for inhalation in the earlier part of the day, as they are mildly stimulating. At night use inhalations of lavender or a bath with a few drops of the oil added. The oil diffused in the bedroom will also help, especially if there is a cough.

Many traditional cold remedies are based on culinary ingredients, highlighting the fact that there is no real difference between medicinal and edible plants. Here is an example of such a treatment. At the first signs of a chill or sore throat, take the following common kitchen spices:

- 1 oz fresh ginger, sliced
- 1 stick of cinnamon, broken
- 1 tsp coriander seeds
- 3 cloves
- 1 slice of lemon
- 1 pint water

Decoct for 15 minutes and then strain off. Sweeten to taste. Drink a cupful of this hot, every two hours.

To prevent and treat colds, include garlic, onions, watercress, and cayenne in the diet and take 1–3 grams of vitamin C daily. Diet plays a part in most cases of catarrh. Dairy products and wheat are known to promote excessive catarrh production in many people and should be excluded for a period by anybody who suffers catarrh frequently, to see whether any improvement is noticed. If so, they may have to be excluded permanently from the diet or included in very small amounts only. Experiment if any other food sensitivities are suspected and adjust the diet accordingly.

Influenza

Severe colds and various unidentified virus infections are often referred to as "flu." Some authorities would argue that true influenza is a much more severe infection that appears in widespread epidemics, often at intervals of approximately ten years. Bacterial secondary infections are the greatest risk incurred by contracting "true" influenza and were responsible for thousands of deaths in past epidemics. The use of antibiotics has dramatically reduced such deaths. Indeed, a really severe infection of this kind is one situation in which the use of antibiotics may well be called for. In this case, do not stop the herbal treatment—it can only be beneficial and will not conflict with more orthodox drug treatment.

As is true for the common cold, there are no miracle cures here, but certain plants can make life much more bearable. These are usually diaphoretics, or sweat-inducing herbs. My own favorite is boneset, an herb that was widely used to ease the pain of the "break-bone fever," a disease that afflicted European settlers in North America. It is a strong infusion drunk *hot* every hour. (Follow the advice given above for the common cold as well, if the symptom picture calls for it.)

■ goldenseal
■ echinacea

Equal parts of tinctures.
Take ½ tsp (2.5 ml every 2 hours).

Treatment is most effective if started at the very first sign of infection. A moderately hot bath with a few drops of antiviral essential oil added will often induce profuse perspiration, followed by a deep, restful sleep. This may be enough to avert a full-blown attack, though it is a good idea to repeat the bathing for the next two or three days. An effective oil for this purpose is tea tree. Some people find this a mild skin irritant and may not be able to tolerate more than three or four drops in a full bath, so it is best to begin with this amount.

Recovery from influenza is often slow, and the convalescent may feel very weak and lacking in vitality. Caffeine-containing herbs should be avoided, as the lift produced thereby is temporary and will slow down recovery. As I have indicated, bitter tonics will speed recovery through their metabolic-stimulating effects. Appropriate bitter tonics include the following:

Boneset: also diaphoretic and anticatarrhal
Gentian: aids the digestion in a number of ways and doesn't taste too bad
Goldenseal: also anticatarrhal and generally tonic
Horehound: also expectorant and anticatarrhal

In addition, the use of adaptogens is often helpful, and attention to diet is essential. It may be helpful to supplement with a multivitamin/mineral formula until appetite and general vitality are back to normal.

Laryngitis

This acute inflammation of the larynx, or voice box, is usually associated with a common cold or overuse of the voice. It is commonly characterized by swelling, hoarseness, pain, dryness in the throat, coughing, and inability to speak above a whisper, if at all. It is usually caused by bacterial or viral infection, which may either be restricted to the larynx or be part of a more general infection of the upper respiratory tract. Where no clear-cut cause is found, such as infection or overuse, skilled diagnosis is called for.

Demulcent and anti-inflammatory remedies will reduce the immediate cause of the distress. Antimicrobial herbs are indicated if there is a causal microorganism involved. Astringents are often effective as a local gargle, especially when the problem has been precipitated by overuse of the vocal cords.

The herbal traditions of the world abound in herbs used for conditions of the mouth, larynx, and pharynx. Osha is an excellent remedy, a small piece of the root being chewed to remove symptoms and promote the body's immune response. In Europe the approach has traditionally been to gargle with astringent herbs. They should not be swallowed, however, as they often constipate—an unnecessary and unfortunate complication! Examples of reliable astringent herbs for such local usage include:

cranesbill	oak bark	yarrow
elder flower	red sage	

An Internal Medication for Laryngitis

- echinacea   2 parts
- osha   2 parts
- goldenseal   1 part

As tincture: take $1/4$ tsp (1 ml) of this mixture every hour.

A Gargle for Laryngitis

- red sage
- chamomile

Equal parts of herbs.
Prepare a strong infusion and gargle often until symptoms subside.

The supplemental and dietary advice given above for sinusitis should be followed. Aromatherapy provides certain oils that ease the inflammation quite effectively. Oil of cypress and bergamot have much to offer, for example. To use as a gargle, put three drops of the essential oil in half a cup of warm water. Gargle hourly and do not swallow.

Sinusitis

The sinuses are four bony cavities behind, above, and at each side of the nose and opening into the nasal cavity. They act as a sound box to give resonance to the voice. Sinusitis is an inflammation of these cavities. Like the nasal passages, the sinuses are lined with mucous membranes, which react to infection by producing mucus to incapacitate infecting bacteria. Because the openings from the nose into the sinuses are very narrow, they quickly become blocked when the mucous membrane of the nose becomes swollen during a cold, hay fever, or catarrh; thus the infection becomes trapped inside the sinus.

Chronic sinusitis may occur if one or more of the drainage passages from the sinuses to the nose becomes blocked. This can cause headache or a dull pain across the face and temple, or around the eyes. If the maxillary sinuses above the cheeks are infected, toothache may be the result. Once the lining of the sinuses becomes swollen, the cilia no longer operate, causing the lining of the sinuses to become permanently thickened and contributing to the retention of phlegm. Sinusitis may be the result of a complication of an upper respiratory infection, dental infection, allergy, a change in atmosphere (as in air travel or underwater swimming), or a structural defect of the nose.

Antimicrobials such as garlic and echinacea are pivotal in the treatment of this often entrenched condition. These herbs will help the body deal with any infection present and also support the immune system in resisting the development of secondary infection. Anticatarrhals will ease the symptomatic discomfort that is characteristic of this problem and also help the body in the removal of buildup in the sinus cavities. Excellent examples are goldenrod and elder flower. Astringents reduce overproduction in the mucous membranes of the sinuses.

■ goldenrod	2 parts
■ elder flower	1 part
■ echinacea	1 part
■ wild indigo	1 part

As tincture: take 1 tsp (5 ml) of this mixture three times a day.

The herbal approach to these problems may be both indirect and direct. The indirect approach sees upper respiratory disease within the context of the whole person. Sometimes overproduction of mucus is an attempt by the body to discharge waste material that is not being properly eliminated by the bowels, kidneys, and skin. In such cases, the herbalist may prescribe bitter tonics to encourage regular bowel movements, or diuretic herbs to encourage kidney elimination of retained fluids and waste materials, or diaphoretic herbs to stimulate skin elimination.

A diet that reduces mucous production is also essential. In particular, a fruit fast for two or three days can help to clear a system clogged and overburdened by toxic wastes. Hot lemon drinks reduce mucous production and so do garlic, onion, and horseradish (grate the fresh root into cider vinegar or lemon juice and eat a little each day). You can also add mustard and aromatic herbs like oregano to your food. Extra zinc and vitamin C will help build up the body's resistance to infection. Certain foods, especially dairy produce and wheat, seem to predispose people toward sinusitis by provoking excessive formation of mucus. During an acute attack of sinusitis, all dairy and wheat-based foods must be excluded for several days, and those suffering from chronic or repeated attacks are advised to exclude these foods completely for several months and then reintroduce them in very small amounts, if at all. Goat's- and sheep's-milk products are sometimes better tolerated than cow's milk.

Sometimes emotional factors such as suppressed grief can lead to blocked upper respiratory passages. In these cases, a good cry can free this blocked energy and alleviate the problem. Finally, some cases of chronic mucus production are due to allergy.

5   The Nervous System

Biology tells us that the brain shrinks and loses thousands of neurons over time. Loss of brain mass does not, however, mean a reduction in mental powers, for we can continue to learn, to create, to reason, and to experience mental and psychological growth for the whole of life. Consider the following:

- The capacity to learn new information does not decline with age. The issue is not ability to learn but motivation!
- The people who age most successfully are those who can shift their focus to mental pursuits if bodily ills cut down their physical activity.
- The brain needs exercise, just like the rest of the body. If the mind is running on "automatic pilot" much of the time, seek stimulation or a challenge.
- It is never too late to take up interesting pursuits. If fostered, cultivation of mental stimulation (outside of your daily work) for learning and creativity will naturally continue into your later years.
- Senility is *not* an inevitable consequence of aging. Anyone who develops the symptoms of senility—marked mental deterioration, memory loss, disorientation—should be checked thoroughly by a physician. These symptoms can be caused by many factors and may be treatable.
- Mild memory loss, common among people as they age, is often regained by some simple mental exercises. Researchers have shown that the mnemonic device called the "method of loci" can greatly boost one's memory power.

The idea is to match information to be remembered with familiar images or objects (household items, for instance).

- Psychologists have developed problem-solving strategies that can be learned at any age. Not only are we capable of learning more than we do; with training we can also use information more effectively.
- To minimize the effects of age-related slowdown in the central nervous system, psychologists suggest continued practice of a skill, such as playing a musical instrument, to keep reaction time sharp.

Several stages of adult development beyond the "midlife transition" have been identified. These distinctive and fulfilling periods of growth include what is termed late late adulthood, which begins around the age of eighty. Many people have experienced tremendous bursts of creativity in this period—think of George Bernard Shaw, Bertrand Russell, Maggie Kuhn, Claude Monet, or Grandma Moses. To quote Shaw, a vegan who lived to be ninety-four: "Your legs give in before your head does."

Herbal Actions

Herbal therapy is uniquely suited to treating nervous system problems. From one perspective, herbs are embodiments of energy and spirit, from another they are packets of biochemicals: a reflection of the human mind/brain itself! The complexities of the mind-body interface that often confuse allopathic physicians concerned with "psychosomatic" illness become an aid in remedy selection to the herbalist.

All of the many herbal nervines have impact on somatic symptoms as well as the mind. A simple example is motherwort, an herb used to treat anxiety and tension. It also has specific affinity for the heart, reducing palpitation reactions and the fear that often accompanies them. Many advances in the field of neurology have come about through the examination of claims for herbal remedies. Most of the areas of concern in neurology can potentially benefit from herbal therapeutics, and, indeed, the science of psychopharmacology itself is largely based on chemicals discovered in plants.

In no other system of the body is the connection between the physical and psychological aspects of our being as apparent as in the nervous system. Clearly, the tissue of the nervous system is part of the physical makeup of the body but, just as clearly, all psychological processes are anchored in the nervous system.

"Dis-ease" on the psychological level will be reflected on the physiological level, and vice versa.

Orthodox medicine tends to reduce psychological problems to a biochemical level and assumes that "appropriate" drugs will sort out or at least hide the problem sufficiently to allow "normal" life to continue. Interestingly enough, some techniques in the field of complementary medicine assume or imply the other extreme: namely, that psychological factors are the cause of all disease. In this view, treatment of the psyche is the only appropriate way of healing and will take care of any physical problem.

By bringing these two reductionist views together, we come closer to the holistic approach. Holism acknowledges the interconnectedness of physiological and psychological factors and regards the nervous system and its functions as a vital element in the treatment of the whole being. To be truly healthy, we have to take care of our physical health through the right diet and lifestyle, but we are also responsible for taking care of our emotional, mental, and spiritual life. We should endeavor to live in a fulfilling, nurturing environment that supports emotional stability. Our thoughts should be creative and life enhancing, open to the free flow of intuition and imagination, rather than conceptually rigid. And we should stay open to the free flow of the higher energies of our souls, without which health is impossible.

Herbal medicine can be an ecologically and spiritually integrative tool, an ideal counterpart on the physical level for therapeutic techniques on the psychological level. Indeed, any successful treatment of nervous system problems with herbs must involve treating the whole body, heart, and mind, not simply the signs of agitation and worry. Of course agitation can be reduced greatly, but the whole system must be strengthened in the face of the storm! Important therapeutic subdivisions and primary herbal examples are listed here:

- *Adaptogen:* ginseng, Siberian ginseng
- *Analgesic:* Jamaican dogwood, valerian
- *Antidepressant:* mugwort, St. John's wort
- *Antispasmodic:* valerian, cramp bark
- *Hypnotic:* hops, passionflower
- *Nervine: tonic*—oats, St. John's wort, skullcap
        relaxing—skullcap, valerian, vervain
        stimulating—cola, guarana

(Adaptogens hypnotics are discussed in the sections on stress and insomnia, respectively: pages 118–21 and 135–38.)

Nervine Relaxants

The nervines included in this group are most important in our times of stress and confusion, alleviating as they do many common symptoms. They should always be used in a broad holistic way, not simply to tranquilize. Too much tranquilizing, even that achieved through herbal medication, can in time deplete and weigh heavily on the whole nervous system.

As can be seen from the list of herbs below, many of the nervine relaxants also have other properties and can be selected to aid in related problems. This is one of the great benefits of using herbal remedies to help with stress and anxiety problems. The physical symptoms that can so often accompany the ill-ease of anxiety may be treated with herbs that work on the anxiety itself.

In addition to herbs that work directly on the nervous system, the antispasmodic herbs, which affect the peripheral nerves and muscle tone, can have an indirect relaxing effect on the whole system. When the physical body is at ease, ease in the psyche is promoted. Many of the nervine relaxants have this antispasmodic action. (Consider also the hypnotics, which in lower dosage will have a relaxing action on the mind and body.) Relaxing nervines have an affinity for each of the following systems:

- *Circulatory system:* Balm, linden, and motherwort, which are all mild sedatives, are helpful to the cardiovascular system. (Most remedies that relax the central nervous system will aid the heart and problems such as high blood pressure because of their calming effect upon the autonomic nervous system.)
- *Digestive system:* All the antispasmodic remedies may be of value to ease colic, but sedatives that actively aid digestion include balm, chamomile, and lavender.
- *Musculoskeletal system:* All relaxing herbs will ease muscular tension and thus relieve pain in this complex system. Remedies to bear in mind are black cohosh, cramp bark, and valerian.
- *Nervous system:* All the remedies mentioned relate here.
- *Reproductive system:* Black cohosh, cramp bark, motherwort, saw palmetto, and wild lettuce all have an affinity for this system.

- *Respiratory system:* Most relaxing nervines will help in problems such as asthma, but, specifically, I can mention black cohosh, bugleweed, lobelia, motherwort, wild cherry bark, and wild lettuce.
- *Skin:* All relaxing nervines may help the skin in an indirect way, but these herbs have a good reputation for addressing skin problems: red clover, pasqueflower, St. John's wort, and black cohosh.
- *Urinary system:* By generally relaxing the body, there may be an increase in water loss. This, however, does not make diuretics of the herbs involved. Saw palmetto is a very gentle sedative that does work on the urinary system.

Nervine Stimulants

Direct stimulation of the nervous tissue is rarely needed in the frantic times we live in. It is usually more appropriate to stimulate the body's innate vitality with the help of nervine or bitter tonics, which seem to augment bodily harmony and so have a much deeper and longer lasting effect than nervine stimulants. In the nineteenth century, much more emphasis was placed by herbalists upon stimulant herbs. (Perhaps it is a sign of the times that our world is supplying us with more than enough stimulants.)

When direct stimulation is indicated, a good herb to use is kola nut, although guarana, coffee, maté, and tea should also be remembered. A problem with these commonly used stimulants is that they have a number of side effects and can themselves cause minor psychological problems such as anxiety and tension. Some of the herbs rich in volatile oils are also gentle stimulants; the most familiar of these are rosemary and peppermint (see page 109).

Nervine Tonics

Perhaps the most important contribution herbal medicine can make in this area is its ability to strengthen and "feed" the nervous system. In cases of shock, stress, or nervous debility, the nervine tonics strengthen and restore the tissues directly. On the other hand, they can contribute directly to the healing of damaged nervous tissue, whether related to a pathological process or to physical trauma. This invaluable group of remedies is best exemplified by oats. Other nervine tonics that have, in addition, a relaxing effect include skullcap, vervain, and St. John's wort. Of these relaxing nervine tonics, skullcap is often the most effective.

Stimulants

The very name *stimulant* has varying connotations depending upon one's assumptions and conditioning. In herbal medicine, it is used to describe an action that quickens and enlivens the physiological activity of the body. This is not necessarily an appropriate action; the needs of the individual and his or her immediate state of health must be taken into account. Debility may be due to overactivity within the body as well as not enough. In such cases, differential diagnosis calls for skill, knowledge, and a certain amount of intuition. Whenever herbal nervine stimulants are used, they are combined with nervine tonics or relaxants to balance any overactivity. As is often the case, the stimulants are chosen based upon their appropriateness for a whole body system.

- *Circulatory system:* This action must be used with care in cardiovascular problems, though stimulation can aid and support an ailing heart. Bayberry, ginseng, prickly ash, rosemary, wormwood, and yarrow may affect this system.
- *Digestive system:* The bitters may be considered as stimulants. Consider balmony, bayberry, dandelion root, gentian, horseradish, mustard, peppermint, rosemary, and wormwood.
- *Musculoskeletal system:* The vital role of ginger and cayenne are reinforced here as stimulants to peripheral circulation. We can add mustard and horseradish.
- *Nervous system:* Nervous stimulants include cola, guarana, coffee, tea, maté, and chocolate.
- *Reproductive system:* Stimulants in this system usually act in the form of emmenagogues and so must be used with care. Pennyroyal, rosemary, tansy, and wormwood can be mentioned here.
- *Respiratory system:* Includes angelica, balm of Gilead, eucalyptus, garlic, horseradish, mustard, peppermint, sage, horehound, and yarrow.
- *Skin:* The wound-healing vulneraries stimulate healing but are not stimulants as such.
- *Urinary system:* Bearing in mind the wide application of cayenne, we can add eucalyptus, gravel root, juniper, and yarrow.

Stress and Its Impact on the Nervous System

There are several ways to define stress. Perhaps the most encompassing is this: Stress is the response of the body to any demand. Just staying alive creates demands on the body for life-maintaining energy; even while we are asleep, our bodies continue to function. By this definition, stress is a fundamental part of being alive and should not be avoided! The trick is to ensure that the degree of stress we experience is such that life is a joy, not a drag.

Any demands made upon us in daily life bring about certain reactions in the body. These same reactions occur under a whole range of different conditions, both physical and emotional—from hot and cold to joy and sorrow. As aware, feeling people, we make a major distinction between the pain caused by the loss of a loved one and the pain caused by a sudden drop in temperature, but the nature of the demand is unimportant at the biological level. To the body it's all the same, because the stress response is always the same. Nerve signals are sent from the brain to various glands, which in turn react by secreting hormones to cope with the task ahead. So stress is not just worry and strain. It is a keynote of life, with all its ups and downs. The range of responses triggered by stress demonstrates the intricate links that exist between the mental and physical components of who we are.

One way to understand stress is to view it as the response to an adverse situation. The physiologist Hans Selye theorized that the stress response is a built-in mechanism triggered whenever demands are placed on us, and is therefore a defense reaction with a protective and an adaptive function. In other words, there is a general physiological reaction to all forms of stress, which usually acts in our own best interests. Selye called this reaction the general adaptation syndrome (GAS). This theory suggests a three-stage process of response:

1. An alarm reaction.

2. A resistance stage, which represents a functional recovery of the body to a level superior to the prestress state.

3. An exhaustion reaction, in which there is a depletion and breakdown of the recovery of stage 2, due to continuation of the stressful situation.

Physiological Responses to Stress

The regulation of physiological responses to stressful demands is handled primarily by the adrenal gland. Immediate response is controlled mainly, though not completely, by the adrenal gland's central medulla, while long-term response is handled by the surrounding cortex. The initial response—preparing the body for what has been called the fight-or-flight reaction—involves increased nervous system activity and the release of adrenaline and/or noradrenalin into the blood stream by the adrenal medulla. These hormones support the nervous system through metabolic activity.

The body's subsequent response to these chemicals includes increased heart rate and blood pressure; surface constriction of blood vessels, so that the blood leaves the skin to provide the muscles with more sugar and oxygen (which is why we go white with shock); and mobilization of the liver's energy reserves through the release of stored glucose.

If the stressful situation is very intense or continues over a long time, the adrenal cortex becomes increasingly involved in the stress reaction. The activity of the cortex is largely controlled by blood levels of adrenocorticotrophic hormone, which is released by the pituitary gland. When information about sustained stress has been "processed" by the central nervous system, a whole range of new bodily responses occurs, and it is these longer-term reactions that can adversely affect the quality of life.

Psychological Responses to Stress

In general terms, the psychological reaction to stress takes the following course:

- The initial reaction is accompanied by emotions such as anxiety or fear.
- Individual ways of coping are activated as we attempt to find a way of dealing with the situation.
- If the coping strategies are successful, the anxiety state subsides.
- If the coping strategies fail and the situation continues, a range of psychological reactions, including depression and withdrawal, may occur.

It is important that we develop our own ways of adapting to and successfully dealing with stressful situations. There are two groups of coping strategies. The first involves attempts to change our unsatisfactory relationship with the environment: for example, escaping from the unpleasant situation (not always possible); or preparing ourselves for situations that we anticipate will be stressful. This might involve thinking ahead of time about the situation and its probable impact, thereby preparing ourselves adequately for the event.

The second group involves palliative strategies that attempt to soften the impact of the stress once it has occurred: for example, denial, the refusal to acknowledge all or some of the threat in the situation; or intellectualization, a form of emotional detachment from the situation.

Both of these strategies serve to protect us and help us maintain a reasonable equilibrium through difficult times. However, there is always the danger that they may make it more difficult to resolve a problem and may become established as part of one's psychological makeup.

No clear solution exists for some stresses—for example, caring for a chronically ill loved one—and in such situations the only way to cope may be to soften the impact of stress. If stress is long-term or particularly severe, marked emotional changes may take place. If our coping strategies don't work, we may regard the situation as insoluble and increasingly see ourselves as unable to control the events of our lives. Hopelessness and helplessness are both likely to give rise to feelings of depression and may even lead to suicidal thoughts. Under the stress of chronic illness, for example, patients (and at times caregivers) may literally give up hope. If this occurs, they may become not only emotionally disturbed but also more vulnerable to further physical illness.

Managing Stress

Much can be done to ease the impact of stress and lessen the weight of anxiety and tension. However, the wide range of possible approaches can itself become a source of stress! Where should we turn for help? Which therapy should we use? These questions, always difficult, are even more difficult to answer when we are not feeling at our best. The different therapies are only ways of helping us find the peace that is in us already. We are all our own healers. The key is an inner attitude of taking responsibility for the quality of our own lives. We can seek aid from "experts," whether medical doctors or herbalists, but our own responsibility for healing can never be handed to another. Healing comes from within and is inherent to being alive. When people are seen as whole beings and not simply as "bodies, with minds on top of them," the deep association between psychology and physiology comes as no surprise. This natural association has profound implications for all illness, not just stress and anxiety.

It is a demonstration of the inadequacies of the dominant scientific approach to health that people are even thought of in terms of the two words, mind and body. There is, in reality, one system that should not be divided. However, since there is no one English term for this system, to talk about it in English, and say what needs to be said, is exceedingly difficult. To help both body and mind, the whole must be treated as a whole. Not only are remedies for specific symptoms needed but a management plan to help us cope with stress is also necessary. This broader view lessens the impact of stress, helps free us, and hopefully creates the space for healing to take place.

Herbs can play a fundamental role in any stress management program. When used in a program that addresses a range of factors, herbs can facilitate a dramatic change in the quality of life experienced by anyone under stress. Holistic medicine reminds us to focus on an individual's unique situation and not simply treat a diagnosed disease syndrome. In the context of this therapeutic ecology, it may be that one person diagnosed with a stress-related problem might recuperate best when treated with dietary advice, herbs, and massage, whereas another would benefit more from tranquilizers and psychoanalysis. Practitioners will often hold firm opinions of the pros and cons concerning one approach or another, but the patient is always more important than any one doctor's belief system.

A well-balanced stress management program will address the various aspects discussed in that model. Herbal remedies will only fulfill some aspects, but they are vital.

- *Bodywork:* All approaches that do something with or to the physical body. Structural factors are focused on as either causing or contributing to illness. This includes the manipulative therapies such as osteopathy, chiropractic, and the varieties of massage, as well as surgery. Personal lifestyle will contribute exercise, dance, or any expression of bodily vitality. Relaxation techniques are invaluable. Herbs will help in an indirect way, as for example when antispasmodics are used as muscle relaxants.

- *Emotions and mind:* This category embraces a whole array of psychological techniques, important for identifying and treating emotional and mental factors in both health and disease. All the branches of psychotherapy are relevant, but especially the more holistically orientated approaches of humanistic and transpersonal psychology. A conscious and free-flowing emotional life is fundamental to achieving inner harmony.

- *Medicine:* Used here to mean anything taken for healing purposes, including those derived from medical herbalism, homeopathy, naturopathy, and drug-based allopathic medicine. All have in common the use of a physical substance that is taken into the body to achieve the therapeutic goal. Herbs act primarily on this level as metabolic agents.

- *Spirituality:* Meditative and prayer-based techniques whereby the person aligns his or her being with a higher spirit, or those in which a practitioner works with the energy body of a patient. Some openness to spirituality is vital, whether it takes the form of being inspired by a sunset, being touched by poetry or art, practicing religion, or simply taking a dogma-free joy in being alive.

Herbs and Stress Management

In the sections that follow, attention is focused on the herbal aspects of such a program, but please do not forget nutrition, relaxation, and all the other factors that must be addressed. Different herbal remedies are identified according to the degree of stress. The best way to approach stress-related problems is to consider both the intensity of the person's problems and the duration of the situation.

DAILY MILD STRESS

If a period of stress can be predicted, it can be prepared for ahead of time, as herbs, diet, and lifestyle changes will minimize the impact. Nervine relaxants can be used regularly as gentle soothing remedies. Those listed below are examples, from which it should be clear that most of the nervine relaxants are appropriate. However, bitter tonics may also benefit some people because of their metabolic toning effects. These herbs can be drunk as teas or cold drinks, infused in massage oil, and used in relaxing foot baths or full baths.

balm	linden blossom	skullcap
chamomile	mugwort	vervain
lavender	oats	

A daily supplement of the B-complex vitamins and vitamin C is also helpful. Besides helping you respond to stress in a healthy way, the use of herbs and improvement in the diet can help soften the impact of the various stressors. Stress relief sometimes seems impossible, but don't put up with something or someone just because they are there. People can change themselves and their lives at any point. It helps to reevaluate your choices:

- Are you doing what you really want to do?
- If not what would you rather be doing?
- Give yourself permission to ask some questions about yourself and your lifestyle, without censoring any of the answers that may come up.
- After pinpointing your inner motivations, choose what you want to do about them.

Relaxation exercises and an honest reevaluation of both lifestyle and life goals are invaluable.

LONG-STANDING STRESS

The line between chronic stress and the daily levels of mild stress we all manage to put up with is fuzzy. A gentle soul with a delicate constitution will cross the line sooner than a stronger person who copes well. Neither of these extremes is "better" than the other; they merely reflect the fact that we live in a world of diversity. That's sometimes a joy and sometimes itself a cause of the stress! The advice given for daily stress relief holds for chronic stress, but in addition adaptogens become important. The two most important remedies, ginseng and Siberian ginseng, will be discussed more fully later.

In addition to adaptogens, every attention must be given to general health. The body often shows its weakening through some somatic symptom. This may be a long-standing complaint that gets worse, an old problem that reappears, or just an acceleration of the aging process.

SHORT-TERM EXTREME STRESS

At times things get to be too much and the pain of existence builds to a crescendo. Immediate herbal relief may be needed in a whole range of traumatic situations, from a car accident to a personal emotional crisis. In all cases, herbs will take the edge off the trauma but will not remove it. At such times herbs can be only an aid, one element of an approach to the difficulties being faced. This approach may also include seeking help from the various caring professions, going on vacation or on a retreat, or even checking into a hospital.

Many plants capable of easing intense stress are considered dangerous in our society, and because they are restricted, they will not be discussed here. However, in addition to the herbs previously mentioned, passionflower, valerian, and wild lettuce remedies might be considered.

One possible prescription for acute stress follows:

■ skullcap	2 parts
■ valerian	2 parts
■ oats	1 part

As tincture: take 1 tsp (5 ml) of this mixture as needed.
As dried herb: infuse 2 tsp to a cup and drink three times a day.

Notice that the dosage is "(5 ml) of this mixture taken as needed." This is a recognition that stress response is cyclical, and each person finds that different times of the day are more challenging than others. As this is largely symptomatic medication, it may be increased until the desired relief is experienced. The dosage may be altered as necessary, varying the time of day and quantity of dose to suit individual needs. For example, a large dose may be taken first thing in the morning, or smaller amounts taken at frequent intervals throughout the day. Individual experience is the guiding principle here.

Stress reactions often have accompanying physical symptoms, so here is one possible prescription for acute stress associated with indigestion and palpitations:

■ skullcap	2 parts
■ valerian	2 parts
■ motherwort	1 part
■ chamomile	1 part
■ mugwort	1 part

As tincture: take 1 tsp (5 ml) of this mixture three times a day.
As dried herb: infuse 2 tsp to a cup and drink three times a day.

Motherwort supports the relaxing of the other nervines but also has a specific calming impact upon heart palpitations.

Relaxation Techniques

When we are tense and on edge, the worst advice anyone can give to us is to "relax and take it easy." That advice is guaranteed to put anyone further on edge as they work at trying to relax! The sad fact is that few people retain the innate skill of relaxation—a skill that must be relearned and practiced.

Many relaxation techniques are available. Some are based on breathing, some on muscle control, some on visualization, and some simply on listening to music. It's a matter of finding which is most suitable for the individual concerned. Of the many possibilities, we will focus here on rhythmic breathing.

RHYTHMIC BREATHING

Breathing is of great value in relaxation, particularly during the initial stages. It is the only automatic body function that we can consciously control and thereby influence all autonomic, and to a certain degree all emotional, responses. When we are tense and anxious, breathing becomes shallower and faster, but when we are relaxed it is deeper, slower, and more rhythmical. By breathing in a relaxed way, we can calm our minds and emotions enough to be able to carry on in spite of the stress life hands us. Rhythmic breathing exercises are very simple and can be done at home or even while in line at the supermarket checkout.

Use common sense to avoid unnecessary distractions. For example: Practice without any background noise, such as the radio or stereo. Unplug your phone or turn off the ringer during your session. Don't practice when you're in a hurry. To avoid drowsiness, do not practice in the late evening or right after meals.

The technique: Ideally, practice rhythmic breathing twice a day for five to fifteen minutes in a quiet room free of disturbance. Avoid distractions such as sunlight, a clock, animals, and so on. Rest on your back with your head and neck comfortably supported, and with a pillow under your knees to take the strain off both them and your back. Sitting in a reclining position may suit you better; try both positions. Place your hands on your upper abdomen, close your eyes, and get comfortable.

The aim is to breathe slowly, deeply, and rhythmically. Take a deep breath; inhalation should be slow, unforced, and unhurried. Silently count to four, five, or six as you inhale. When inhalation is complete, exhale through the nose, letting your chest fall naturally and slowly. Again, count to four, five, or six as when breathing in. The exhalation should take as long as the inhalation.

There should be no sense of strain. If at first you feel you have breathed as deeply as you can by the count of three, don't worry. Gradually try to extend the inhalation until a slow count of five or six is possible, with a pause of two or three between inhaling and exhaling. This pattern of breathing should be repeated fifteen to twenty times. Since each cycle can take up to fifteen seconds, the whole exercise should take a total of about five minutes.

Once the mechanics of this technique have been mastered, introduce thoughts at different parts of the cycle. For example, on inhalation you might try to sense a feeling of warmth and energy entering your body with the air, and on exhalation, you might try to sense a feeling of sinking and settling deeper into the surface that supports you.

When you have completed the exercise, do not get up immediately, but rest for a minute or two, allowing your mind to become aware of any sensations of stillness, warmth, heaviness, and so on. Once mastered, this exercise can be used in any tense situation with the certainty that it will defuse the normal agitated response. It should thus result in a far greater ability to cope with stress.

Stress and the Adaptogens

A range of herbal remedies are coming to light that increase nonspecific resistance to damaging man-made factors as well as illnesses. Russian scientists have coined the term "adaptogens" to describe herbs that produce this wonderful increase in resistance and vitality. The two readily available herbs that can be considered adaptogens are ginseng and Siberian ginseng.

Pharmacological research suggests that the active principle of these plants is their complex glycosides, which increase the general resistance of the body to a whole range of diverse chemical, physical, psychological, and biological factors. However, it comes as no surprise to the herbalist that the extracted chemicals cannot reproduce the effects of the whole plant.

Siberian ginseng, one of the most remarkable of these plants, has a broad action range and very low toxicity. A great deal of excellent clinical and laboratory research has been conducted in Russia, where Professor L. L. Brekhman and his team in Vladivostock have studied the herb for over twenty years. Large-scale clinical trials have been undertaken on both healthy and sick people resulting in more than one thousand published research papers. The safety of Siberian ginseng and its ability to increase the resistance of the human body to extreme conditions make it a remedy of great importance.

These studies of Siberian ginseng provide some of the best clinical trials of herbal medicines so far. Large numbers of people were involved, using control groups and long-term study. The results were favorable and sometimes very noticeable. Concern with production and efficiency is very evident in the findings, whereas quality of life and individual health are only touched upon as factors in economic equations. However, the results speak for themselves.

Reduction of total disease incidence. Between the years 1973 and 1975, 1,200 drivers at the Volga Automobile Plant were given 8 to 12 mg of Siberian ginseng extract daily for two months each year in the spring and autumn. By the end of the experiment, the total disease incidence had decreased by 20 to 30 percent. In the winter of 1975, the authorities at the factory undertook a mass program of preventive medicine with the herb. It was included in the diet as Siberian ginseng sugar at a dose of 2 ml. Altogether, 13,096 persons took part in the experiments. Disease incidence dropped by 30 to 35 percent in comparison with a control group that did not use the remedy.

Reduction of influenza and acute respiratory disease. Siberian ginseng is an adrenal stimulant, not an antiviral herb. However, the Russians have accumulated much data on its anti-influenzal effect. Such findings imply that it either possesses an invigorating and tonic action on natural immunity, or has direct antiviral activity. In the Primorye region of Pacific Russia, a group of 180 men were given the herb every other day during March. As compared with the control group, the incidence of influenza and acute respiratory disease decreased from 17 to 12.7 percent In the winter of 1972–73, about 1,000 workers received 22 ml of Siberian ginseng extract daily for two months. The incidence of influenza and acute respiratory disease dropped almost 2.4 times versus the control group (the same number of workers at a shop with the same working conditions). In 1973 the number of days lost because of acute respiratory disease per 100 workers was 282; in 1979 it had dropped to 11.

Reduction of hypertension and ischemic heart disease. The test group were 1,200 drivers at the Volga Automobile plant. In 1973 the number of cases of hypertension at the motor transport administration was approximately the same as at the whole plant. After prophylactic treatment with the herb in 1975, the number of hypertensive drivers went down 3.5 times. The number of cases with worsening of heart disease was 6.7 per 100 workers in 1973; in 1978 it dropped to 0.2.

Reduction in disease under environmental stress. During long-term navigation in the tropics, where high temperature and humidity affect endurance, sailors were given an extract from the root of Siberian ginseng. The herb substantially reduced unpleasant changes in the central nervous system, cardiovascular system, and thermoregulation that characterize physiological stress under such conditions. It promoted an increase in physical and mental endurance, improving vision and the ability to think analytically.

An ever increasing number of pathologic conditions have been demonstrated to improve with the use of this adaptogen, including neurasthenia, chronic gastritis, diabetes, atherosclerosis, tuberculosis, brain injuries, and infectious disease.

Some of the published papers deal with surgery. Apart from the actual findings of these studies, they demonstrate the open approach of orthodox medicine in other parts of the world to herbal therapy. The provisional results indicate that Siberian ginseng speeds postoperative recovery. When used in postoperative treatment of oncological patients, it ameliorates the stress response that can aggravate metastasis. Furthermore, prognosis was improved if Siberian ginseng was used *with* the orthodox techniques in the treatment of lip cancer and breast cancer. Its ability to potentiate antitumor immunity has been discovered only recently: it brings about an increase in the activity of a group of antineoplastic white blood cells, called "natural killers." It also induced the synthesis of *y*-interferon. It is well known that stress decreases the activity of the immune system and particularly that of the natural killers. A clear biochemical association exists between stress, immune function, and the herb.

In these times of pollution and exposure to dangerous chemicals, this fascinating plant may prove helpful, as it also reduces the toxic impact of many chemical compounds as shown in laboratory tests with mice and rats.

Siberian ginseng exerts a range of specific effects on the metabolic and physiological mechanisms of the general adaptation syndrome, prolonging the resistance phase while reducing the alarm reaction and exhaustion stages.

From all of this, Siberian ginseng starts to look like a very special remedy indeed. It can increase individual resistance to the whole spectrum of factors that contribute to stress reactions and exhaustion, whether the stress is caused by extremes of weather or psychological problems. Its universal properties make this herb one of the most efficacious and promising medicines for increasing nonspecific resistance.

Nervous System Problems

Alzheimer's Disease and Dementia

Alzheimer's disease, named after Alois Alzheimer in 1906, is a progressive, degenerative, and irreversible neurological disease with no known cure, affecting an estimated four million American adults. The actual onset of Alzheimer's disease is unclear, but symptoms can appear most frequently around the age of sixty-five. Approximately half of men and women over the age of eighty-five have Alzheimer's disease. Nearly one hundred thousand people die of complications from Alzheimer's annually, making it the fourth largest killer of adults in the United States.

The cause is unknown but there are common clinical features. These include impaired memory, impaired thinking, impaired behavior, and difficulty in grasping or expressing thoughts. The loss of memory, by making it difficult to perform familiar tasks, has an adverse influence on all aspects of life. As the disease progresses a person may experience decreased judgment, disorientation, impairment in abstract thinking, changes in mood, abnormal behavior, and personality changes. One of the characteristic changes is the loss of memory, accompanied by the laboratory finding of reduced levels of the neurotransmitter acetylcholine from neurons of the brain. This understanding has led to medications for the treatment of the dementia associated with Alzheimer's that seek to replace the depleted levels of acetylcholine in the brain.

Neurotransmitters are chemicals that are used to relay, amplify, and modulate electrical signals between a neuron and another cell. Each neuron contains a particular transmitter. There are well over fifty of these chemical signals, which include glutamate, gamma-aminobutyric acid (GABA), and acetylcholine. The glutamate and GABA signals are the principal excitatory and inhibitory transmitters that "drive" the system. Superimposed on this framework are the modulatory transmitters that govern the mode of the system. Acetylcholine is concerned with attention and memory.

Because of the reduced acetylcholine levels that are found in various forms of dementia, therapeutic approaches have been developed to facilitate what is called "cholinergic replacement." However, acetylcholine is inactive if taken as a medicine so other methods must be developed to achieve a therapeutically meaningful elevation. So rather than using the neurotransmitters themselves as drugs, the approach has been to get more of these vital signal molecules released into the synapse, or to block the enzymes that break them down once they have done their job. Either way, you keep more neurotransmitters in the synapse for longer, improving communication between the cells.

Increasing levels of acetylcholine can be achievable using substances known as acetylcholinesterase inhibitors. Acetylcholinesterase is the enzyme responsible for the breakdown of acetylcholine, so by inhibiting its activity, existing levels of acetylcholine are maintained and even increased. For this reason, inhibitors of the enzyme acetylcholinesterase have attracted attention as potential treatments of Alzheimer's disease. Clinical trials show that these drugs can stabilize or improve cognition, global assessment scores, mood, and behavior in people with Alzheimer's disease. Unfortunately, as the disease progresses, there are fewer and fewer cholinergic neurons and so there is less potential for these drugs to work. Thus the drugs only slow the symptomatic progression of the disease and don't alter the underlying disease process.

HERBS AND ACETYLCHOLINE

"Sage will retard that rapid progress of decay that treads upon our heels so fast in latter years of life, will preserve faculties and memory more valuable to the rational mind than life itself."

JOHN HILL, THE BRITISH HERBAL (1756–1757)

Many of the drugs used today for the treatment of disorders of the mind/brain work by altering neurochemical signaling pathways. However, long before these complex brain mechanisms were discovered, herbal medicines have been used to treat these various central nervous system (CNS) conditions, for example belladonna for Parkinson's disease, the opium poppy for pain, and valerian for anxiety/stress. Herbs have a long history of use in specifically treating memory-related disorders. An example is Ashwaganda *(Withania somnifera),* used in Ayurvedic medicine to "attenuate cerebral functional deficits, including amnesia, in geriatric patients."

It turns out that many plants contain anticholinesterases, and physostigmine from the Calabar bean *(Physostigma venenosurn)* was one of the first to be isolated and used clinically. Further examples of plant-derived anticholinesterases are huperzine A from *Huperzia serrata* (currently in phase II clinical trials sponsored by the National Institute on Aging) and galantamine (approved by FDA for treating Alzheimer's) found in the bulbs of snowdrops *(Galanthus nevalis)* and daffodils (*Narcissus* spp.).

The club moss *Huperzia serrata* is the Chinese folk medicine *Qing Ceng Ta*. This herb is found chiefly in southern China, where it grows in moist places in hilly regions. The decoction of dried whole plant has been used to treat trauma, fractures, scalds, hematuria, and infections of the skin and subcutaneous tissues. However, the herb is also a component of a tea administered to elderly people in China. The alkaloid huperzine A was isolated from the moss, and shown to be a potent acetylcholinesterase inhibitor. There is some clinical evidence that huperzine A may compare favorably in symptomatic efficacy to cholinesterase inhibitors currently in use. Additionally huperzine A has antioxidant and neuroprotective properties that suggest that it may be useful as a disease-modifying treatment for Alzheimer's disease. It is currently available as a nutraceutical in the United States.

Several plants have been investigated for their memory-enhancing activity and have yielded compounds that may be of clinical relevance in Alzheimer's management. In Europe a number of herbs have been used historically for memory enhancement. Balm *(Melissa officinalis),* rosemary *(Rosmarinus officinalis),* and especially sage *(Salvia officinalis)* are documented as "strengthening the brain" or enhancing memory. Although many plants exist that could possess memory enhancing properties, sage is of especial interest because it is a common culinary herb and can therefore be assumed to be relatively safe.

Recent research has gone a long way to substantiate such historical use of sage for memory enhancement, as anticholinesterase activity has been found in both the essential oils and extracts in human brain tissue (postmortem). This could account, at least in part, for its memory-enhancing reputation. The Latin name for the sage genus is *Salvia* and comes from the Latin *salvare* meaning "to be saved." *Salvia* (with over seven hundred species) is the largest genus in the Mint family and, although not all have been researched pharmacologically, many have actions on the central nervous system. The genus features prominently in the pharmacopoeias of many countries throughout the world, particularly in China where the amount of their best tea was three times that traded for European sage tea. European sage and Chinese sage have been widely investigated phytochemically and a vast array of biological activities have been identified, many of which are relevant to CNS disorders.

Animal research has found that sage oil inhibits acetylcholinesterase in select parts of the brain, specifically the striatum and hippocampus but not the cortex. This inhibition in the striatum may be of relevance to Alzheimer's disease as this part of the brain is thought to participate in emotional and motivational behavior. One of the primary symptoms of Alzheimer's is short-term memory loss and the hippocampus plays a major role in short-term memory. This laboratory evidence that sage inhibits striatal and hippocampal acetylcholinesterase, provides a basis for the traditional observation that it improves cognitive function particularly. Also since the striatum is a major site of pathology in Parkinson's disease, targeting this area may be important in the treatment of Parkinson's disease.

Additional research has shown that, in addition, sage has antioxidant and anti-inflammatory properties, all actions considered to be valuable in Alzheimer's therapy. Many diseases of the nervous and nonnervous systems involve free radical damage due to excess reactive oxygen species. Cellular damage due to lipid, protein, and DNA caused by free radicals is associated with a number of disorders. Of relevance here is its contribution to neuronal cell damage in neurodegenerative disorders as well as the general aging process. Free radical damage has been described in the pathological changes that occur in Alzheimer's and limiting this by antioxidants is considered to be an important therapeutic strategy. Common to many *Salvia* species is their antioxidant ability. Antioxidant components of sages are carnosol, methyl carnosate, and carnosic acid. This implies that the memory-enhancing reputation of sage may thus be due to a combination of actions.

The herb industry and the supplement manufacturers are making such dramatic claims for ginkgo in the treatment of dementia and Alzheimer's disease that it is worthwhile to review some of this research on ginkgo, much of it coming from France. While the herb has a classical reputation as an antimicrobial and antitubercular agent, new research has also shown a profound activity on brain function and cerebral circulation. It has been clinically shown to be effective in patients with vascular disorders, in all types of dementia, and even in patients suffering from cognitive disorders secondary to depression (because of its beneficial effects on mood).

Of special concern are people who are just beginning to experience deterioration in their cognitive function, for it appears that ginkgo may delay deterioration and enable such people to maintain a normal life. The earlier the treatment begins, the better the prognosis, especially in Alzheimer's. Even in advanced cases, however, improvement may begin almost immediately and continue over many months. This property is important because every cell of the body will suffer when there is an inadequate supply of blood, leading to lack of energy, susceptibility to infection, decreased mental and physical function, and other problems. Indeed, dementia in the elderly is usually related to inadequate circulation.

Laboratory studies of ginkgo show it to reduce vascular, tissue, and metabolic disturbances as well as their neurological and behavioral consequences. Several membrane mechanisms seem to be involved, including protection of the membrane ultrastructure against free radicals.

The uniqueness of the pharmacological properties of ginkgo lies in the fact that it focuses its effects on tissue that is experiencing a lack of oxygen, by increasing the flow of blood into ischaemic tissue. According to recent research,* ginkgo may work by:

- Raising levels of glucose and ATP in the cell, thus maintaining energy levels.
- Stabilizing cellular membranes including the blood-brain barrier, thus reducing any cerebral edema and hypertension.
- Slowing the onset of dementia resulting from sclerosis of cerebral arteries.
- Ameliorating the effects of progressive cerebral circulatory insufficiency due to age.
- Decreasing the consumption of insulin, thus being of potential use in diabetic angiopathy. Because it has minimal impact on glucose metabolism, ginkgo is especially appropriate for diabetics (who generally suffer from insufficient circulation).
- Being hypotensive and peripherally vasodilating, and thus offering a treatment for hypertension as an aid in recovery from coronary thrombosis and intermittent claudication.

Ginkgo has marked effects on neurophysiology, but it also seems to concentrate in the vascular and endocrine systems that strongly affect the function of the

---

*F. Clostre, "From the body to the cell membrane: the different levels of pharmacological action of *Ginkgo biloba* extract," *Presse Med* 15/3, no. 1 (Sept. 25, 1986): 1529–38.

nervous system. This is especially so in the adrenal gland, which is responsible for producing dopamine, epinephrine, and norepinephrine as well as intermediary products required in the formation, activity, and metabolism of other neurotransmitters. Ginkgo is also, through its effects on blood flow, able to improve the availability of acetylcholine, another important neurotransmitter. These effects include:

- Stimulation of the synthesis of important neurotransmitters, which increases the capacity for physical activity in the way of both voluntary and involuntary functioning (e.g., digestion, blood pressure regulation, hormone secretion, blood sugar regulation).
- Increase in the flow of blood to the brain and stimulation of the growth of receptor sites. These effects lead to increased cerebral capacity, manifested by improved memory and reasoning power, improved mood, improved reaction time, alertness, and speech.
- Inhibition of synaptic breakdown of neurotransmitters, which in effect increases their availability during neural stimulation. This, in turn, increases the efficiency of the nervous system, and thus improves mood, memory, and self-mastery.

Ginkgo is prescribed European orthodox medicine in several neurological and behavioral disorders, in peripheral vascular deficiency, and in some functional disorders of the ear, nose, throat, and eye. Controlled clinical trials have been conducted to justify this use, and these excellent clinical findings are in agreement with pharmacological data currently available. Ginkgo extract has been found to act on cerebral circulation, on neuronal metabolism threatened by a lack of oxygen, on neurotransmission, and on neurone membrane lesions caused by free oxygenated radicals.* Improvement of the functioning of the auditory nerve of the ear through use of ginkgo is discussed further in the section on tinnitus (see page 140).

The herb offers much hope as a treatment in all types of dementia and even in patients suffering from cognitive disorders secondary to depression, because of its beneficial effects on mood. Of special concern are people who are just beginning

---

*Gautherie et al., "Vasodilator effect of *Gingko biloba* extract determined by skin thermometry and thermography," *Therapie* 27/5 (Sept.-Oct. 72): 881–92.

to experience deterioration in their cognitive function. Ginkgo may delay deterioration and enable these subjects to maintain a normal life. Anyone can benefit from the use of ginkgo, whether he or she is already experiencing the effects of aging on mental function or is just approaching that point. In addition, the herb is quite safe even in doses many times higher than those usually recommended.*

From experimental and clinical findings it appears that ginkgo may affect a number of major elements involved in both Alzheimer's and dementia. The theorized causes of Alzheimer's disease include free radical damage, vascular insufficiency, ischemia, and cholinergic and noradrenergic dysfunction. Ginkgo has been clinically shown to be active on circulatory functions, on neuronal and metabolic consequences of ischemia and hypoxia, on neurotransmission, and on membrane resistance to free radical damage. All clinical studies so far confirm that the diverse physiological effects of ginkgo lead to positive effects on behavior, an increased sense of well-being, decreased need for hospitalization, and improved capacity for self-sufficiency.

Free radicals have been implicated in the aging process and degenerative disease. The flavonoids of ginkgo, including quercetin, are extremely potent oxygen scavengers. With its particular affinity for the central nervous system as well as the adrenal and thyroid glands, the herb is ideal for protecting the heart, blood vessels, and brain against the destructive impact of free radicals.

- In one in vitro study, ginkgo was seen to destroy free radicals, blocking their formation and inhibiting membrane lipid peroxidation, a destructive effect for which free radicals are partly responsible. The herb also stimulates the biosynthesis of prostanoids, vasodilators having a hypotensive effect.
- One of the side effects of diabetes in rats is the gradual impairment of eyesight, thought to be due to free oxygenated radicals damaging the retina. Ginkgo significantly prevented the onset and severity of this damage.
- Ginkgo improved visual acuity in patients suffering from senile macular degeneration, a condition that involves free-radical damage.
- A protective effect against argon laser-induced damage of retinal cells was found. Pretreatment with ginkgo, by capturing free radicals, prevented significant tissue damage.

---

*D. M. Warburton, "Clinical psychopharmacology of *Ginkgo biloba* extract," *Presse Med* 15/31 (Sept. 25, 1986): 1595–604.

Clearly ginkgo could be an important herbal contribution to the treatment and prevention of Alzheimer's disease. The French scientists suggest that this herb fulfills the conditions laid down by the World Health Organization concerning the development of effective and safe drugs against cerebral aging.* Here again the plant kingdom may be supplying our needs.

Depression

Depression is a state of mind familiar to almost everyone, but this very familiarity becomes problematic in the treatment of depressive states. In ordinary usage, the word refers to a mood state that the medical world knows as *dysthymia* (as contrasted with the normal mood state of *euthymia,* and the opposite state of *elation*). Depression is defined by a standard set of symptoms. As described in the American Psychiatric Association's *Diagnostic and Statistical Manual of Mental Disorders,* they are:

- agitation, or retardation, of movement and thought
- diminished ability to think or concentrate, or indecisiveness
- fatigue and loss of energy
- feelings of worthlessness, self-reproach, or excessive or inappropriate guilt
- insomnia, or increased sleep
- loss of interest or pleasure in usual activities or decrease in sexual drive
- poor appetite and significant weight loss, or increased appetite and significant weight gain
- recurrent thoughts of death or suicide, or suicide attempts

Not all these symptoms occur in each individual who becomes depressed. For purposes of psychiatric treatment, a person is considered to have experienced a major depressive episode if he or she exhibits a loss of interest or pleasure in all or almost all usual activities and shows at least four of the above symptoms nearly every day for at least two weeks.

Herbs have much to offer this condition, but, unfortunately, they will rarely replace appropriate drugs in cases of major depressive illness. Herbs can be used

---

*M. Allard, "Treatment of the disorders of aging with *Ginkgo biloba* extract: From pharmacology to clinical medicine," *Presse Med* 15/31 (Sept. 25, 1986): 1540–45.

in conjunction with medications to good effect and in mild depression herbs will often be enough. Nervine tonics are the basis of herbal support for long-term change, to help the person cope with life and make necessary adjustments. Oats and St. John's wort are the herbs of choice here. Nervine relaxants may be called for in the short term or if the depression has an agitated and hyperactive aspect to it. The stronger nervines should not be used, as this might trigger a more entrenched depression. The strongest to consider are skullcap, vervain, or motherwort; in fact milder herbs such as linden, lavender, and chamomile are often adequate. Avoid the use of hops altogether in treating depression. Stimulants help occasionally but not predictably. If some form of stimulation is appropriate, it is better to use the bitter tonic stimulants.

Bitters often bring about changes in experience of oneself and one's life. This appears to occur through a generalized stimulation of metabolism and a general "lift" of the body. A nervine bitter such as mugwort is often used, as is the more directly digestive bitter gentian. Antispasmodic herbs will alleviate any muscular tension that may manifest as a bodily expression of the psychological depression. Adaptogens help the adrenals to combat the stress that the whole body is going through. Hepatics can be very important in supporting the liver's detoxification work, especially if the patient has been using prescription psychopharmaceuticals.

As far as I am concerned, there are no clear-cut specific antidepressive herbs. St. John's wort has a long tradition of use in Europe, but while it sometimes gets remarkable results, it also sometimes does nothing! It must be taken regularly for at least a month for any effects to be seen.

Antidepressive Formula

- St. John's wort   2 parts
- oats   1 part
- lavender   1 part
- mugwort   1 part

As tincture: take 1 tsp three times a day for at least one month.
As dried herb: infuse 2 tsp to a cup and drink three times a day.

When dealing with depression, the whole gamut of therapeutic issues touched upon in this chapter must be taken into account. From green salads to relaxation, from spinal adjustments to changing the music one listens to, the list is endless. Exercise is especially important. The *Textbook of Natural Medicine* suggests the following nutritional supplements:

> **B vitamin complex:** 50 times the recommended
>   daily allowance (RDA)
> **vitamin C:** 1 g three times daily
> **folic acid:** 400 mg daily
> **vitamin B$_{12}$:** 250 mcg daily
> **magnesium:** 500 mg daily

Headache

Headache is one of humanity's most common afflictions. In the United States alone, up to fifty million people seek medical help for headaches every year, and about half a billion dollars is spent on headache remedies annually! Interestingly enough, however, most headaches are caused by fatigue, emotional disorders, or allergies, with only about 2 percent of all headaches resulting from organic disorders.

The brain itself is insensitive to pain, as is the bony covering of the cranium. Headache pain results from the stimulation of such pain-sensitive structures as the membranous linings of the brain and the nerves of the cranium and upper neck. This stimulation can be produced by inflammation, by the dilation of normal or abnormal blood vessels of the head, or by muscle spasms in the neck and head.

Headaches brought on by muscle spasms are classified as tension headaches; those caused by the dilation of blood vessels are called vascular headaches. A more specialized classification, by the International Headache Society, further divides headaches into fourteen categories for research purposes! A system designed to help the phytotherapist select the appropriate remedy groups headaches as follows:

- *Dietary:* possible allergy to certain foods or additives
- *Environmental:* caused by pollutants, poor body posture, lighting, sound, etc.
- *Stress:* physical, emotional, or mental in origin
- *Organic:* disease (hypertension, etc.)

Many plants exist that may be considered "headache" herbs. Unfortunately, not all will always work for all people.

balm	lavender	skullcap
cayenne	marjoram	thyme
chamomile	peppermint	valerian
elder flower	rosemary	wood betony
Jamaican dogwood	rue	wormwood

If a clear-cut underlying pathology exists, this will naturally serve as the focus of treatment. If none has been found, herbs should be selected that will ensure good elimination, support liver function, and address any obvious general health needs.

Various essential oils can be used to relieve headaches. Particularly effective oils are lavender, rosemary, and peppermint, either separately or in combination. Lavender can be rubbed on the temples or made into a cold compress and applied to the temples, the forehead, or the back of the neck. Equal parts of lavender and peppermint may be even more effective, for lavender has the ability to enhance the action of other oils when it is used in blends. It is also worth noting that while lavender is a sedative, peppermint is a stimulant, and that many commercial headache remedies combine a stimulant (usually caffeine) with one or more analgesics. This is because painkilling drugs often have a slightly sedative (sometimes even a depressant) effect; hence caffeine is included to counteract this. Lavender and peppermint will produce a similar effect without the risks inherent in synthetic drugs.

If the headache is caused by catarrh or sinus infection, inhalations with lavender, peppermint, rosemary, or eucalyptus will usually be very effective in both relieving the headache and clearing the underlying congestion. All these oils are antiseptic and will combat the nasal infection as well as give immediate symptomatic relief.

The National Headache Foundation has developed the following tips to help control headaches:

- Avoid aged cheeses, citrus fruits, and chocolate.
- Compose a list of all the foods that cause you discomfort, and avoid them.

- Eat regular meals.
- Sleep well. Try to wake up the same time every day and avoid sleeping late on your days off.
- Choose your environment. Avoid bright or glaring lights and wear tinted glasses if necessary. Avoid smoke- and perfume-filled rooms.
- Lean to relax. Practice relaxation and stretching techniques to release built-up tension.
- Don't overexert or take on more than you can handle; practice saying no.
- When traveling, give your body time to adjust to new surroundings.
- Drink plenty of water and eat lots of foods high in complex carbohydrates, such as pasta.
- Try to avoid all alcoholic beverages. If you are going to drink, limit your intake to one or two drinks.
- Beware of medications that may aggravate your headaches.

MIGRAINE

Orthodox medicine considers the underlying cause of migraine headaches to be unknown. Yet the herbalist (like other holistically orientated therapists) can achieve excellent results by focusing on certain factors—which would seem to suggest causal links. Indeed, specific herbal remedies can prove exceptionally successful if used in a holistic context, so that the whole body and environment of the patient are addressed. About 8 percent of all headaches treated by the family doctor can be classified as migraine or one of its variants, with some sixteen to eighteen million Americans affected.

The immediate basis of migraine appears to be spasmodic activity in the muscular walls of the blood vessels of the brain and scalp. In about 30 percent of all cases, migraine attacks are preceded by warning signs such as scintillating visual effects, blind spots, zigzag flashing lights, numbness in parts of the body, and distorted visual images. These signs of an imminent attack are probably due to intracerebral vessel constriction, while the head pain is linked to dilation of scalp arteries. All such symptoms may clear just before the onset of pain or merge into it. The pain may be unilateral or generalized but tends to follow a pattern in each particular person. Attacks may occur daily or only once every several months. Untreated attacks may last for hours or days and are often accompanied with nausea, vomiting, and photophobia.

Possible causes that should be considered include those listed below; however, rarely will *all* be involved in any one individual.

- *Food sensitivity:* This category can include anything, but the common triggers are dairy products, especially cheese; chocolate; eggs; wheat and wheat products; peanuts; citrus fruits; tomatoes; red meat and shellfish; alcohol (especially red wine and spirits).
- *General "toxicity":* Any tendency to constipation, liver problems, or general "congestion" will be a marked trigger in some individuals.
- *Hormone levels:* Occasionally, changes of certain hormone levels may trigger an attack.
- *Stress and fatigue:* Will undoubtedly compound the problem and may be a clear trigger.
- *Structural:* Cranial and spinal misalignments may be involved, as may poor posture, even when not associated with overt skeletal problems.

Feverfew is the only herb used by European herbalists that is known to be specific for the treatment of migraine. It is also the best example of a remedy well known to medical herbalists that has recently been accepted and used by allopathic medicine. Historically, feverfew has long been used as a bitter tonic and remedy for severe headaches. Through wide media coverage in recent years, the herb has gained a well-deserved reputation as a "cure" for migraine. Clinicians at the London Migraine Clinic observed that patients were reporting marked improvements when they took the herb. Fortunately for migraine sufferers, these doctors had the enquiring and open minds of true scientists and so started their own investigations into the claims for feverfew. Clinical observations were soon being reported in medical journals.

An example is the work of Dr. D. M. Hylands and colleagues. Seventeen patients who regularly ate fresh leaves of feverfew daily as prophylaxis against migraine were invited to participate in a double-blind placebo-controlled trial of the herb. Of these, eight patients received capsules containing freeze-dried feverfew powder, and nine a placebo. Those taking the placebo had a significant increase in the frequency and severity of headache, nausea, and vomiting as well as the reemergence of untoward effects during the early months of treatment. The group given capsules of feverfew, on the other hand, showed no change in the lack of symptoms of migraine. This clear evidence of effectiveness led the researchers to strongly suggest its use by migraine sufferers who have never treated themselves with this herb before. Long-term users often report beneficial side effects such as relief from depression, nausea, and arthritic pain due to inflammation.

The venerable English herbalists John Gerard and Nicholas Culpeper would hardly have been surprised at these findings! It is a pity that the patients given the placebo had to go through the renewed migraine attacks to demonstrate something already well known by herbalists as well as by the patients themselves.

Pharmacologists are directing much attention to this humble weed in their search for a new class of effective antimigraine and analgesic drugs. As the dried or fresh leaf of the plant itself is an excellent formulation, why not just suggest it to patients? It raises social, political, and economic issues as well as the obvious medical ones. To overtly recommend an herbal remedy means that the allopathic doctor is relinquishing a measure of power to the patient, for the patient in herbal therapy is no longer totally dependent upon the expert skills of the professional therapist but is actively involved in his or her own healing. The pharmaceutical industry may also not be too happy about the possible outcome, as the plant is grown by nature free of charge and is nonpatentable—in other words, there is no profit in it for them! This is not to deny the value of pharmacological research and exploration of herbal therapeutics, rather to question the ends to which this information is used.

Quite often a very simple herbal approach will suffice, used in the context of the dietary and environmental suggestions I have given above. The herbal component could take this form:

Migraine Remedy I

■ feverfew
125 mg of dried herb once a day.

■ lavender
Massage oil into temples at the first sign of an attack.

Here is one possible prescription for migraine associated with stress and hypertension:

Migraine Remedy II

- hawthorn
- linden blossom
- skullcap
- cramp bark

Equal parts of herbs or tinctures.

As tincture: take 1 tsp (5 ml) of this mixture three times a day.

As dried herb: infuse 2 tsp to a cup and drink three times a day.

Insomnia

Various herbs are reputed to be effective sleep remedies, but there are no legal plants that actually render a person unconscious! The key to any successful treatment of insomnia, of course, is to find the cause and deal with it: this may be anything, from grief to constipation. Psychological issues often need attention, as do health problems causing pain or discomfort. Dietary indiscretions must be identified, as must environmental factors (be it freeway noise or a snoring spouse). Insomnia can push the practitioner's diagnostic skills to the limit, making the free and easy prescribing of benzodiazepine sleeping medications at least understandable!

HERBAL HYPNOTICS

Hypnotics are herbal remedies that can help to induce a deep and healing state of sleep. They have nothing at all to do with hypnotic trances! They work in a variety of ways, from mild muscle relaxation through the use of essential oils that ease psychological tensions, to remedies that contain strong alkaloids that work directly on the central nervous system. Some of the most effective plant hypnotics are illegal for the very degree of their effectiveness. However, the remedies I will list here are entirely safe and have no addictive properties. These herbs should be used in a context that also involves relaxation, dietary advice, and lifestyle reevaluation.

Often the key to successful treatments lies in focusing upon some part or function of the body that is experiencing problems. Hypnotics and nervines can be used within the context of such treatments. These can be selected by the role they play in the system in question and not simply according to their strength as hypnotics.

- *Circulatory system:* Here we can mention motherwort, linden, and balm.
- *Digestive system:* The relaxing nervines and canninatives are important, such as chamomile, balm, hops, and valerian. The antispasmodic herbs will help with intestinal colic: examples are hops, Jamaican dogwood, passionflower, and valerian.
- *Musculoskeletal system:* All hypnotics reduce muscle tension and associated pain. They may be used internally or as lotions. Especially useful are Jamaican dogwood and valerian.
- *Nervous system:* All the following remedies work on the nervous system.
- *Reproductive system:* Hypnotics are important here when used as muscle relaxants.
- *Respiratory system:* All the hypnotics can help as antispasmodics in conditions such as asthma, if used at the right dose. Wild lettuce eases irritable coughs.
- *Skin:* Chamomile and cowslip are active healing agents; otherwise the value of hypnotics here is to ensure that the body has a good recuperative rest each night.
- *Urinary system:* Hypnotics are important here when used as muscle relaxants.

The many sleeping remedies can be categorized according to their strength (but bearing in mind the very subjective nature and individual variability of human response to these herbs). We can very roughly identify three groupings:

- *mild:* motherwort, chamomile, balm, linden, and red clover
- *medium:* pulsatilla, mugwort, motherwort, skullcap, and vervain
- *strong:* California poppy, hops, wild lettuce, passionflower, Jamaican dogwood, and valerian

By selecting herbs to address specific health problems that compound the sleep difficulties, better results are obtained than by simply selecting a powerful hypnotic. For example, the presence of palpitations might suggest use of motherwort. The following mixtures will show how a basic mixture for sleep can be adjusted to suit specific needs.

A Possible Prescription for Insomnia

- passionflower
- valerian

Equal parts of tinctures.

Take 1–2 tsp 30 minutes before bedtime.

A Possible Prescription for
Insomnia Associated with Menopause

- passionflower
- valerian
- motherwort

Equal parts of tinctures.

Take 1–2 tsp 30 minutes before bedtime; administer in addition to appropriate daytime treatments (please refer to the chapter on the reproductive system).

A Possible Prescription for
Insomnia Associated with "Indigestion"

- passionflower
- valerian
- mugwort
- balm

Equal parts of tinctures.

Take 1–3 tsp 30 minutes before bedtime; administer in addition to appropriate daytime treatments (refer to the chapter on the digestive system).

An infusion of chamomile, linden, or balm at night would also be helpful.

> ### A Possible Prescription for
> ### Insomnia Associated with Depression
>
> - passionflower
> - valerian
> - St. John's wort
> - mugwort
>
> Equal parts of tinctures.
> Take 1–3 tsp 30 minutes before bedtime; administer in
> addition to appropriate daytime treatments (refer to the
> chapter on the cardiovascular system).

CAUTION: Avoid the use of hops in depression.

Peripheral Neuropathy

Peripheral nerve problems are caused by a range of factors, including physical trauma, arthritic and metabolic diseases, microorganisms, toxic agents, nutritional deficiencies, and malignancies. Appropriate treatment is based on accurate diagnosis, which is often problematic in this complex of conditions. The therapeutic approach suggested here is a basic one, ideal for traumatic neuritis and may be of symptomatic value in any of the syndromes mentioned above. Traumatic neuritis may be induced by injury, pressure paralysis, exposure to cold, and radiation.

Nervine tonics are important, as they will "feed" the traumatized nerve tissue, while the nervine relaxants ease any associated tension. Anti-inflammatories will help reduce the inflammatory response; antispasmodics will alleviate any muscular tension developed in response to the discomfort. Adaptogens will support coping with both the stress of the pain and any stress-related causes.

> ### For Internal Use
>
> - St. John's wort
> - skullcap
> - oats
> - Siberian ginseng
>
> Equal parts of herbs or tinctures.
> **As tincture:** take 1 tsp (5 ml) of this mixture three times a day.
> **As dried herb:** infuse 2 tsp to a cup and drink three times a day.

> ### For External Use
>
> - peppermint oil
> - St. John's wort oil
>
> Apply either oil liberally over affected area.
>
> - colloidal oatmeal
>
> Use as a dusting powder to reduce skin irritation.

The internal prescription may be made stronger by the addition of valerian or Jamaican dogwood. However, these analgesics can be too sedating at an effective painkilling dose. It may be appropriate in such cases to recommend prescription analgesics. Stress management techniques accompanied by good quality nutrition are essential. The B-complex vitamins must be given as supplements.

Shingles

Shingles is a viral infection of sensory nerve cells caused by the same virus *(Varicella zoster)* that causes chicken pox. The virus remains latent in the dorsal root ganglia of the spinal cord after the initial attack of chicken pox. The condition is characterized by pain along an affected nerve and its branches and the eruption of blisters over skin areas supplied by the nerve. An attack is usually preceded by a few days of intense pain in the affected areas. Many extremely painful and itchy blisters develop, normally lasting seven to fourteen days. These eventually form crusty scabs and fall off. The pain may continue for months even when the blisters are gone. The disease occurs most frequently in people over fifty.

Nervine tonics help to nourish the traumatized nerve tissue. Nervine relaxants may ease the associated pain and will lessen associated anxiety. Anti-inflammatories reduce the inflammatory response. Antimicrobials help the body to deal with the intransigent viral infection. The following approach has proven useful.

> - oats
> - St. John's wort
> - echinacea
> - skullcap
>
> Equal parts of herbs or tinctures.
> **As tincture:** take 1 tsp (5 ml) of this mixture three times a day.
> **As dried herb:** infuse 2 tsp to a cup and drink three times a day.

Peppermint oil applied topically may reduce the pain through a mild local numbing effect. Do not attempt this if the skin is extremely sensitive. Colloidal oatmeal powder can be dusted on the affected skin to act as a dry lubricant that may help to reduce pain from irritating contact with clothes.

Good nutrition and support of general health are crucial. Pain relief medication containing acetaminophen (e.g., Tylenol) may actually prolong the illness. Pharmacological research suggests that capsaicin from cayenne may act as a pain reliever, and thus capsules of cayenne may be helpful. The following supplementation is recommended:

> **vitamin B complex:** 100 mg three times a day with food
>
> **vitamin C:** 2 g twice a day
>
> **lysine (an amino acid):** 500 mg twice a day

TINNITUS

One person out of ten has some type of hearing impairment or ear problem, and of these 85 percent have some associated tinnitus (a sensation of noise in the ear). The most common causes of tinnitus are noise-induced damage and age-related hearing loss. Because tinnitus is not a disease but a symptom, it often serves as an important marker for other conditions such as concussion, cranial or cervical fracture, whiplash, and problems with the temporomandibular joint (the hinges of the jaw). In hyperthyroidism, an increased heart rate and consequent increased blood flow through the ear may cause ringing. Tinnitus is also a symptom of Ménière's disease. A transient tinnitus can follow a cold or influenza, but it generally subsides two to four months after the infection.

Whatever the underlying cause, tinnitus tends to be exacerbated by muscle spasms, stress, and tension. Substances that can accentuate it include nicotine and caffeine. Some people under stress will begin to notice ringing in their ears, often because they clench or grind their teeth. Reducing stress and relieving temporomandibular joint dysfunction improves the tinnitus. Unfortunately, by the time most people realize that they have suffered noise-induced tinnitus or hearing loss, hair cell damage in the inner ear is irreversible. The distress can be minimized, however, by use of herbs and avoidance of aggravating factors.

My training in Britain suggested the use of black cohosh and goldenseal for tinnitus. In my work with patients from industrial South Wales who suffered from noise-induced tinnitus, these herbs proved gratifyingly helpful. Since then I have also become aware of the research on ginkgo for a range of vascular disturbances of the inner ear. This seems so clear that I have included that herb in the suggested prescription. The brief review of the research given here is from a collection of core research papers translated from French and Italian into English.*

Problems of the inner ear resulting from a disturbance in blood supply may be helped with ginkgo.† Such problems include tinnitus, vertigo, and some forms of hearing loss (deafness resulting from head injuries, sonic damage, or vascular problems of recent origin). Clinical research found that many people with vertigo experienced total recovery taking ginkgo daily for several weeks. For example:

- Disturbances of the inner ear resulting from an underlying vascular defect have been successfully treated with ginkgo. One study of hearing loss due to old age, tinnitus, or vertigo found an improvement of hearing by 40 percent of the patients. Most of the tinnitus patients experienced significant improvement within ten to twenty days.
- An 88 percent success rate was found in patients suffering from hearing loss, tinnitus, vertigo, and labyrinthitis. The researchers concluded that the herb is effective in neurosensory diseases of the inner ear of vascular origin that manifest themselves by ringing in the ear, vertigo, and headache.

However, once hair cells are damaged, no medication will eliminate tinnitus completely.

The following formulation may be helpful if taken over an extended time:

- black cohosh
- goldenseal
- ginkgo

Equal parts of herbs or tinctures.
As tincture: take 1 tsp (5 ml) of this mixture three times a day.
As dried herb: infuse 2 tsp to a cup and drink three times a day.

---

*Fünfgeld, E. W. (ed.). *Rökan, Ginkgo biloba. Recent Results in Pharmacology and Clinic* (Berlin: Springer-Verlag, 1988).

†Stange et al., "Adaptational behaviour of peripheral and central acoustic responses in guinea pigs under the influence of various fractions of an extract from *Ginkgo biloba*," *Arzneim Forsch* 26/3 (1976): 367–74.

A number of other issues can be addressed in the attempt to alleviate tinnitus. If stress is an issue, this can be treated with the use of herbs, as well as relaxation techniques or other methods (see pages 112–18). The majority of patients experience their tinnitus as mild annoyance or are not aware of it most of the time. However, the constant noise can be upsetting and may lead to depression. By treating the depression, these patients sleep better, feel better, and find that the tinnitus is not as distracting. St. John's wort is the main herb to consider.

Ear protection is important, especially in the presence of potentially harmful noise. If occupational noise is a problem, the patient should try to reduce the noise level or change the working environment to avoid exposure. This is not always easy! Tinnitus can often be masked with a background noise. Background music or "white sound" may be more tolerable than the internally generated tinnitus, especially for older patients with high-frequency hearing loss.

6 The Urinary System

The importance of the urinary system cannot be overemphasized, as the physiological functions fulfilled by the kidneys are fundamental to health and well-being. As major organs of elimination of waste from the body, the kidneys work in conjunction with the liver, the lungs, the skin, and the bowels in ensuring a healthy internal environment. Excess water, metabolic waste, and inorganic salts are disposed of in the form of urine. Because of their excretory function, the kidneys are also largely responsible for maintaining the water balance of the body and the pH balance of the blood. They also play important roles in other body activities, such as in releasing the protein erythropoietin (which stimulates bone marrow to increase the formation of red blood cells) and in helping to control blood pressure. Certain drugs or their metabolites are also eliminated via the kidney.

The production of urine is a complex and quite wonderful process. Far from being a simple removal of water from the body, it is a process of selective filtration that removes waste and potential toxins from the blood while retaining essential molecules.

To keep the kidneys running smoothly it is essential to drink water regularly. As approximately 50 percent of the body's water supply is gained from solid food and as the average person's caloric intake declines with age, it is particularly important that people, as they age, drink plenty of fluids. Nutritionists recommend between six and eight glasses a day. In addition, avoid excessive amounts of protein. The kidneys must rid the body of nitrogen from any protein the body does not use and can be overtaxed thereby, which in turn creates a potential for disease. Finally, it is important to detect kidney disease early so that treatment may begin immediately.

Signs of Kidney Disease

The most prominent warning signs of kidney disease are

- a burning sensation while urinating or difficulty in urinating;
- more frequent need to urinate, especially at night;
- excretion of blood-tinged urine;
- persistent pain in the small of the back just beneath the ribs;
- puffiness around the eyes or swelling of the hands and feet; and
- high blood pressure.

High blood pressure can mean trouble for the kidneys, and conversely, kidney problems can sometimes cause high blood pressure. The National Kidney Foundation reports that of all cases of kidney failure, some 10 to 20 pecent are caused by high blood pressure.

Nature has been abundant in the provision of plants that have a beneficial impact upon the urinary system. It is often difficult to explain the mechanisms at work, but it is a relatively straightforward task to reach therapeutic conclusions concerning indications and contraindications. The most important group are known as the *diuretics*—an often missused term in the herbal world.

Herbal Actions

Diuretics are agents (herbs or drugs) that help the body to rid itself of excess fluids by increasing the rate of urine production by the kidneys. The accumulation of excess fluid in tissues, known as edema, is symptomatic of a wide range of disorders of the heart, kidney, liver, and other organs. Such disorders must be specifically addressed, but diuretics may be used to alleviate edema in conjunction with other herbs that treat the underlying condition. Many diuretics alter the excretion of electrolytes by the kidneys; these electrolytes (such as sodium and potassium salts) are involved in many processes, including the regulation of blood pressure, nerve impulse transmission, and muscle contraction. In the tradition of herbal medicine, the term *diuretic* has come to imply an herb that has some sort of beneficial action on the urinary system. Thus, references to this category may include not only true diuretics but also demulcent and anti-inflammatory remedies—which may lead to confusion when selecting remedies for a particular individual. If we limit ourselves to diuretics in the strict sense, there are two broad groups: those that increase kidney blood flow and those that reduce water reabsorption in the nephrons of the kidney.

The *first group* includes not only herbal diuretics such as broom but all herbs that are cardioactive and circulatory stimulants. These increase blood flow in the kidney by stimulating effects on the heart or elsewhere in the body. Because there is more blood passing through the kidney, more urine is produced. Caffeine-containing herbs such as kola, guarana, tea, and coffee also have this effect.

Diuretics of the *second group* may work in any of various ways. Some cause diuresis because some portion of their constituents are secreted by the kidney and possibly change the osmotic balance, causing more water to be lost. This appears to be the case with dandelion leaf, couch grass, and corn silk. Others work by irritating the reabsorption mechanism through volatile oils, saponins, or alkaloids they contain.

The herbal remedies that are sometimes referred to as "diuretics," but whose primary effect is other than diuretic in the strict sense, include demulcents and anti-inflammatories for inflammation reduction; astringents for reducing any associated bleeding; antimicrobials for treatment of infection; and antilithics for treatment of conditions associated with stone formation. These include the following:

- *Anti-inflammatories:* celery seed, cleavers, corn silk, couch grass, and gravel root
- *Antilithics:* gravel root, hydrangea, and stone root
- *Antimicrobials:* bearberry, buchu, couch grass, juniper, and yarrow
- *Astringents:* agrimony, bearberry, broom, horsetail, and yarrow
- *Demulcents:* bearberry, corn silk, couch grass, and stone root

Keeping the Kidneys Healthy

Like so many factors that contribute to human health and wholeness, kidney function is taken for granted and often given little attention by therapists except for the occasional prescription of a diuretic. In fact, the range of remedies available does provide certain therapeutic options beyond the simple increase in diuresis so dramatically produced by dandelion leaf.

The urinary system is not served by all-around tonics equivalent to hawthorn for the cardiovascular system or oats for the nervous system, which can be administered to create many unique options of toning. Instead, each herbal practitioner will have his or her own favorite gentle tonics for the urinary system. These will vary from one region to another, but remedies that might be considered common for such purposes include cleavers, couch grass, and yarrow.

Here the emphasis is on nourishing the tissue and helping the normal functioning of the various organs and tissues involved. Attention to certain simple principles will help maintain health and avoid the development of illness in the whole of the urinary system.

- Drink adequate amounts of water, about six to eight glasses a day.
- Too much protein in the diet will tend to overload the kidneys, because they must deal with much of the nitrogen-rich metabolic waste produced by protein molecules. Under normal conditions this is, of course, not really a problem. However, anyone with kidney problems should be on a low-protein diet whereby protein is obtained primarily from vegetable sources, such as peas, beans, lentils, mushrooms, and asparagus.
- Good personal hygiene is essential.
- Avoid dietary irritants, especially foods containing oxalic acid, such as rhubarb and spinach, and coffee and tea in excess. Plant volatile oils taken internally can be damaging to the delicate tissue of the nephrons.

Urinary Problems

Cystitis

This inflammation of the wall and lining of the bladder may be due to bacterial infection or to mechanical abrasion from microcrystals in the urine. Symptoms of cystitis include frequency, painful urination, and cloudy or bloody urine, with pain and tenderness in the lower abdomen. The urine itself may be cloudy because it contains pus or blood and may also have an unpleasant odor. These symptoms must be distinguished from those caused by vaginitis, sexually transmitted diseases, and irritations of the urethra.

Acute urinary tract infections are very common, involving at least 15 percent of all women at some point in their lives. They occur at any age and are about twenty times more common in women than men. This is because the urethra is much shorter in women than in men, so that infective organisms have far easier access to the bladder. Such "ascending" infections are usually announced by discomfort at the urethral opening; as the condition progresses, the irritation travels upward. The infection is usually caused by the rod-shaped bacterium called *Escherichia coli*. This is a normal bacterium found in the bowel, and after a bowel movement they can be wiped on to the urethral opening. Less commonly, infection from the bloodstream and the kidneys descends into the bladder. These "descending" infections are usually associated with backache, headache, tiredness, and pain in the abdomen.

A number of predisposing factors are known:

- *Antibiotics.* Overuse of these potentially lifesaving drugs will select for resistant bacteria, often leading to cystitis.
- *Chemical factors.* Antibacterial soaps, sprays, douches, feminine deodorants, and contraceptive jellies and creams alter the vaginal environment and may cause irritation that makes the tissue susceptible to infection. In addition, barrier contraceptive devices such as the diaphragm may cause mechanical irritation of the urethra. Some forms of interstitial cystitis may be caused by food contaminated with pesticides.
- *Diabetes.* Diabetics and those with high consumption of sugar are predisposed to cystitis.
- *Gender.* The female urethra is prone to colonization due to its proximity to the anus, its short length (about 4 cm), and its termination inside the labia. Friction during intercourse may cause minor inflammation of the urethra, predisposing to infection, and organisms may even be moved into the urethra.
- *Hormonal changes.* Oral contraceptives may initiate infection in some individuals.
- *Pregnancy.* Pregnant women may be more susceptible to infection because of hormonal changes resulting in dilation and reduction in tone of the ureters. Pressure of the uterus on the bladder and local venous congestion and pressure may also be factors in precipitating cystitis in pregnancy.

- *Retention of urine.* Anatomical deviations such as uterine malpositions may result in retention of urine and thus potentiate infection.
- *Stress.* Stress results in the production of hormones such as ACTH, gluco-corticoids, and aldosterone, all of which reduce circulating white blood cell counts and contribute to the susceptibility for infection. Many who experience recurrent infection can relate stress (chemical, physical, emotional) to the onset of symptoms.

Herbs can be very effective in the treatment of cystitis, but sometimes the key to success lies in finding the right combination for the individual concerned. Antimicrobial diuretics will help the body control and then clear bacterial infection. However, many of the well-known antimicrobial remedies (such as echinacea) do not fulfill the herbalist's hopes in the case of cystitis. It is important to use plants that are specifically active in the urinary tract. Thus antimicrobials with essential oils, such as bearberry and buchu, are indicated here as the oil is excreted from the body via the kidney, thus directing to the site of infection in the bladder. Anti-inflammatories will soothe the pain and discomfort. However, the symptomatic relief they produce must be applied in the context of removing the infection that causes the inflammation. Antispasmodics may be necessary if there is much pain.

Many plants are traditionally reputed to be effective in the treatment of cystitis, yet their efficacy will often vary from fresh to dried samples, time of year they were picked, and so on. In Wales, freshly picked yarrow, preferably from sea cliffs, had a dramatic effect even for intransigent cases. Unfortunately, tincture or infusion made from the same plants dried did not replicate such results.

■ corn silk	2 parts
■ bearberry	2 parts
■ buchu	1 part

As tincture: take 1 tsp (5 ml) of this mixture three times a day.
As dried herb: infuse 1–2 tsp to a cup and drink three times a day.

Following is a possible prescription for cystitis associated with much pain and discomfort:

■ corn silk	2 parts
■ bearberry	2 parts
■ black haw	1 part
■ valerian	1 part

As tincture: take 1 tsp (5 ml) of this mixture three times a day.
As dried herb: infuse 2 tsp to a cup and drink three times a day.

Hot infusions will ease symptoms dramatically. As an example, consider a combination recommended by British medical herbalist Annie McIntyre. Combine the following dried herbs:

■ marshmallow root	2 parts
■ corn silk	2 parts
■ couch grass	2 parts
■ horsetail	2 parts
■ bearberry	2 parts
■ buchu	1 part

Add 1 tsp of this mixture to a cup of boiling water. Let infuse for 10–15 minutes.
Drink hot four to five times a day.

A number of nonherbal considerations can be taken into account. The following list of factors will provide a broader context of treatment:

- Avoid tampons, as they contain additives that can injure the lining of the vagina.
- Discontinue use of diaphragm, oral contraceptives, or any chemicals used in the vaginal area.
- Discontinue use of deodorant soaps. These soaps are irritating to the skin and will destroy normal external bacteria, which are then replaced by more virulent, less easily killed pathogens.
- Increase intake of water to at least eight to twelve glasses per day. This will help to flush out the bacteria and will often reduce dysuria (painful urination).

- Acidify the urine by drinking unsweetened cranberry juice. Avoid or reduce intake of foods that are alkaline-forming such as dairy products, citrus juices, sodas.
- Eat a light diet consisting of grains and nonsweet vegetables.
- Eliminate bladder irritants such as coffee, black tea, alcohol.
- Discontinue all intake of foods high in sugar including sweet vegetables and fruits, sugar, and honey. Chocolate is also a bladder irritant.
- New studies show that ascorbic acid irritates the bladder; thus vitamin C must be obtained in the form of calcium ascorbate, which is relatively buffered. Avoid vitamins containing aspartate, as it is a bladder irritant.
- Supplement with vitamin E (400 to 600 IU day) and vitamin B_6 (300 mg/ day).

Kidney Stones

Three percent of all Americans will suffer from a kidney stone at some time in their life, and half of these people will suffer recurrences over the following ten or more years. It is thus a disease that touches a significant portion of the population. It rarely causes permanent loss of kidney function if properly treated and is almost never fatal in the absence of complications.

The most important kinds of kidney stones are calcium oxalate stones, calcium phosphate stones, and uric acid stones. The vast majority contain calcium in some form. Exceptions to this are the uric acid stones, which account for less than 10 percent of all stones.

Normal urine contains predictable amounts of calcium, magnesium, uric acid, and other by-products of metabolism. Normally these substances are in solution and pass into the bladder. However, under certain conditions of high saturation, and in a complex chemical environment that is not yet completely understood, the chemicals may crystallize and form a stonelike particle in the kidney. Once formed, it stimulates continued crystallization. If the stone remains in the wide open spaces of the kidney, symptoms may be entirely absent, although there may be microscopic signs of blood in the urine. Once a piece of the stone breaks off and enters the ureter leading to the bladder, spasms occur promptly, leading to painful symptoms.

An infection of the urinary tract can cause cellular debris to act as a focus or "seed" on which crystals can form. Bacterial action makes the urine more alkaline, resulting in the deposit of phosphates, which form calcium phosphate stones. Excessive uric acid, increased excretion of calcium by the kidney, combined with an increased insolubility of calcium in the urine, can also cause stones to form. Long-term confinement to bed or even a chronic lack of exercise may encourage mobilization of calcium from the bones into the blood and so increase calcium levels in the urine. Similarly, steroids can increase blood and urine calcium levels. An inherited genetic attribute and excess weight can also predispose you to kidney stones.

The pain of a kidney stone comes on suddenly. Classically, there is severe, excruciating pain in the flank on the side of the stone, coming in waves, radiating around to the lower abdomen and into the groin, scrotum, or vagina, and occasionally into the upper thigh area. The intensity is as severe as most people ever experience.

Along with the pain caused by kidney stones, there may or may not be blood in the urine. There may be nausea, vomiting, and profuse sweating. After anywhere from minutes to days or even longer, most stones pass into the bladder, and the pain is gone. The small, usually brown or black stone may be identified in the urine and should be kept for analysis. If fever is present, it may indicate that infection has formed behind the stone in the stagnant urine.

Antilithic remedies are the core of any herbal treatment of kidney stones. These herbs in some way facilitate the passing of the stone or gravel. How they work is not at all understood, yet they can be very effective. Anti-inflammatories are indicated to lessen the irritation caused by the passage of hard material along the delicate tissue of the whole system. Such remedies will thus lessen the pain and discomfort to some degree. Antispasmodics are essential to help reduce muscle spasms along the urinary tract as peristalsis moves the stone. Unfortunately, the antispasmodic herbs that are legally available are not strong enough to deal with the problem in acute cases.

Several plants have a long tradition of use in Europe, such as these important examples:

couch grass	nettle	pellitory
goldenrod	parsley	piert
hydrangea		

To these can be added the North American plants gravel root, stone root, and corn silk.

■ stone root
■ gravel root
■ corn silk
■ wild yam
■ black haw

Equal parts of herbs or tinctures.
As tincture: take 1 tsp (5 ml) of this mixture three times a day.
As dried herb: infuse 2 tsp to a cup and drink three times a day.

Drink 1 cup of an infusion of nettle regularly.

Profuse sweating or low fluid intake can make the urine more concentrated, causing urinary salts to solidify and stones to form. Avoid dehydration, especially after exercise but even during routine days, by drinking large amounts of fluid. Drink four to six pints of fluid a day and one pint of fluid before going to bed. Drink enough to ensure that the twenty-four-hour urine output is never less than three pints. Ideally, the patient should be drinking enough to cause routine awakening at night to urinate. Some dietary guidelines have been proposed depending upon the makeup of the stones involved.

- *Calcium oxalate stones:* Avoid foods containing oxalates such as spinach, rhubarb, beets, parsley, sorrel, and chocolate. Those who have a tendency to form oxalate stones often secrete too much calcium in their urine, which reacts with oxalic acids to form the stones. For this reason, it is also advisable to restrict intake of dairy products, which are rich in calcium. Drink mineral waters that are rich in magnesium to increase the solubility of calcium. Both vitamin B_6 and folic acid are thought to restrict the amount of calcium formed in the body.
- *Calcium phosphate stones* are usually formed when there is a urinary infection. The urine is alkaline, so eat foods to acidify the urine such as meat, fish, and eggs. Avoid dairy products.

- *Uric acid stones:* Here the urine will be acid. To "dissolve" these stones, eat an alkaline diet, including potatoes, green vegetables, and fruit (not citrus). Reduce your protein intake, since protein tends to increase uric-acid levels. In particular, avoid liver, kidneys, fish roe, and sardines. Also, drink alkalinizing mineral water.

Frequent Urination

Increased frequency of urination without an increase in the volume of urine passed is a common symptom indicating that the bladder cannot hold as much fluid as usual. A range of processes can cause this, and such causes must be identified and treated if possible. Infection, foreign bodies, stones, or tumors can all injure the tissue of the bladder wall and in turn give rise to inflammation.

Antimicrobial diuretics will help the body to rid itself of any pathogens present, thus reducing inflammation and its resulting symptoms. If there is no infection present, diuretic anti-inflammatories will soothe the inflamed tissue and so reduce the local muscle spasm. Diuretics will often help simply because they usually have one of the above effects. A number of diuretic demulcent remedies work well, though it is difficult to say whether they act by reducing inflammation by some cellular effect or primarily act as demulcents that soothe the cell surface. The best example here would be corn silk, followed by couch grass and marshmallow leaf.

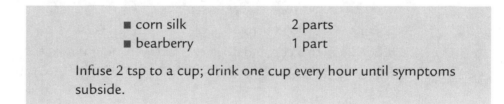

■ corn silk	2 parts
■ bearberry	1 part

Infuse 2 tsp to a cup; drink one cup every hour until symptoms subside.

A traditional approach for soothing the urinary tract is barley water, which has been used in Britain and Ireland, much as cranberry juice is used in North America. The two work in different ways but achieve similar results. Barley water may be used in all cases where frequency, pain, or other distressing urinary symptoms occur (see recipe on page 154).

> ### Barley Water
> Boil 4 oz (100 g) whole barley in a little water, then strain off the water.
>
> Pour 1 pint (500 ml) of water over the cleaned barley and add $^1/_2$ oz (15 g) of peel of a well-washed lemon (preferably organic).
>
> Simmer until the barley is soft, then remove from the heat and allow to cool until lukewarm.
>
> Strain and add a little honey; drink several cups a day.

Painful Urination

This important symptom can appear in conjunction with a wide range of conditions; hence knowledge of an approach to its relief can be very useful. However, successful alleviation will depend upon accurate diagnosis accompanied by appropriate treatment. Antimicrobials, anti-inflammatories, and diuretics will usually ease the pain because of the reduction in inflammation and combine well with antispasmodics, which reduce the muscular spasms that often accompany urinary tract problems.

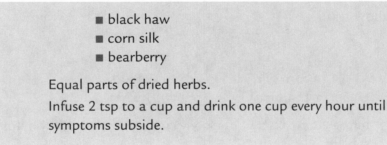

> - black haw
> - corn silk
> - bearberry
>
> Equal parts of dried herbs.
> Infuse 2 tsp to a cup and drink one cup every hour until symptoms subside.

Water Retention

Abnormal accumulation of fluid in the spaces between the cells of body tissues may be associated with liver or kidney disturbance, pregnancy, premenstrual syndrome, and heart failure. Because it is such an important diagnostic sign, water retention should *never* be treated without identifying its causal factors. Here we are faced with one of the paradoxical problems associated with the current use of herbs: too often they are used successfully to address symptoms while the more fundamental healing work that they can promote is ignored. The undoubted value of herbal diuretics in helping rid the body of excess water is a prime example. The practitioner who simply offers dandelion leaf whenever edema is part of the patient's symptom picture is probably missing an opportunity to identify and treat the specific underlying condition.

By far the most effective diuretic herb is dandelion leaf, its effects being comparable to that of the drug furosemide. Moreover, dandelion leaf has added benefits as a rich source of potassium. The usual effect of stimulating kidney function is a loss of vital potassium from the body. This will have an impact on a range of body functions, but most crucial is the electrolyte balance in the heart muscle. If the diuretic is being prescribed to treat edema associated with congestive heart failure, any reduction in potassium availability will aggravate the cardiac symptoms. With dandelion, however, we have one of the best natural sources of potassium, replacing all that is flushed from the body via diuresis. It thus makes an ideally balanced diuretic that may be used safely wherever such an action is needed, including in cases of water retention due to heart problems.

■ dandelion leaf

$1/2$ tsp of tincture three times a day or 1 tsp of tincture when needed, but not at night (it works too well!).

7 The Reproductive System

It should come as no surprise to us that nature is rich in plants that nurture or address in some way the process of conception and birth. After all, this creative process is the very keynote of life. However, the phytotherapist is faced with an unfortunate twentieth-century dilemma. Some of the primary remedies for the female reproductive system used by American medical herbalists of past centuries are now seriously endangered species, particularly false unicorn root *(Chamaelirium luteum)*, lady's slipper (*Cypripedium* spp.), and beth root (*Trillium* spp.).

One sign of the ecological holocaust that humanity has wrought on our world is that healing plants of this importance have become endangered to such a high degree. Although they are still occasionally abundant locally, their ecological range has been dramatically diminished.

The following section refers to these plants, especially *Chamaelirium,* because they offer such profound healing possibilities. However, I caution the reader against buying them unless they have been cultivated, which in the case of *Cypripedium* is extremely difficult. Collecting in this case would be an ecological crime.

For more information about endangered plants and conservation issues that relate to your geographical area, please consult local conservation groups or native plant societies. A good source for addresses of such groups is *The National Wildflower Research Center's Wildflower Handbook.*

The Female Reproductive System/Female Sexuality

As a woman ages, her body goes through many changes, menopause being the primary passage. But menopause, or the "change of life," is a normal part of life, just like puberty. Menopause is the cessation of menstruation and the termination of fertility, which are not the same thing and may occur at different times. Climacteric is defined as the transitional phase, that lasts for 15 to 20 years, during which time ovarian function and hormone production decline and the body readapts. Menopause is simply one event within this climacteric process. Although technically it is the time of the last menstrual period, symptoms can begin several years before that and can last for months or years after. This stage, called the *perimenopause,* often begins several years before the last menstrual period. It lasts for one year after that last period, the point in time known as *menopause.* A full year without a period is needed before a woman has been "through menopause." *Postmenopause* follows menopause and lasts the rest of the woman's life.

Menopause doesn't usually happen before the age of forty, but it can happen any time from the thirties to the mid-fifties or later. The average age is fifty-one. Interestingly, smoking can lead to early menopause.

Grasping the difference between menopause and climacteric is important, as it is the key to successful treament of problems that might arise as these events unfold. Neither of these two natural processes is a health problem, but rather a natural part of the process of human life. Either may be accompanied by problems, and these should be addressed, but assumptions about our humanness and the role of women are as much a problem here as the biology of the process. In our "civilized" society this time is approached with dread by many women as a time when one's role as a woman (mother, lover, wife)—and hence one's socially defined persona—inevitably becomes devalued.

From another perspective, menopausal changes can be seen as a great gift in a woman's life—an initiation into a new time, a liberation from earlier roles. This rite of passage presents the opportunity to reevaluate one's purpose in life, perhaps to change in many ways and to see change not as something to fear but as something to embrace.

Advancing age does bring inexorable changes in ovarian and menstrual function. The average length of a woman's monthly cycle gradually shortens from about twenty-eight days at the age of twenty to just over twenty-six days at the age of forty. The ovaries then begin to lose their ability to produce mature eggs, estrogen, and progesterone. Thus, there is a sharp drop in fertility among women in this age group. The regular intervals between periods that typify menstruation for most women become interspersed with increasing numbers of cycles of short and long duration. Finally, the interval between periods lengthens and menstruation ceases.

Differences between Menopause and Climacteric

Menopause	Climacteric
Counterpart of menarche	Counterpart of puberty
One biological event	A series of changes
Cessation of periods	Transition period in which ovarian function and hormone production decline
Termination of fertility	
Lasts 1 to 7 years	Lasts 15 to 20 years
Occurs between ages 48 and 52	Occurs between ages 40 and 60

Herbal Actions for the Female Reproductive System

There is much confusion in modern herbalism when remedies for the reproductive system are considered. The problem is not the herbs or the herbalists but semantics! Most books concerned with herbalism have lumped together remedies that produce a range of effects under the umbrella term *emmenagogue*. Yet the term has a very specific meaning—that of stimulating the menstrual process. To clarify matters, I have therefore grouped the remedies into the following more specific categories.

Emmenagogues

Of the many plants that can stimulate the menstrual process, some have a tonic effect on the system as well. Of the emmenagogues listed, some work through bitter stimulation, others through localized irritation or other action. The following herbs will also nourish the system to some degree:

false unicorn root	partridgeberry
mugwort	yarrow

Hormonal Normalizers

A number of plants have a direct impact upon hormonal levels in the body. Of course, there are many human hormones, and only a few affect reproductive function. Unfortunately, little endocrinological research has been undertaken on these herbs; of those with an observable influence, the herbalist tends to talk in terms of "hormonal modulators" or "normalizers." The most important such herb in European phytotherapy is *Vitex agnus castus* (chasteberry), which will tend to move the body back to normal function regardless of which female sex hormone is deficient or in excess. How this works is a matter of conjecture. The uterine tonics and bitters may have a similar effect because of some more generalized toning influence, but these are not as predictable as with chasteberry.

Nervines and Antispasmodics

By using the appropriate nervine or antispasmodic, much can be achieved in terms of correcting functional tone. Valuable remedies in this category include:

black cohosh	cramp bark	pasqueflower
black haw	motherwort	

Uterine Astringents

Various herbs reduce blood loss from the uterus, whether in excessive periods (menorrhagia), bleeding between periods (metrorrhagia), or bleeding associated with organic disease such as fibroids. An important but unanswered question is how they work, since no astringent tannin can reach the tissue from the gut. It is possible that a hormonal process is involved with some (but not all) of these plants. Of the many valuable remedies listed as astringents at the beginning of this chapter, the most toning are beth root and yarrow.

Other important uterine astringents that are not included above as "emmenagogues" are

American cranesbill	periwinkle
lady's mantle	shepherd's purse

Uterine Demulcents

Here again, it is unclear exactly how the remedies work, but there is no question that they soothe inflamed tissue. The most toning is blue cohosh.

Uterine Tonics

These plants have a toning, strengthening, nourishing effect upon both the tissue and functioning of the female reproductive system. The hows and whys are usually unknown, but this should not belittle their remarkable therapeutic value. Important examples are:

black cohosh	false unicorn root	raspberry
blue cohosh	life root	partridgeberry

Selecting Appropriate Herbal Actions

With regard to menopausal changes and the herbal actions listed above, hormonal normalizers will help endocrine control mechanisms balance activity in the face of menopausal changes. Uterine tonics will help the various organs and tissues involved to move through the changes with a minimum of trauma. Nervine relaxants are often indicated for the anxiety and tension that may accompany menopausal changes. (The nervines selected should ideally be tonics as well.) Antidepressants will be called for if the woman develops such a tendency. Bitters will help in general ways and may be taken as part of the diet.

Among European herbalists, chasteberry and St. John's wort are reputed to ease the symptomatic distress that may accompany the hormonal changes experienced by women during this time. St. John's wort can lessen depression; North American herbalists seem to use life root in a similar way. Motherwort helps to relieve the distressing palpitations that often accompany hot flashes.

A number of excellent books explore holistic approaches to menopausal problems. For a detailed examination of nutrition, supplements, and relevant exercises, see, for example, Linda Ojeda's *Menopause Without Medicine*.

Problems Specific to Women

Premenopausal Problems

UTERINE FIBROIDS

Fibroid tumors are benign muscle tumors that cause enlargement and distortion of the uterus in premenopausal women. They may make menstruation painful and heavy, possibly leading to anemia. This is the most common reason for hysterectomy, but unless the fibroids are causing significant problems, it is best to avoid such a drastic step. Fibroids rarely become malignant. As they are dependent on estrogen for their growth, they will shrink at menopause. If surgery is necessary, consider the new laser-based techniques rather than removal of the whole womb.

An herbal contribution to the treatment of fibroids is based upon uterine tonics and hormonal normalizers. Together they will help the general health and vitality of the uterus. If needed, uterine astringents will reduce blood loss. Alteratives are often found to help in health problems associated with benign growths. Antispasmodics will lessen the cramping pains, while lymphatics will support drainage of fluid from the womb.

Internal Medication for Uterine Fibroids

■ blue cohosh	2 parts
■ periwinkle	2 parts
■ chasteberry	1 part
■ black cohosh	1 part
■ wild yam	1 part
■ cleavers	1 part

As tincture: take $^1/_2$ tsp of this mixture three times a day.

As dried herb: infuse 1 tsp to a cup and drink three times a day.

Attention to general health and well-being is vital. A whole range of issues must be addressed to ensure that one can be at ease with both one's body and one's life.

- *Diet:* Eat a well balanced and nutritious diet rich in fresh green vegetables.
- *Bodywork:* Explore approaches that will engender an experience of bodily ease and relaxation. This may be aromatherapy massage, walks by the ocean, dancing, and so on.

- *Peace of mind:* Relaxation exercises, meditation, or counseling may be appropriate.
- *Lifestyle:* Reevaluation of work and home environments, relationships, and personal goals will often clarify areas of positive growth and transformation.

Menopausal Problems

Among many possible physical problems associated with menopause are the following:

- Some atrophy of vagina, cervix, uterus, and ovaries.
- The vaginal wall shortens, thins out, and loses muscle tone.
- The labia majora become thinner, paler, and less elastic.
- Supporting structures lose muscle tone (sphincter muscles, bladder, and rectum).
- Secretion of cervical mucus is reduced.
- Breast size, firmness, and shape changes.
- Body hair gets thinner in most cases; occasionally it increases.
- Wrinkling and loss of skin tone occur.
- Body fat is redistributed
- Bone mass is lost.
- Metabolic rate becomes slower.

A series of specific symptomatic problems may arise through this process, or other health problems may be compounded. The herbal therapist will want to support the menopausal changes as well as treat the particular symptom.

GENITOURINARY SYMPTOMS

During menopause and climacteric, falling hormone levels cause the vaginal tissues to shrink and atrophy, and there is a loss of support due to weakening of the pelvic tissues. Especially in women who have borne multiple children, the relaxation of the supporting tissues may be severe enough to allow the uterus to drop down into the vagina. With decreased production of natural lubricating substances, the vagina becomes dry and irritated. Itching and painful sexual intercourse may result. See page 165 for an internal remedy as well as page 166 for a soothing topical ointment.

HOT FLASHES

The most common symptoms resulting from the menopausal decline in estrogen secretion are hot flashes, flushing, feelings of warmth, and sweating. About 85 percent of all women over age fifty are affected. The onset is sudden, and when associated with palpitation, dizziness, or faintness, this can be a frightening experience. Emotional stress, exercise, alcohol, and certain foods can be triggers in some individuals. Typically, they occur several times a day and last a few minutes at a time. Chasteberry is an effective remedy for this often distressing symptom. See page 164 for a suggested remedy.

HYPERTENSION AND ATHEROSCLEROSIS

Heart disease and "hardening of the arteries" are less prevalent among premenstrual women than they are among men, although in the years after menopause, these differences between the sexes gradually disappear. Women who have their ovaries surgically removed prior to natural menopause are known to have a higher incidence of heart attack and atherosclerosis. While estrogen deficiency is believed to play a role in the development of atherosclerotic heart disease, postmenopausal estrogen replacement therapy has not yet been proven to be of benefit for this indication. See page 165 for a suggested remedy for anxiety and heart palpitations.

INSOMNIA, FATIGUE, AND DEPRESSION

Menopause is often a time of emotional upheaval. Depression, insomnia, anxiety, and questions about self-worth and sexual inadequacy may develop as attention is drawn toward physical ailments and declining health. The problem may be compounded by fears about what to expect from menopause. Other contributing factors may be marital discord and changing family relationships as one's children grow and leave home. Although some women note that their desire for sexual activity wanes after menopause, decreased estrogen secretion has no direct effect on libido. As long as vaginal symptoms are effectively treated, there is no reason why postmenopausal women should not be able to enjoy a satisfying sex life. In general, the emotional symptoms associated with menopause are caused by situational factors, not hormone deficiencies. See page 164 for a suggested remedy.

OSTEOPOROSIS

This disorder is characterized by a slow but progressive thinning and loss of the calcium content of the bones. Although the process actually begins in the fourth decade in both sexes, it is accelerated in women after menopause. Thin, white, inactive, female smokers are predisposed. With time, their bones become brittle and more susceptible to fractures from seemingly minor injuries. Even coughing, sudden movements, or everyday activities may break a bone when the disease is advanced. Wrist and hip fractures and collapse of the spinal vertebrae are especially common. The latter results in a loss of height and a forward curvature of the spine. Estrogen deficiency plays a role in postmenopausal osteoporosis by diminishing the intestinal absorption of calcium as well as increasing its loss from the bony skeleton. Other hormonal factors are also known to be important. See below for a suggested remedy.

TREATMENT OF MENOPAUSAL COMPLAINTS

As discussed, while menopause is not a disease, a series of specific symptomatic problems may arise throughout the process. In addition, other health problems may be compounded. These should be approached within the context of treating particular symptoms while supporting the menopausal changes.

In terms of tonic support, the reproductive, endocrine, nervous, and cardiovascular systems should all be taken into consideration. Of course, there is also a fundamental need for uterine tonics.

Here is a remarkably effective herbal approach to general menopausal symptoms:

A Prescription for Easing Menopause Symptoms

- chasteberry   2 parts
- St. John's wort   1 part
- life root   1 part

As tincture: take 1 tsp (5 ml) of this mixture three times a day.
As dried herb: infuse 1–2 tsp to a cup and drink three times a day.

When menopausal symptoms are accompanied by anxiety and palpitations, consider:

> ### A Prescription for Menopause Symptoms with Anxiety and Heart Palpitations
>
> | | |
> |---|---|
> | ■ chasteberry | 2 parts |
> | ■ motherwort | 2 parts |
> | ■ St. John's wort | 1 part |
> | ■ black cohosh | 1 part |
> | ■ life root | 1 part |
>
> **As tincture:** take 1 tsp (5 ml) of this mixture three times a day.
>
> **As dried herb:** infuse 1–2 tsp to a cup and drink three times a day.

Postmenopausal Problems

ATROPHIC VAGINITIS

Atrophic vaginitis is an inflammation of the vagina caused by lack or loss of estrogen. This distressing condition commonly occurs after menopause or after surgical removal of both ovaries. The lining of the vagina becomes thin, dry, and increasingly susceptible to infection. Common symptoms include itching, burning, and painful intercourse. Herbal treatment has a number of goals:

- *Reducing discomfort.* The treatment that gives the most immediate help is the use of soothing, topical applications of anti-inflammatories.
- *Addressing the hormonal imbalance.* This is not always possible, especially if the ovaries have been removed. The hormonal normalizers are not themselves sources of estrogen but either stimulate its production or contain molecular precursors that facilitate its synthesis by the body.
- *Guarding against secondary infection,* either by general support of immunity or by topical application of antimicrobial herbs. Topical use should not be the initial approach, however, as many antimicrobials can be irritating to the overly dry vaginal lining.

> ### Internal Treatment
>
> | | |
> |---|---|
> | ■ chasteberry | 2 parts |
> | ■ echinacea | 1 part |
> | ■ goldenseal | 1 part |
> | ■ wild yam | 1 part |
>
> **As tincture:** take 1 tsp (5 ml) of this mixture three times a day.

> ### Topical Soothing Emollient
>
> - 1 tbsp grated beeswax, packed
> - 2 tbsp coconut oil
> - ¹/₄ cup almond oil (or calendula oil)
>
> Melt the oils gently over very low heat, just until wax melts. Cool in refrigerator until edges begin to congeal. Meanwhile, have ready in a blender ¹/₂ cup rosewater or orange flower water, 2 tbsp aloe vera juice or gel, ¹/₄ tsp vitamin E oil, 10 drops or so essential oil (lavender, geranium, or lemon is nice; a drop or so of peppermint makes a wonderful, refreshing foot cream!).
>
>   When the oils have cooled, set blender on high and add the oils slowly in a steady stream (as if you were making mayonnaise). Scrape out all of the oil/wax mixture with a spatula. Store in a cool place.

The Male Reproductive System/Male Sexuality

If you are a middle-aged man, what can you do to maintain and enhance your sex life? Obviously, no simple answer will do. For one thing, it is not a matter for you alone, but involves your partner or partners as well. You should be reassured by the fact that recent studies of aging lovers report wide variation in the frequency and the kinds of sexual experience sought by older people. "Normal" appears to be everything from holding hands at midnight to frequent, wholehearted sexual activity.

Keep your head clear, your mind open, and your senses alive, and you'll be able to make as much love as you want for years to come. If you know about the changes that will occur, you are less likely to worry. As men age, the following changes may be noted:

- It takes longer to get an erection, and the penis may require direct stimulation before the erection occurs.
- Longer periods of stimulation are needed to reach orgasm.
- The period of "ejaculatory inevitability," or emission, becomes briefer and eventually disappears, thus reducing the two-stage aspect of a young man's orgasm to one shorter orgasmic period.
- The force and volume of the ejaculation diminishes.

- After ejaculation, the refractory period increases. A late middle-aged or older man may need from twelve to twenty-four hours before another erection is possible.

If a man is not ill and does not suffer from psychological blocks, his ability to have an erection will not be impaired by age. However, certain factors can cause a transitory loss of function. These factors are:

- *Alcohol:* As a depressant alcohol can numb the senses and cause temporary impotence.
- *Mental stress:* A man preoccupied with problems at work or problems in his relationships may lose both the desire for sex and the ability to attain an erection.
- *Physical fatigue:* Physical activity in a well-conditioned man does not interfere with sexual interest. However, unaccustomed physical activity for the out-of-condition older man can cause loss of sexual responsiveness for twenty-four to forty-eight hours.
- *Psychoactive drugs:* Recreational drugs (marijuana, LSD, cocaine, and others that are sometimes taken to heighten sexual experience) can interfere with erection in men and orgasm in both men and women.
- *Therapeutic drugs:* Medications such as tranquilizers, high-blood-pressure drugs, and antidepressants can interfere with sexual function.

A man's general vitality and continuing sexual activity in middle age seem to be the most important indicators of what his sex life will be like in later years. The man who engages in sex on a regular basis between the years of forty and sixty is most likely to have a satisfying sex life after sixty.

A number of herbs are currently being touted as aphrodisiacs or "male tonics." In fact, there are some remedies that can be effective when male sexuality problems relate to debility or exhaustion, but do little when the man is constitutionally well. These include yohimbé and damiana. Yohimbé stimulates the nerves that control erection, but care is needed to avoid inflammatory response. Because of its alkaloid content, it should not be used in conjunction with alcohol or antihistamines (or indeed with any drug). General tonics for the male reproductive system include sarsaparilla and saw palmetto.

Herbal Actions for the Male Reproductive System

As is true for the female reproductive system, certain herbs will act as tonics for the organs and functioning of the male reproductive system. Ideas about appropriate tonics vary from one herbalist to another, but all would agree on saw palmetto, sarsaparilla, and ginseng. General genitourinary tonics that have additionally valuable actions should be used as well, including mild astringents and diuretics such as yarrow, horsetail, hydrangea, couch grass, and cleavers. Urinary system antimicrobials are appropriate even when there are no obvious symptoms of infection. Examples are echinacea, bearberry, and buchu. Soothing demulcent remedies that can be used to ease symptomatic discomfort include couch grass, corn silk, and marshmallow leaf.

Internal Medication

■ saw palmetto	2 parts
■ hydrangea	2 parts
■ sarsaparilla	1 part
■ damiana	1 part
■ corn silk	1 part
■ bearberry	1 part

As tincture: take 1 tsp of this mixture three times a day.

Strong Infusion for a Sitz Bath

■ horsetail
■ couch grass
■ bearberry

Equal parts of dried herbs.
Use 2 oz of the mixture to each pint of water.

If symptoms are not markedly impairing the patient's life and if recurrent, serious, or resistant infections or kidney damage are not present, conservative therapy may be adequate for some time. This consists of:

• prompt treatment of infection
• occasional massage of the gland through a rectal exam to relieve excessive congestion

- frequent ejaculations on the patient's part for the same purpose
- avoidance of drugs that reduce bladder tone, such as antidepressants, certain tranquilizers, and antihistamines.

In addition, James Green, in *The Male Herbal,* suggests addressing the following factors:

- Relaxation of musculature in the genital region. This is best achieved through stress management and relaxation techniques but may also involve the use of relaxing nervines.
- Drink plenty of pure water and chew up to one half cup of pumpkin seeds daily.
- The following supplements are recommended:

> **vitamin E:** 800 IU daily
>
> **calcium/magnesium combination:** 400–600 mg daily
>
> **zinc picolinate:** 20–50 mg daily

Problems Specific to Men

Benign Prostate Enlargement

The prostate gland, present in all males from birth, assumes importance when fertility is achieved. It produces the fluid that accompanies the sperm during ejaculation. Located deep within the pelvis, it sits on top of the urethra, the tube connecting the penis to the bladder. As it achieves adult size, the prostate wraps itself around the urethra, into which its secretions empty. The gland is normally about the size of a chestnut, but because of its location, if it becomes inflamed or enlarged, it may exert pressure on the urethra or block the outlet to the bladder, thereby obstructing the flow of urine. This can cause interrupted or difficult urination, or urgent or frequent urination, especially at night. Urination may also be painful.

As the swelling progresses, flow through the urethra decreases, and the bladder grows thicker and stronger to compensate for the increased resistance it has to overcome. Eventually, the bladder is no longer able to overcome such forces completely and emptying becomes incomplete; urine thus stagnates in the bladder. If the obstruction becomes severe, pressure backs up to the kidneys causing damage. When the bladder is unable to empty itself of all its contents, the occasional bacteria present in the urinary tract are able to multiply, and urinary infection occurs. This, in turn, can worsen the swelling already present in the prostate.

Congestion and overgrowth of the prostate gland is virtually universal in men over the age of sixty. Why this happens is not understood, but theories suggest hormonal responses of glandular cells as androgen and other hormone levels vary with age. Many older men do not in fact experience problems as a consequence (although the others who are not so lucky take little consolation in that fact).

WARNING: A small number of enlarged or inflamed prostates may be cancerous. Any symptoms suggesting prostate trouble call for proper medical investigation.

Prostatitis

This is an inflammation or infection of the prostate gland which can lead to inflammation of the urethra and ultimately the bladder. The common symptoms of an inflamed, infected, and/or enlarged prostate gland are similar: aching pain in the area of the prostate; pain on sitting; frequent dribbling; difficult urination, both at first and in emptying the bladder; blood may appear in the urine; chills and fever are often present.

Antimicrobials that work well in the urinary system are fundamental to achieving success. Examples include bearberry and buchu. Prostate tonics should be used as in benign prostatic enlargement. Important examples are saw palmetto and hydrangea. Diuretics help the bladder and kidneys to void urine; however, they may be contraindicated where there is marked blockage due to prostate swelling. Demulcents that soothe the urinary system help alleviate symptoms.

Prostatitis Remedy

- bearberry
- couch grass
- buchu
- echinacea
- saw palmetto
- corn silk

Equal parts of tinctures.
Take 1 tsp (5 ml) of this mixture three times a day.

Diuretic

- corn silk
- yarrow

Equal parts of dried herbs.

Infuse 1 tsp of this mixture to a cup and drink throughout the day.

The same factors mentioned by James Green in relation to prostate enlargement (see page 169) should be addressed here.

8 The Musculoskeletal System

Once we are open to the premise that most of the biological needs of humanity and the other animals are met by our evolutionary environment, the wealth of anti-inflammatory herbs provided by the plant kingdom will come as no surprise. Although such herbs are rarely as powerful as steroid drugs, it can also be said that they are very rarely as dangerous. The steroidal anti-inflammatory drugs were developed themselves from plant material and are still largely synthesized from saponins such as diosgenin, from the Mexican yam.

Inflammation occurs in response to various traumas ranging from sunburn and wounds to infection and autoimmune conditions. Whatever the cause, the process is basically characterized by four physical signs; warmth, redness, swelling, and pain. Warmth and redness result from dilation of the small blood vessels in the injured area and increased local blood flow. Because blood vessels become more permeable during inflammation, a protein-rich exudate escapes from blood plasma to the damaged tissue and causes swelling. Pain is believed to result from such chemical substances as serotonin or from tension of tissue over the inflamed area. Thus inflammation in autoimmune conditions such as rheumatoid arthritis is fundamentally the same as that of simple infections; what triggers the reaction is, however, very different.

The biochemistry and pathology of this complex process might suggest that chemistry is the medical answer. Yet herbalists around the world know of many plants with inflammation inhibiting properties. These plants as whole medicines can reduce and soothe inflammation whether we know their biochemistry or not.

Whether it be bogbean, nettle, or the Kalahari Desert herb known as "devil's claw"—they work.

Herbal Actions

Herbal "Antirheumatics"

Various herbal actions will prove helpful in cases of musculoskeletal illness. Often, however, the specific insights that such remedies can provide are clouded over because they are lumped together under the general heading "antirheumatic." The fact that these remedies have been observed to relieve many patients' experience of rheumatic problems is not to say that they have a specific effect upon the disease or even necessarily upon musculoskeletal tissue itself. The term refers to outcome rather than process, and as such is very limited in its applicability. The following are the main examples familiar to Western herbalists:

angelica	dandelion	parsley
arnica	devil's claw	poke
bayberry	feverfew	prickly ash
bearberry	ginger	rosemary
birch	gravel root	sarsaparilla
black cohosh	guaiac	white poplar
blue cohosh	horseradish	wild yam
blue flag	juniper	willow bark
bogbean	kelp	wintergreen
boneset	meadowsweet	wormwood
burdock	mugwort	yarrow
cayenne	mustard	yellow dock
celery seed	nettle	
cramp bark	Oregon grape	

To help choose the most appropriate remedy in any individual case, the herbs listed above can be subdivided as follows:

- *Antirheumatic/alterative:* Herbs that gradually restore proper functioning of the body, increasing health and vitality. Some alteratives support natural waste elimination via the kidneys, liver, lungs, or skin; others stimulate digestive function, are antimicrobial, or work in some other way. Blue flag, feverfew, kelp, guaiac, celery seed, blue flag, bogbean, poke, yellow dock, sarsaparilla, and nettle.

- *Antirheumatic/anti-inflammatory:* These soothe inflammation or reduce inflamed tissue. Angelica, celery seed, birch, wild yam, meadowsweet, wintergreen, guaiac, devil's claw, bogbean, white poplar, willow, and feverfew. (For a detailed discussion of some of these important herbs, see below.)
- *Antirheumatic/antispasmodic:* The antispasmodics alleviate muscular tension, either generally throughout the body or in specific systems or organs, and (as many are also nervines) may ease psychological tension as well. Black cohosh and cramp bark.
- *Antirheumatic/circulatory stimulant:* Horseradish, mustard, cayenne, bayberry, rosemary, prickly ash, and ginger.
- *Antirheumatic/diuretic:* These herbs may actually increase the production and elimination of urine or may simply have a beneficial action on the urinary system, helping the body to eliminate waste and support the whole process of inner cleansing. Celery seed, yarrow, bearberry, boneset, gravel root, juniper, parsley, and dandelion.
- *Antirheumatic/other action (or basis unclear):* Arnica, wormwood, mugwort, and blue cohosh.

Herbal Anti-inflammatories

Orthodox medicine places much emphasis on chemicals that work to reduce the symptoms of inflammation and ease suffering in many diseases. This symptomatic alleviation is not the ideal way to use herbal anti-inflammatories, and although they are certainly safe to use for the relief of pain and discomfort, they are best used in combination with other remedies to address the underlying problem.

They reduce inflammation in a number of different ways but rarely inhibit the natural reaction. Rather they support and encourage the work the body is doing. It is important to know that inflammation is a normal bodily response to infection or other problems; through local biochemical and tissue changes, the inflammatory reaction will often bring about the changes necessary to heal the area of disease and restore health. It is a mistake to inhibit this response (except, of course, in life-threatening situations). For example, simply suppressing symptoms of inflammation in the stomach to relieve the discomfort will not change underlying causes possibly leading to the development of a stomach ulcer. We have become conditioned into seeing inflammation as always something to suppress rather than to work with. As in all health matters, balance is called for.

Herbal anti-inflammatories fall into five groups according to the way they are thought to work. (It cannot be overemphasized, however, that the action of any plant is always more than the action of any specific constituent chemical.)

- *Oil-containing:* Many of the aromatic herbs with their wonderful essential oils have an anti-inflammatory action. Two of the best of these remedies are balm and chamomile. Calendula and St. John's wort also contain oils that soothe and reduce inflammation.

- *Resin-containing:* Some resin-containing plants reduce inflammation but will often cause inflammation in the stomach. This obviously limits their use, but they are irreplaceable in the treatment of arthritic conditions. Examples are bogbean, devil's claw, and guaiac.

- *Salicin-containing:* Many plants contain natural aspirin-type chemicals called salicylates. It is worth noting that all the aspirin drugs were originally isolated from plant sources; indeed, the name aspirin comes from the old botanical name for meadowsweet, *Spiraea,* and salicylate derives from the Latin name for willow, *Salix.* In significant quantities these herbs have a marked effect without the adverse side effects of aspirin itself. In fact, meadowsweet (which is especially rich in salicylates) can be used to staunch mild stomach hemorrhage—a condition that synthetic salicylates actually cause! Other plants rich in these constituents include willow bark, wintergreen, birch, many of the poplars, and black haw.

- *Saponin-containing:* The steroids themselves were first isolated from plant material, and some herbs contain saponins, safe compounds that are metabolized by the body into its own inflammation-fighting steroidal molecules. Such plants will aid in reducing certain kinds of inflammation. Examples are licorice and wild yam.

- *Other types of anti-inflammatories:* Various valuable anti-inflammatories have no clear-cut chemical basis for their action (serving as another reminder that there is more to health and well-being than pharmaceutical chemistry!). Of the many remedies in this group, we can mention black cohosh.

For each system of the body, plants that are particularly suited to that system will also work as anti-inflammatory remedies. This natural correspondence allows the herbalist to nurture the health of a particular system that is suffering while reducing any inflammation present.

- In the *circulatory system,* a number of herbs may be used to reduce inflammations in blood vessels, including linden, hawthorn berries, horse chestnut, and yarrow.
- As the remedies go directly to the *digestive system,* they can be of use especially in conditions ranging from stomach ulcers to colitis and hemorrhoids. Such herbs include chamomile, wild yam, licorice, goldenseal, calendula, and peppermint. The demulcent remedies (e.g., marshmallow) can soothe and reduce inflammation through local contact.
- A number of herbs soothe the tissue of the *urinary system* directly as their anti-inflammatory constituents pass through the kidneys and bladder. Plants that soothe the tissue and reduce infection will also have an anti-inflammatory action. Specific urinary anti-inflammatories are goldenrod and corn silk.
- For the *reproductive system,* many tonics and other specific reproductive remedies often act to reduce inflammation. Lady's mantle and blue cohosh are two examples.
- For hardworking and abused *muscles and bones,* the salicylate-containing remedies come into their own. Willow bark, meadowsweet, white poplar, and birch are excellent. Others to consider are bogbean, devil's claw, black cohosh, feverfew, and wild yams.
- Although the *nervous system* may seem to "need" anti-inflammatories, the best remedies for an inflamed state of mind are the herbal relaxing nervines. The only true anti-inflammatory for nervous tissue is St. John's wort, which helps in the recovery of damaged nerves. However, nervines such as oats and valerian are very useful here.
- Many remedies act to reduce inflammation on the *skin*. These gifts of the natural world include marigold, St. John's wort, myrrh, goldenseal, arnica, chickweed, and plantain.

Additional Herbal Remedies

There are a range of remedies appropriate for musculoskeletal problems, each having its distinct area of application. Consider first the following herbs:

angelica	celery seed	willow bark
birch	devil's claw	wild yam
black cohosh	meadowsweet	
bogbean	nettle	

Stronger remedies may be found useful in more intransigent conditions, but these should be reserved for cases where the gentler herbs have not produced the results desired. Again, the herbalist has the gift of toning herbs for use in these problems.

The emphasis on toning throughout the book is especially applicable to muscle and joint problems. There is often no need to resort to intense treatment, as the milder antirheumatics are often effective, given time. This is not to say that such treatment will completely clear osteoarthritis in someone who has had it for years, and whose body has sustained structural damage; but he or she will assuredly feel better and will be in the best situation possible.

External Applications

External applications of various kinds can often help to relieve the discomfort caused by musculoskeletal problems. The following brief list, drawing on numerous sources, is organized by primary herbal component.

BLACK MUSTARD *(BRASSICA NIGRA)*

Mustard seeds are used externally to ease acute local pain, sciatica, and gout. A poultice may be prepared by mixing the powdered seeds with warm water to form a paste. Spread onto brown paper and apply to affected area. In cases of rheumatic pain, mustard oil, a powerful local irritant, may be incorporated into liniments and applied.

CAYENNE (*CAPSICUM* SPP.)

A stimulating application for arthritis and rheumatism can be found on the next page.

- cayenne pepper   1 part
- mullein leaf   }
- slippery elm powder   } equal parts
- apple cider vinegar to
  dampen the mixture

Make a poultice. If the application of cayenne gives too much of a burning sensation, apply vegetable oil to coat the surface of the skin.

Equal parts of cayenne and glycerin can be shaken together and applied to painful joints. Cayenne powder or tincture can also be rubbed on swellings and inflammations for added relief.

CHICKWEED *(STELLARIA MEDIA)*

Chickweed may be applied in the form of a poultice, fomentation, or ointment to give relief in certain cases of rheumatism and for many types of skin problems.

The following poultices may be effective for stiffness:

- chickweed   1 oz
- cabbage leaves   1 tsp
- thyme leaves and flowers 1 tsp
- cayenne pepper   1 tsp

Blend above ingredients with 1 oz powdered slippery elm and 1 tbsp fenugreek; moisten with hot cider vinegar until mixture has the desired consistency. Spread on a cloth and apply warm. Cover poultice with plastic to retain warmth.

- 1 lb freshly cut chickweed
- 1 1/2 lbs vegetable shortening
- 2 oz beeswax

Place ingredients in a stainless steel pot; cover and bake in oven for 3 hours at 200°F. Strain; when cold, it is ready for use. Apply as needed.

LAVENDER *(LAVANDULA OFFICINALIS)*

A small amount of essential oil of lavender added to bland oils makes a useful anti-inflammatory in the treatment of rheumatic conditions.

LOBELIA *(LOBELIA INFLATA)*

For cramps, relief of rheumatism, or inflammation, the following antispasmodic tincture has been recommended:

- 1 oz lobelia, mixed crushed seed and powdered leaves
- 1 oz skunk cabbage
- 1 oz skullcap
- 1 oz gum myrrh
- 1 oz valerian
- $^{1}/_{2}$ oz cayenne

Infuse dried herbs for one week in a closely corked quart of brandy. Use a wide-necked bottle and shake well daily. After one week, strain and press out the clear liquid. Rub on affected areas.

MULLEIN *(VERBASCUM THAPSUS)*

Mullein combines well with black cohosh and lobelia in liniments. For swollen joints and to relieve the aches and pains of arthritis and rheumatism, rub mullein oil in well or apply on saturated cotton and cover. It may be prepared with two ounces each of mullein flower and olive oil. However, do not use on any swellings where it would be injurious to have a deposit absorbed. To treat painful and swollen joints, cover a small quantity of mullein with boiling vinegar, cover, simmer slowly for twenty to thirty minutes, strain, and add a little tincture of cayenne and lobelia.

For arthritis, stiff joints, and rheumatism, the following is helpful:

- 2 oz mullein
- $^{1}/_{2}$ oz lobelia leaves
- 1 tsp cayenne
- 2 qts apple cider vinegar

Simmer for 15 minutes, strain, and foment as warm as is convenient over the affected parts.

MYRRH *(COMMIPHORA MOL-MOL)*

A liniment has been recommended in treating rheumatism.

> - 1 part myrrh, tincture
> - $1/4$ part cayenne, tincture
> - 2 parts echinacea, tincture
>
> Mix thoroughly; 10–15 drops in plenty of water applied externally.

SASSAFRAS *(SASSAFRAS ALBIDUM)*

A traditional liniment for rheumatic problems can be made thus:

> - 1 oz sassafras, tincture
> - 1 oz prickly ash, tincture
> - 1 oz cayenne, tincture
> - 1 oz myrrh, tincture
> - 1 oz camphor, tincture
> - 8 oz distilled water
>
> Shake the ingredients together well and apply to the affected parts.

WHITE MUSTARD *(BRASSICA ALBA)*

Poultices made with mustard flowers, bread crumbs, and vinegar are used in treating rheumatic and sciatic pains. In making such applications, the white seeds may be mixed with the black and although this may redden the skin, it is very stimulating and efficient.

Placing the feet in a bowl of hot water with mustard seed or powder will greatly alleviate rheumatic pain and may even prevent impending rheumatic conditions if this remedy is employed as soon as possible after symptoms are first noticed.

The remedy on the next page is an example of a poultice combination mentioned in many sources.

> ### Fleshbone Poultice
>
> - 3 g powdered plantain
> - 3 g powdered comfrey
> - 1 g powdered marshmallow root
> - 1 g powdered lobelia
> - $\frac{1}{8}$ g powdered cayenne
>
> Relieves painful, swollen joints. The poultice may be applied throughout the day and night.

Nonsteroidal Anti-inflammatory Drugs

More than thirteen million people take nonsteroidal anti-inflammatory drugs (NSAIDs) to alleviate the pain or reduce the inflammation caused by arthritis, sore muscles, tendonitis, headache, or menstrual discomfort. Because arthritic conditions become more common with age, most long-term NSAID users are older people. They are also the people most sensitive to drugs and most predisposed to illness caused by medical treatments. Most of these drugs are prescription items, but in 1984 ibuprofen was licensed for sale over the counter and subsequently became one of the most used medications in the United States.

However, NSAIDs do pose risks, especially to older people, or those with impaired kidney function or vulnerable stomach linings. Researchers have reported that hospitalization for gastrointestinal problems is six times greater for older patients taking NSAIDs to treat rheumatoid arthritis than for similar patients not using these drugs. It is estimated that gastric bleeding from NSAIDs is the most frequent and severe drug side effect in the United States, causing twenty thousand hospitalizations and twenty-six hundred deaths each year in patients with rheumatoid arthritis alone. The number of yearly fatalities associated with long-term NSAIDs use in the United States is said to be between ten and twenty thousand.

NSAIDs relieve pain, lessen inflammation, and lower fevers by inhibiting the synthesis of prostaglandins in the body. Although prostaglandins are not the cause of inflammation, they are a crucial part of the process. Prostaglandins are small molecules that diffuse short distances from one group of cells to another. NSAIDs limit the body's ability to produce not only the inflammatory prostaglandins but also other types. In the kidney, prostaglandins play a vital role in maintaining the flow of blood and regulation of blood pressure; in the stomach they help to protect the lining from the acid of digestive fluid. Their inhibition leads to the following primary side effects:

- *Kidney function.* In disease or dehydration, the body restricts the amount of blood circulated in peripheral tissues, but the kidneys must maintain their circulation so as to continue clearing the blood of wastes. They can partially override a general reduction in blood flow by secreting prostaglandins, which in turn dilate the internal vessels of the kidneys. After the fourth decade of life, renal blood flow declines approximately 10 percent per decade and so an older person has a greater potential for kidney harm from drugs that decrease this blood flow further. Here, diuretic remedies will promote urine production, while circulation stimulants and tonics will ensure adequate blood flow through the kidneys.
- *Stomach irritation.* Like aspirin, NSAIDs in high doses damage the lining of the stomach, typically producing multiple, small, superficial patches of erosion, but large ulcers can also result. The cause of this damage is the reduction of prostaglandin secretion by cells in the stomach lining that stimulate production of mucus to cover the surface exposed to digestive fluid; these cells also promote secretion of bicarbonate, which neutralizes acid, into the mucus. Prostaglandins also speed the rate at which cells of the stomach lining repair damage. They are thus a crucial link in the stomach's defense against self-digestion. (Incidentally, these functions directly point to the relevance of demulcent remedies, which mimic the coating properties of the stomach's mucus and thereby reduce inflammation.)

All these facts highlight the relevance of using herbal alternatives to the "safe" anti-inflammatory medicines. At times NSAIDs may be needed, when herbs are not effective enough, but they should not be the first line of defense.

Musculoskeletal Problems

Rheumatism

This vague and misused term refers generally to aches and pains in the musculature of the body. As such symptoms are characteristic of the early stage of many infections and a range of autoimmune conditions, careful diagnosis may be called for. A safe guideline is that if symptoms cannot be eased to some degree within two weeks, consider the problem more deeply. Efficacious herbal therapy must take into account the underlying issues and not simply attempt to stop the discomfort. For example:

- If it is the result of long-standing sports injuries, then connective tissue must be strengthened, while antispasmodics are given to ease the musculature.
- If there is a history of digestive problems, the use of appropriate digestive tonics is indicated.
- Cardiovascular tonics should be used if hypertension or even overt heart disease is present. Creating a balance between herbs for active treatment of rheumatism and those for cardiovascular treatment calls for professional skill.
- Long-term stress may lead to tight muscles and, in turn, tightly-held joints. Over the years, this can develop into "wear and tear" arthritis, but even short-term tension can cause pain and stiffness.

The antirheumatics all help here, but they should be selected based upon their fundamental properties (usually anti-inflammatory, alterative, or antispasmodic). Diuretics can be surprisingly effective in easing vague rheumatic aches and pains. Circulatory stimulants help through increasing local circulation in muscles and associated tissue and are usually best used in the form of liniments. Rubefacient herbs generate a localized increase in blood flow when applied to the skin. Stimulating circulatory activity, they promote removal of tissue waste and the local supply of oxygen and nutrients. Pain-relieving analgesics are of limited symptomatic use. (This is discussed in more depth below.)

The salicylate-containing anti-inflammatories are the core of treatment among the various folk traditions of the world. Especially important are meadowsweet, wintergreen, white poplar, and willow. In addition we can add angelica, celery seed, and in fact all the antirheumatics mentioned above! Some kind of external applications will often help; these may be rubefacient, circulatory stimulants, salicin-containing oils, or even antispasmodics, depending upon the individual's response. An example of a commonly used European approach follows.

Internal Remedy for Rheumatism

- willow   2 parts
- angelica   1 part
- nettle   1 part

As tincture: take 1 tsp (5 ml) of this mixture three times a day.

As dried herb: infuse 2 tsp to a cup and drink three times a day.

Muscle-relaxing Antispasmodic Rub

- lobelia
- cramp bark

Equal parts of tinctures.

Rub mixture into the painful muscles as needed.

The internal treatment provides a basic range of antirheumatics that give salicylate anti-inflammatory action along with support for the digestive process as well as a more generalized alterative. External treatments are so numerous that it is as much a matter of cultural preference as that of therapeutic judgment.

Dietary factors must be considered. A careful review of one's lifestyle will help clarify issues of posture, work conditions, stress, and so on. Chiropractic, osteopathy, aromatherapy, massage, and attention to appropriate exercise may prove useful.

Arthritis

Among the most common inflammatory conditions to affect humanity are the varieties of arthritis, and throughout the world herbal medicine is used in its treatment. *Arthritis* is a general term for over one hundred known diseases that produce either inflammation of connective tissues, particularly in joints, or noninflammatory degeneration of these tissues. The word *arthritis* literally means "joint inflammation," but because other structures are also affected, these disorders are also called *connective tissue diseases*. The causes of these disorders range through immune-system reactions to the normal wear and tear of aging.

Herbal medicine works with the body's natural processes in promoting amelioration of the specific condition while alleviating pain and discomfort. Anti-inflammatory and antirheumatic remedies alone will not suffice here, however: therapy must focus on liver function, circulation, and elimination as well as the patient's quality of life. Such technical therapeutic considerations go beyond the range of this book, but there is much that can be done simply and safely.

OSTEOARTHRITIS

Osteoarthritis (degenerative joint disease) is the most common form of arthritis, affecting about one in six Americans, including 80 percent of all people over seventy. Most have few associated symptoms, and the disease is diagnosed only because X-rays of the spine show characteristic spurs or because some joints in the fingers become knobbed by bony proliferations. In some, the bony spurs pinch nerves as they emerge from the spinal canal. In others, the changed joints are a source of ligament strain and muscular tension. The result is pain that becomes worse as the day goes on. These degenerative processes are in part caused by wear and tear and affect weight-bearing joints, joints subject to trauma or to malpositioned anatomy. Joints damaged by other forms of arthritis are prone to later degenerative joint disease. Physical trauma produces microscopic fractures in the cartilage that lines the moving surfaces of joints, thus exposing underlying bone. The bone cells then release enzymes that destroy the protein and polysaccharide components of bone.

A number of predisposing factors can hasten this degenerative process, even in young people. If they are recognized as present in an individual's life, preventive measures can be undertaken. These factors include:

- obesity (which puts more physical stress on weight-bearing joints)
- bone deformities (which generate abnormal mechanical forces affecting the joint)
- previous cartilage injury
- joint infection
- certain types of inflammatory arthritis, especially rheumatoid arthritis and gout
- diabetes mellitus
- acromegaly (a condition caused by excess growth hormone)
- repetitive occupational or exercise-related joint movements (which induce unusual physical strain on the joints concerned)

Osteoarthritis, or OA, is usually experienced as aching joints and stiffness. The pain is aggravated by movement and by weight-bearing. Although swelling may occur, warmth and redness usually imply an actively inflammatory type of arthritis. The hips, knees, ankles, neck, lower back, and hands are the most common joints affected. Hip pain can be especially severe, making walking difficult. The fingers often develop a knobby and gnarled appearance. Osteoarthritis of the spine is a common cause of chronic pain and decreased neck and back mobility. In some cases, large bone spurs may compress the spinal cord or "pinch" its nerves. Osteoarthritis differs from rheumatoid arthritis (RA) in several ways:

- The duration of stiffness described for OA is shorter than RA—usually minutes as opposed to hours.
- Pain in OA is associated with activity, whereas pain in RA often exists at rest.
- Although both conditions commonly have joint swelling, those with redness and warmth are typically associated with RA.
- OA does not usually occur in symmetrically opposite joints.

How can the herbalist proceed in cases of osteoarthritis? Antirheumatics will usually help, hence their name, but their selection must be based upon a sound therapeutic rationale, based upon various important considerations.

- *Alteratives* are the key to approaching any underlying systemic problem that may be present. If the OA has its roots in physical wear and tear, they will not be quite so relevant. Of the many possible herbs here consider bogbean, devil's claw, nettle, and sarsaparilla.
- *Analgesics* will ease discomfort but must not replace appropriate treatment.
- *Anti-inflammatories* are fundamental. Their use will not only ease the symptom picture but will help arrest degenerative changes to bony tissue. In OA, the salicylate-containing herbs such as meadowsweet and willow bark are especially helpful.
- *Antispasmodics* such as black cohosh and cramp bark lessen the impact of friction on the joints.

- *Circulatory stimulants* will further the healing process through an increase in the flow of blood through the tissue involved. Prickly ash is often used.
- *Hypnotics* will promote sleep in the face of pain. The healing power of restfull sleep cannot be overemphasized! Consider valerian, Jamaican dogwood, and passionflower.
- *Nervines* are usually relevant because of the many ways in which a person under stress can benefit from such support. Nervine relaxants also act as antispasmodics, while nervine tonics will help the person deal with the constant stress of the pain and discomfort. Important herbs here are black cohosh, valerian, celery seed, and skullcap.
- *Rubefacients* can help in the form of liniments; they provide local stimulation of circulation.

The herbalist should also ensure that the whole *digestive process* is working well and is not damaged by reactions to nonsteroidal anti-inflammatories. Bogbean can be considered here. The main drawback is that its use has been almost forgotten in North America, so that it is now difficult to find. Nettle is a traditional remedy throughout Europe, used internally and externally as a rubefacient. This external use, with fresh raw leaf, is not a treatment for the fainthearted!

■ bogbean	2 parts
■ meadowsweet	2 parts
■ black cohosh	1 part
■ prickly ash	1 part
■ celery seed	1 part
■ angelica	1 part
■ yarrow	1 part

As tincture: take 1 tsp (5 ml) of this mixture three times a day.

Nutritional factors are very important in the successful treatment of OA. There are many ideas about which foods or supplements to use for any condition, but the simplest approach is to let the person with OA identify and avoid any foods that clearly aggravate arthritic problems. Such diets produce best results in the earlier, more painful stages of this disease. In the extreme of long-standing OA, a balance must be struck between nutritional dogma and one's daily eating habits. For optimal benefit, the diet should exclude the following:

- artificial additives, flavorings, and preservatives
- berries rich in fruit acids (gooseberries, red and black currants)
- carbonated drinks
- coffee (regular or decaffeinated)
- food or beverages known to trouble the individual patient
- processed foods
- red meat of any kind in any form (pork is a red meat, regardless of what the advertisers would have us believe!)
- red wine, port, and sherry
- refined white flour and its products
- refined white sugar and its products
- shellfish
- vegetables that contain high levels of plant acids (e.g., tomatoes, rhubarb)
- vinegar and anything cured in vinegar (e.g., pickles); apple cider vinegar *may* be an exception

Attention must be given to physical aids for the patient who is becoming disabled by this disease. A wealth of simple devices are available to ease the simple daily tasks of life, from specially designed kitchen cutlery, can openers, and faucet grips, to brushes with extended handles and adaptations to telephones. These ADL (Activities of Daily Living) devices belong to the realm of occupational therapists and other specialists. More information can be obtained through the publications of the Arthritis Foundation (see page 318) and your local official agencies on aging.

RHEUMATOID ARTHRITIS

Rheumatoid arthritis (RA) is a chronic inflammatory condition that involves not only the joints but other connective tissue as well. Three times as many women as men are affected. Some individuals are more susceptible than others, and a familial pattern is commonly observed, suggesting a genetic association.

A disorder of the body's immune system is suspected to be the culprit. One important laboratory finding is the presence of rheumatoid factor, a special antibody that reacts against the normal antibodies present in the bloodstream. Why it develops is unknown, but current theories point toward an exaggerated immune response to long-term stimulation by infectious agents or "foreign substances." Rheumatoid factor itself is not directly responsible for the inflammatory process but acts as a marker for the disease.

The joint destruction that occurs with severe RA results from inflammation of the synovia, the thin, smooth membrane or capsule lining the joints. As part of the immune response to the unknown stimulus, white blood cells and antibodies infiltrate the synovial membranes, causing them to proliferate and fold over on themselves.

Persistent or recurrent inflammation eventually causes permanent damage to the joint cartilage, bones, ligaments, and tendons. The widespread inflammatory process also involves other tissue such as blood vessels, skin, nerves, muscles, heart, and lungs. The result is painful joints, loss of mobility, and generalized soreness and depression. The various signs and symptoms of RA are as follows:

- Joint pain, aching, and stiffness come on gradually.
- This is followed in a few weeks by joint swelling, redness, and warmth.
- The hands, wrists, shoulders, elbows, feet, ankles, and knees are usually involved on both sides of the body, but inflammation of a single joint may be the initial presentation.
- Symptoms tend to be worst in the morning, diminishing with activities of the day.
- Small firm lumps beneath the skin (rheumatoid nodules) appear in some patients, especially around the elbow.
- There is often distressing fatigue in the early afternoon, and difficulty in sleeping.
- RA can affect other organs. Vasculitis (inflammation of the blood vessels) may cause skin rashes, ulcers, or gangrene. Other manifestations include scarring of the lungs, inflammation of the membranes surrounding the heart and lungs (pericarditis, pleurisy), nerve damage, dry eyes and mouth (Sjögrens syndrome), and enlargement of the spleen and lymph nodes.

In about 5 to 10 percent of people with RA, the disease is mild or limited to one or two episodes. Another 25 percent will have an erratic pattern of prolonged remissions and periods of relapse. In the majority, however, the clinical course is progressive with intermittent flare-ups. Most sufferers continue to function well in the world despite some pain and discomfort, but about 10 percent of RA patients progress to severe permanent joint deformities, limitation of movement, and disability.

Herbal therapy offers much in the treatment of this distressing problem but cannot provide a miracle cure. Treatment takes time and may well be undertaken in conjunction with orthodox therapy. The considerations to be taken into account are similar to those described for OA, with certain exceptions and additions.

- *Alteratives* have a beneficial impact on immune system functioning (see page 217). They are the safest way to address the underlying systemic problem, as more active immunostimulating plants may aggravate the condition. Consider bogbean, devil's claw, nettle, and sarsaparilla.
- *Anti-inflammatories* are very important, as much of the symptom picture is the direct result of the inflammatory process. The saponin-containing anti-inflammatories come into their own, but the salicylate herbs are helpful as well. Consider wild yam, meadowsweet, and willow bark.
- *Antispasmodics* such as black cohosh and cramp bark will ease associated muscular tension.
- *Circulatory stimulants* are not as important for RA as for OA but should still be considered. This difference reflects the role of the blood in both conditions. Prickly ash is often used.
- *Nervines* are especially relevant, considering the acknowledged "psychosomatic" nature of this problem.
- *Rubefacients* rarely help.

There are no specific herbal remedies for rheumatoid arthritis (which is entirely understandable when the multifactorial nature of this type of immunological condition is taken into account). Of special relevance are the alterative-based anti-rheumatics. This includes bogbean, celery seed, sarsaparilla, and blue flag. Guaiac and wild yam are especially useful as anti-inflammatories. Feverfew can be very helpful in some cases. Remedies using combinations of these herbs can be found on the following page.

Anti-inflammatory for Rheumatoid Arthritis

- bogbean   2 parts
- meadowsweet   1^1/$_2$ parts
- wild yam   1^1/$_2$ parts
- guaiac   1 part
- valerian   1 part
- black cohosh   1 part
- celery seed   1 part
- angelica   1 part
- St. John's wort 1 part

As tincture: take 1 tsp (5 ml) of this mixture three times a day.

For Sleep and Pain Relief

- valerian
- Jamaican dogwood
- passionflower

Equal parts of tinctures.

Take 1–3 tsp (5–15 ml) half an hour before retiring.

The digestive system must be working well, so treat any stomach irritation as a priority. This combination does not take such problems into account. As with OA, if there is any stomach tenderness due to the harshness of the bogbean or guaiac, add marshmallow. The general suggestions given above for the broader context of treatment in OA are equally pertinent here; it may be worthwhile to consider some variety of counseling, or at least a stress management program.

Bursitis and Tendinitis

A bursa is a pocket of connective tissue adjacent to a joint. Lined by a smooth inner surface, it facilitates the gliding movements of muscles and tendons over bony prominences. Bursitis, or inflammation of a bursa, causes pain, tenderness, stiffness, and in some cases swelling and redness. Any bursa can be affected, but involvement of the shoulder, elbow, hip, and knee are most common.

Although the cause of this condition is unknown, one predisposing factor may be repetitive direct pressure on a bursa. In particular, certain activities or occupations are associated with specific forms of bursitis because of the nature of the physical stress placed on the bursa: examples are housemaid's knee (kneeling) and student's elbow (leaning). Shoulder bursitis, the most common type, is characterized by an aching pain localized on the outside of the top of the shoulder. Pain is intensified by lifting and back-rotating the arm. Typically there is morning stiffness, which diminishes with the application of heat or through carrying on with routine activities.

Tendinitis occurs either spontaneously or in association with an injury, work and sports activities, certain types of arthritis, or infection. As with bursitis, the shoulder is most commonly affected. The attachment of the biceps tendon at the shoulder is especially susceptible. Bicipital tendinitis manifests as an ache along the biceps muscle that radiates up to the shoulder and down to the forearm. Pain is worse with movement. Other common locations for tendinitis are the elbow, wrist, hand, knee, and ankle.

Herbs can be effective in treating these conditions if selected appropriately. Anti-inflammatory, antirheumatic herbs provide symptomatic relief. Antispasmodics help in easing associated local muscular tension. Circulatory stimulants contribute by increasing local blood circulation. Analgesics may help. However, pain relief is best achieved through the use of anti-inflammatories and antispasmodics.

- *Antispasmodic:* lobelia, cramp bark, and celery seed
- *Circulatory stimulant:* prickly ash
- *General anti-inflammatory:* celery seed
- *Salicylate anti-inflammatory:* willow bark and meadowsweet

Internal Remedy for Bursitis and Tendinitis

■ willow bark	2 parts
■ cramp bark	2 parts
■ celery seed	2 parts
■ prickly ash	1 part

As tincture: take 1 tsp (5 ml) of this mixture three times a day.

As dried herb: infuse 2 tsp to one cup water and drink three times a day.

Antispasmodic Rub

- ■ lobelia
- ■ cramp bark

Equal parts of tinctures.
Rub into the painful muscles as needed.

Gout

The inflammatory process in gout is caused by deposition in the joints of uric acid. In acute gouty arthritis, needlelike crystals of the deposited uric acid are ingested by white blood cells, which in turn release enzymes that evoke inflammation. In extreme cases the gouty process results in tophi, or large deposits of uric acid, around the joints.

Classically, gout occurs acutely as intermittent attacks of joint pain swelling, redness, and warmth. However, in some individuals, it is a progressive, crippling chronic disease that also damages the kidneys. Gout is twenty times more common in men than women. Obesity, high blood pressure, and atherosclerotic heart disease are often associated. A familial pattern is observed in 5 to 15 percent of cases.

To understand gout it is necessary to have a grasp of the chemistry of uric acid. This naturally occurring substance is a product of the chemical breakdown of the purine bases that compose the genetic material DNA. As cells die and release DNA from their chromosomes, purines are converted into uric acid, which is then excreted in the urine and (to a lesser extent) the intestinal tract.

The level of uric acid dissolved in the bloodstream is directly related to this delicate balance between uric acid production and the body's ability to excrete it through urine. High blood concentrations of uric acid are commonly due to an underexcretion of uric acid by the kidneys. However, although sudden swelling and pain in a joint (especially the big toe) suggests a diagnosis of gout, many other arthritic conditions and some infections present themselves in a similar manner.

Diuretics play the pivotal role in any therapy that attempts to go beyond symptomatic relief, as they can help flush urates from the body. Antirheumatics will help to some degree, but only those herbs that have marked diuretic properties. The antilithic and diuretic remedies are often considered. Colchicine, from the autumn crocus, is a specific allopathic drug. However, it is very unsafe to use the whole plant due to its inherent toxicity. An example of a safe, gentle, and effective combination of herbs to soothe the symptoms of gout can be found in the remedy on the next page.

■ gravel root	2 parts
■ couch grass	2 parts
■ celery seed	2 parts
■ guaiac	1 part

As tincture: take 1 tsp (5 ml) of this mixture three times a day.

As dried herb: infuse 2 tsp to a cup and drink three times a day.

A strong infusion of nettle should be drunk often.

To augment the efficacy of the herbs, follow these dietary suggestions:

• Eat raw fruit, vegetables, grains, seeds, and nuts. Especially recommended are cherries and strawberries.
• Preferably eat no meat, which is rich in uric acid-forming components.
• Drink six pints of fluid a day. Slightly alkaline natural spring water is recommended.
• Avoid purine-rich foods: anchovies, asparagus, crab, fish roe, herring, kidney, liver, meat gravies and broth, mushrooms, mussels, peas and beans, and sardines.
• Avoid rapid weight loss diets, which can lead to increased uric acid levels in the blood.
• Avoid all alcoholic drinks.

Osteoporosis

In osteoporosis, slow progressive thinning and loss of calcium content of the bones occurs and the skeleton becomes brittle and susceptible to fractures from seemingly minor injuries or even everyday activities. It is a major health problem affecting about twenty million Americans.

Ninety-eight percent of the body's calcium is deposited in the skeleton along with other minerals; the rest is found in the tissues and bloodstream involved in blood clotting and the activity of muscle and nerve cells. The skeleton reaches its peak mass around the age of thirty-five, and after the fourth decade bone content is lost at the rate of 1 to 2 percent annually. This process accelerates after menopause so that by the age of sixty-five most women have lost 30 to 50 percent of their skeletal mass. Men are affected to a lesser degree.

To sustain life, the level of calcium in the bloodstream must be kept within a very narrow range. This is accomplished by a homeostatic mechanism that adjusts for diet, intestinal absorption, excretion, and hormonal functions as well as growth, physical activity, and disease. Under the influence of vitamin D and parathyroid hormone, skeletal calcium is kept in a state of equilibrium with the circulating blood pool. A slight drop in blood calcium stimulates the release of calcium from the bones and its absorption from the intestine and decreases its loss into the urine. The process is reversed and bone mineral content is continuously being replenished and reformed through the actions of vitamin D, calcitonin, and estrogen and other hormones.

Clearly, treatment of osteoporosis is not simply a matter of taking calcium supplements. Many factors are involved in calcium absorption, including the following:

- Genetic makeup (e.g., inherited bone disease).
- Certain diseases that affect retention of calcium (e.g., overactivity of the thyroid or adrenal gland).
- Estrogen level (estrogen enhances calcium absorption; postmenopausal bone loss is the most common cause of osteoporosis).
- Calcium absorption declines with increasing age in both men and women, but decline comes earlier in women.
- Exercise increases absorption; prolonged bedrest or inactivity decreases it.
- Medications (e.g., corticosteroids, anticonvulsants, antacids containing aluminum, diuretics), drugs, smoking, caffeine, and certain foods impede absorption, increase excretion of nutrients, and decrease their utilization.
- Chronic stress depletes both the immediate supply and stored levels of calcium.
- Lack of other specific nutrients will deter absorption, especially vitamins D, C, and K and the minerals magnesium and phosphorous.

Herbal and nutritional treatment cannot eliminate osteoporosis but can certainly slow the process. A North American tradition calls for horsetail, oat straw, and alfalfa for the long-term treatment of osteoporosis. They do not contain particularly high levels of calcium—despite traditional claims that have been made—but they are often effective! Herbal hormonal normalizers may also be helpful if started early enough. Antirheumatics will help joint and muscle pain, and anti-inflammatories will similarly reduce discomfort.

Gout Remedy

- chasteberry   2 parts
- horsetail   1 part
- celery seed   1 part
- oats   1 part
- alfalfa   1 part

As tincture: take 1 tsp (5 ml) of this mixture three times a day.

As dried herb: infuse 2 tsp to a cup and drink three times a day.

Regular exercise, avoidance of tobacco, and maintenance of normal body weight are advised. The addition of the following daily supplements may prove beneficial:

calcium: 1,000 mg before menopause; 1,500–2,000 mg thereafter
magnesium: 500 mg before menopause; 750–1,000 mg thereafter
vitamin C: 1,000 mg
vitamin D: 400–800 IU

9 The Skin and Hair

The body's largest organ, the skin, consists of a thin outer layer, the epidermis, and a much thicker inner layer, the dermis. Beneath the dermis is a layer consisting of tiny lobes of fat bound together by tough fibers extending down from the dermis. Between the epidermis and dermis is the basement membrane, to which both layers are attached. This characteristic layering of cells, from the live and actively replicating cells of the stratum germinatum to the dead flakes on the surface, provides the unique setting for skin disease.

The Skin and Its Functions

A number of important functions are fulfilled by the skin:

- It is the interface between the body's internal structures and the environment, serving as a protective coat against mechanical injury and attack by bacteria, fungi, viruses, and parasites; the pigment melanin protects against ultraviolet radiation.
- It is a major organ of elimination (through sweat).
- It plays a vital role in temperature regulation. Heat is lost through the skin by transfer from the dermis capillaries to the cooler epidermal cells; the amount lost varies through constriction or dilation of the dermal blood cells. Sweating cools the epidermis by evaporation. The amount of heat conducted from the depths of the body is modified by the layer of insulating fat.

197

- The five sensations arising from stimulation of skin nerves include touch, pain, heat, cold, and pressure. Other skin sensations, such as vibration, are composites of these basic sensations. In hairy skin, the only nerve endings are simple, threadlike, naked terminals. In nonhairy skin, there are several types of specialized nerve endings. Although they appear the same, each nerve ending is capable of responding to only one of the five basic types of sensation.
- A number of immunological responses, such as hives, occur in the skin.
- It is the interface between the individual's consciousness and the outside world, being the vehicle through which we express, communicate, and perceive. Thus, the psychological and spiritual aspects of an individual will impact and be impacted by the skin.

This array of functions highlights the complexity of relationships between skin, internal organs, and psychology and suggests that effective herbal treatments of skin disease are best achieved through internal medication, not simply from topical applications.

The Aging Skin

Below the layers of the skin, muscles begin to deteriorate and lose their tone. Although much depends on activity, progressive loss of muscle and muscle tone generally goes along with age. Skin sags and creases as the muscles beneath it decrease in both volume and tone.

Fat in the innermost layer of the skin also deteriorates. Loss of this fat affects the skin in the same way as loss of muscle. In the skin's innermost level, the number of capillaries bringing oxygen and nutrients to the skin decreases, arteries and veins become less efficient, and less blood is pumped throughout the body. As the skin consequently gets less and less nourishment, it loses its glow and takes longer to repair itself.

In the middle layer of cells, the netting of fibers that gives the skin its strength and elasticity gradually weakens, resulting in stiffer, less pliable skin. Oil glands become increasingly inactive. Without the lubricating substance produced by the oil glands, the skin becomes dry and leathery. The sweat glands shrink, producing less and less sweat—our best natural moisturizer. Less sweat also means that the skin is a less efficient regulator of body temperature.

In the skin's top layer, new skin cells are not produced as quickly. Healing takes longer; there will be thinner skin, offering less protection against the environment. The top layer of skin loses some of the pigment cells that protect us from the sun's ultraviolet rays. From our late twenties to our mid-sixties, 20 percent of pigment cells are lost each decade. Without the dark shield of melanin, the skin's inner layers become increasingly vulnerable to damage. When the rays penetrate to the middle layer of skin, they destroy the elastic fibers that give the skin its strength and stretchability. The damage is both cumulative and irreversible.

Decades of the pull of gravity leave their mark. Life itself produces wrinkles. We grin, grimace and glower, furrow our forehead, crinkle our nose, curl our lip. Each time we make a face, the skin folds and creases in a certain pattern. As we repeat the patterns, we gradually "iron" in the creases. In our thirties, as our skin becomes less resilient, we begin to experience the facial fallout from millions of smiles. The road map of our common expressions is etched on our faces.

Herbal Actions

As skin problems are often a manifestation of internal systemic conditions, therapy will involve any of a wide range of herbs, depending upon the particular symptoms. Most important among these are the alteratives. These herbs gradually restore proper functioning of the body, increasing health and vitality. While their mode of action on the body is not yet clearly understood, the value of alteratives in holistic health care cannot be doubted. In broad terms, they act to alter the body's processes of metabolism so that tissues can best deal with the range of functions from nutrition to elimination. Many herbs in this category improve the body's ability to eliminate waste from the body through the kidneys, liver, lungs, or skin. Others work by stimulating digestive function or are antimicrobial; still others just work!

The popular term "blood cleanser" hints at much, yet says little. In fact, if the blood were indeed in need of cleansing there would be a major medical emergency afoot. Still, immunological research on secondary plant products has begun to provide some interesting suggestions for the basis of the alterative action. Saponins, plant constituents that have a soaplike effect in water, are known to have many properties, including that of immunomodulation. They appear to have a profound if little-understood modulating effect upon the cells that make up the immune system and the white cell macrophages of the mononuclear phagocyte system (MPS). It is the MPS that removes much of the waste matter from the blood—in other words, it actually does "cleanse" the blood. Saponin-containing herbs have also been shown to stimulate the production of interferon in the body. Interferon is a protein that affects the development of viruses, bacteria, and cancer cells. Remember, however, that the specifics of plant activity are the result of the whole plant upon the human body and not simply that of specific "active ingredients."

A wide range of remedies are appropriate for aging people with skin problems, each having a distinct area of application. Some remedies are for external use only: many of the essential oils, for instance, are helpful as topical applicants. The major herbs are these:

blue flag	figwort	plantain
burdock	goldenseal	pokeweed
calendula	heartsease	red clover
chaparral	motherwort	sarsaparilla
chickweed	nettle	St. John's wort
cleavers	Oregon grape	yellow dock

Skin Problems

Dry Skin

Dry skin is a common complaint among people as they age; fortunately, the plant world has much to offer to augment or replace commercial moisturizing products. Some essential oils gently stimulate the sebaceous glands, helping them to work more efficiently. (In addition, any internal herbal treatment that promotes general health will improve skin tone, especially if the problem is related to conditions such as an underactive thyroid gland.)

Pleasant oils that can be safely used include rose, chamomile, jasmine, rose geranium, and neroli. It is important to use the best quality available; avoid synthetic substitutes.

Eczema

The terms *eczema* and *dermatitis* are the cause of much confusion, but here I shall use them synonymously to mean a superficial inflammation of the skin. The most important subdivision is between those cases where the cause is an internal one and those with an external cause. In the latter cases, it is possible to solve the problem by simple avoidance of the surface irritant, if it can be identified! Common causes of such conditions, which are often referred to generally as "contact dermatitis," include the following:

- industrial solvents
- dyes
- nickel or other metals
- leather-tanning chemicals
- some soaps

Here eczema is the final result of a complex chain of internal reactions to exposure to allergens and irritants. It often accompanies other allergic diseases such as hayfever and asthma, but it may also occur alone. The rash is a very itchy, peeling, thickened, sometimes weepy area, typically noted in the creases of joints and in the trunk area. The rash may fluctuate both seasonally and over the course of the day. Scratching may lead to bleeding and infection.

In the treatment of eczema, like other skin conditions, certain herbs are taken internally while others are used topically. The alterative herbs are the classic remedies for internal treatment of eczema; how they work is unclear, but they are often dramatically effective. Relaxing nervines help with the commonly associated problem of anxiety and will often ease skin discomfort because of their relaxing effect upon the peripheral nerves. This will reduce itching and even inflammation to some extent. General health should be a priority here, so all the herbal actions that facilitate elimination of waste and internal metabolic harmony can be helpful. This might involve, for example, diuretics and hepatics.

For internal use, the leafy alteratives are often considered the closest remedies we have to treat this often intransigent condition. These also often act simultaneously as diuretics and lymphatic remedies. Herbs in this group include:

cleavers	heartsease	red clover
figwort	nettle	

The rooty alteratives tend to be more active on the liver and are often too strong for eczema, aggravating rather than healing the problem. For intransigent cases that prove unresponsive to the herbs above, however, stronger remedies are indicated. Blue flag, feverfew, and goldenseal are effective for severe eczema.

Application to the skin will alleviate symptoms. Antipruritics—remedies that reduce the sensation of itching—are indicated to lessen the intense irritation that characterizes some cases. This is not simply to make the patient feel better, but to reduce the degree of physical trauma caused by scratching. Anti-inflammatories applied topically and taken internally will speed the curative work of the alteratives but do not replace them. Vulnerary herbs will support the healing of skin lesions when applied topically but do not replace appropriate internal treatment. Astringents, used topically, will reduce any "weeping," or oozing of fluids.

Relevant herbs for topical use abound, but bear in mind that the actual healing of eczema is based upon internal medication, not on surface application of salves. Select remedies based upon the actions most appropriate for the individual's specific symptoms.

- *Anti-inflammatory:* Plantain, calendula, St. John's wort, chamomile, and the anti-inflammatory essential oils, such as lavender, can all be used.
- *Antimicrobial:* Essential oils are all antimicrobial, most notably thyme, eucalyptus, and tea tree. Also consider myrrh and goldenseal.
- *Antipruritic:* Chickweed is an extremely effective remedy for the relief of itching (except in cases of jaundice). It is most effective in a nongreasy form such as a bath, fomentation, poultice, lotion, or cream. Distilled witch hazel is another effective application.
- *Astringent:* Witch hazel and yarrow
- *Vulnerary:* Comfrey

A Possible Prescription for Eczema

- cleavers
- nettle
- red clover

Equal parts of herbs or tinctures.
As tincture: take 1 tsp (5 ml) of this mixture three times a day.
As dried herb: infuse 2–3 tsp to a cup and drink three times a day.

- nettle *or* cleavers

Drink an infusion of the *fresh* herb two or three times a day.

> ## A Possible Prescription for Persistent Eczema, Unresponsive to Mild Alteratives
>
> - cleavers
> - blue flag
> - figwort
>
> Equal parts of herbs or tinctures.
>
> **As tincture:** take $^1/_2$ tsp (2.5 ml) of this mixture three times a day; build up to 1 tsp (5 ml) three times a day.
>
> **As dried herb:** infuse 2–3 tsp to a cup and drink three times a day.
>
> - nettle
>
> Drink an infusion of the *fresh* herb two or three times a day.

Care should be taken with figwort initially, as it can produce the opposite of the desired effect in some patients. If there is a flare-up of the skin eruption, stop the figwort and try again.

If dietary triggers can be identified, it is essential to avoid them completely. Often the specific food restrictions that are called for can be a challenge to adhere to. Even if there are no obvious food triggers, it is always worth excluding milk and milk products. Goat's milk, sheep's milk, and soy milk rarely trigger allergy problems. Common eczema triggers that are relatively easy to exclude include cow's milk, eggs, cheese, some fish, and food additives. Supplements suggested for inclusion in a broad therapeutic approach to the treatment of eczema by Drs. Pizzorno and Murray in their *Textbook of Natural Medicine* include:

> **vitamin A:** 50,000 IU daily
>
> **vitamin E:** 400 IU daily (mixed tocopherols)
>
> **zinc:** 50 mg daily as picolinate (decrease as condition clears)
>
> **quercetin:** $^1/_8$-$^1/_4$ tsp three times a day
>
> **evening primrose oil:** 2–4 capsules eight times a day. As patient improves, switch to the less expensive flaxseed oil.

Other authorities have recommended additionally supplementing with vitamin C and vitamin B complex.

Fungal Skin Infections

Fungal infections of the skin are very common and a result in a range of health problems. Caused by microscopic fungal organisms that normally live on the skin surface without causing symptoms, they start to grow more rapidly and invasively under the right conditions of moisture, warmth, irritation, or minor skin injury. Certain underlying conditions (e.g, some endocrine disorders and immune diseases) other than the above may also lead to fungal infections, and these should be considered when the infection is highly recurrent or resistant to treatment.

Such infections are especially prevalent in tropical environments, where the heat and humidity allow the fungi to thrive.

TINEA

The most common group is made up of the varieties of tinea. Tinea is characterized by an itchy red scaly patch that spreads outward as it grows. Hairs in the area may fall out or break. Sometimes the skin may crack and become secondarily infected with bacteria. The fungus is spread by brushes, clothes, and other personal contact. Common varieties are tinea capitis, involving the scalp or neck, tinea barbae, affecting the beard; tinea corporis, in the nonhairy parts of the body; tinea cruris, involving the groin; and tinea pedis, affecting the feet.

ATHLETE'S FOOT (TINEA PEDIS)

Athlete's foot is characterized by an itchy, scaly, odorous rash between the toes. Cracks, irritation, redness, and bacterial infections may complicate the picture. Certain forms of the infection cause yellow blisters and can involve the soles and sides of the feet. Athlete's foot is not limited to sports enthusiasts! Hot weather and wearing shoes that do not allow the feet to "breathe" are two predisposing factors. Most susceptible are people who have previously had the infection, adult men, those whose feet perspire, and those with a weakened immune response; children, women, and people who go barefoot do not often contract it. Internal treatments do little unless the cause is related to immune system problems.

Fungicidal essential oils are the most effective topical treatment. Examples are myrrh, tea tree, and garlic (which can be both dramatically effective and malodorous).

A combination of equal parts of lavender and myrrh is a traditional treatment among aromatherapists in Britain. Myrrh is fungicidal, while lavender acts as an anti-inflammatory and vulnerary. If the skin is deeply cracked and painful, calendula oil is especially valuable. Initially, use the oils dissolved in alcohol for a few days until the moistness of the skin has dried out. Then continue treatment with an ointment or cream containing between 3 and 5 percent essential oils until the skin is completely clear. In addition, the following hygiene pointers are important:

- Clean repeatedly around toenails and fingernails, as the minute fungal mycelium often lodges under the nails and causes repeated infections.
- Keep the feet dry, especially between the toes.
- Wear open-toed shoes or sandals when you have to have any footwear on at all. Avoid vinyl uppers and athletic shoes with rubber soles. Cotton socks are better than synthetics.
- Wash your feet and soak them in a vinegar-water solution (2–4 tablespoons per pint) for twenty minutes, three times daily. Herbal vinegars would be best.

Psoriasis

This common skin disease of unknown cause affects up to 3 percent of the population. Onset is usually before the age of twenty, but all age groups are affected. The severity of this condition can vary from one or two lesions to a bodywide spread, from a benign cosmetic source of annoyance to a physically disabling and disfiguring affliction. General health is not usually affected unless the condition is associated with arthritis. In extreme cases, psoriasis may be physically, emotionally, and economically debilitating.

Psoriasis usually develops slowly, following a typical course of remission and recurrence. The characteristic plaques are sharply demarcated, usually not itchy, red, and raised, and are covered with silvery scales that easily bleed. These lesions will heal without leaving scar tissue or affecting hair growth. The nails may develop pitting. Certain patients have a tendency to develop psoriasis at the sites of physical trauma or irritation. Some cases are associated with a severe arthritis (psoriatic arthritis) that is much like rheumatoid arthritis. This common skin problem is not contagious in any way.

In normal skin, the time necessary for an epidermal cell to go from creation to shedding or scaling is about twenty-eight days; psoriatic cells complete the process in three or four days, almost nine times faster than usual. However, there appears to be no loss of normal regulatory mechanisms of cell division. Thus there can be an enormous buildup, inadequate maturation, and finally plaque formation from the affected cells. Much of psoriasis therapy is directed toward nontraumatic removal of the plaques as well as easing any attendant discomfort.

The underlying cause of this characteristic rapid cell turnover is not known. Theories abound: some practitioners view it as having a mainly nutritional cause, others invoke stress and psychological factors, still others put it down to genetics. There is undoubtedly some immune system involvement, leading some authorities to describe psoriasis as an autoimmune condition. It is common for a flare-up or worsening to accompany infection (especially upper respiratory). Environmental factors such as injury, stress, and climate are important in some patients. About one third of all patients experience spontaneous remission of the disease.

Psoriasis is a classic example of a disease requiring a holistic perspective, which explores as many aspects of the individual's life as possible. As in the case of eczema, alteratives are important, but in practice often the rooty "hepatic alterative" herbs work best The other actions to consider are very similar to those described for eczema above.

Many herbs have been cited as specific for this common skin problem, depending upon local botany and cultural preferences. However, it must be said that there are probably no true specific remedies here—as is only to be expected, considering the multifactorial, systemic roots of psoriasis. Some people respond wonderfully well to one herb while others have no reaction at all. This can prove a frustrating challenge to the practitioner, let alone the patient!

The woody, hepatic alteratives that work so well here include:

blue flag	sarsaparilla
feverfew	yellow dock

Of course, any of the other alteratives may prove equally helpful for any one individual. Of the leafy alteratives, remember:

cleavers	figwort	nettle
chapparal	heartsease	red clover

Many herbs are suitable for topical application. An important factor is the lifting and removal of scales along with reduction of local inflammation. This often means that the form of the application, such as whether it is an oily salve or a water-based lotion, is as important as any remedies it contains. Choice of topical form should be governed to some extent by the personal preference of the patient, a point that often necessitates experimentation. Plants that are widely used for this purpose include:

calendula	chickweed
plantain	western hemlock

A Possible Prescription for Psoriasis

- blue flag
- yellow dock
- cleavers
- skullcap

Equal parts of herbs or tinctures.

As tincture: take 1 tsp (5 ml) three times a day.

As dried herb: decoct 1–2 tsp to a cup and drink three times a day.

- nettle *or* cleavers

Drink an infusion of the *fresh* herb two or three times a day.

A Possible Prescription for Psoriasis Associated with Severe Anxiety and Tension

- blue flag
- yellow dock
- cleavers
- valerian
- vervain

Equal parts of herbs or tinctures.

As tincture: take 1 tsp (5 ml) three times a day.

As dried herb: decoct 1–2 tsp to a cup and drink three times a day.

- chamomile

Drink an infusion as desired.

> ### A Possible Prescription for Intransigent, Unresponsive Psoriasis
>
> - blue flag   2 parts
> - yellow dock   2 parts
> - sarsaparilla   2 parts
> - poke   1 part
> - valerian   1 part
>
> **As tincture:** take 1 tsp (5 ml) of this mixture three times a day.
>
> **As dried herb:** decoct 1–2 tsp to a cup and drink three times a day.
>
> - nettle *or* cleavers
>
> Drink an infusion of the *fresh* herb two or three times a day.

Psoriasis is a condition in which self-determination becomes vital. Patients carry around the label *psoriasis sufferer*—and suffer they do! They are often told little about the range of simple nursing techniques that help reduce itching and scale removal and so make their skin experience easier. As an interface between the person and his or her world, the skin senses and expresses. Psoriasis affects the individual's experience of being in the world in two broad ways. The physical distress makes being at ease difficult and the psychological trauma of feeling "disfigured" may lead to social isolation and depression. Stress management is crucial and will ideally be part of the patient's reevaluation of his or her lifestyle, personal goals, and vision.

For the majority of people with psoriasis, exposure to sunlight can alleviate the condition or even clear it. Yet unfortunately we have disrupted our environment such that this natural treatment is no longer to be recommended due to potential damage from ultraviolet light let through by the depleted ozone layer.

Much of the nutritional guidance for this condition is contradictory; I have seen some patients respond well to a grapefruit fast and others to a no-citrus diet! It is almost impossible to generalize here; specifics of diet must be based upon the individual, not the pathology.

Herbal "First Aid" for the Skin

Herbs can help in the treatment of many of the minor physical traumas and crises of daily life. To be effective, however, they must be used in the context of competent first aid. Some herbal suggestions are given below, but a good basic first-aid guide is irreplaceable. See, for example, the *AMA Handbook of First Aid and Emergency Care.*

Traditional herbalism abounds in recipes for topical applications of the wound-healing, or vulnerary, plants. Making these time-tested formulations involves simple techniques that can be easily reproduced at home. (See pages 245, 246, 247, and 248 for detailed instructions for preparing compresses, ointments, oils, and poultices, respectively.)

Many types of herbs can be used to heal wounds, soothe burns, stop itching, and so on. The most reliable and easiest to find are listed below with their main topical uses.

- *Arnica:* The primary remedy to be used externally for treating bruises, sprains, and other injuries. The one precaution to be noted is that arnica should not be taken internally or used on wounds where the skin is broken in any way.

- *Calendula:* Almost a medicine chest in itself! Its range of indications include wounds (new or slowly healing), bruises, burns, ulcerations, inflammations of the skin, and bacterial and fungal infections. It may be applied in the form of an ointment, poultice, compress, or even ingested as a simple infusion. Its value, efficacy, and safety cannot be overstated.

- *Chickweed:* This very common garden "weed" may be the best remedy available for itching. The only time it appears to be powerless is when the cause of itching is jaundice.

- *Comfrey:* Its other name in Britain is knitbone, acknowledging its value as a healer. Research has shown it to contain allantoin, a chemical that stimulates cell division in the basal layer of the epidermis. Hence it speeds wound healing quite dramatically. However, comfrey should not be used on deep puncture wounds because the surface may heal over before healing has occurred inside, which can lead, in turn, to abscess formation.

- *Plantain:* This very common herb is an excellent wound healer, emollient, and anti-inflammatory agent for the skin.

- *St. John's wort:* In addition to the internal uses of St. John's wort for treating the nervous system, it has some special healing effects upon the skin. It may be used for cuts and scrapes, mild burns, and sunburn. It has also been found helpful in some cases of eczema, especially those that respond well to sunlight.

Burns

Minor burns are common household injuries that require prompt attention and conscientious care to reduce scarring and speed healing. Because normal skin acts as a protective barrier against bacteria, burn wounds are particularly susceptible to infection. A first-degree burn (e.g., normal sunburn) involves only the superficial layer of the skin: redness, pain, and minimal swelling occur. Second-degree burns have blisters and are more painful. Third-degree burns involve the full thickness of the skin with charring and damage to deeper tissues. They heal by scarring unless a skin graft is applied. Many burns are combinations of all three types.

A burn that has affected a small area and damaged only the outer layer of skin can be treated safely at home; *anything more extensive, or a burn caused by chemicals or electricity, calls for immediate medical advice.* If the burn is a minor one, cold aloe vera gel or the content of a freshly picked aloe leaf will reduce burn damage, speed recovery, and soothe the wound immediately. Adding lavender oil (four ounces of aloe gel to twenty drops of lavender oil) will help.

Bruises

Bruises, or "black and blue" marks, represent bleeding from the small blood vessels beneath the surface of the skin. They are almost always caused by injuries from direct blows. Older people, those with bleeding disorders, and individuals taking cortisone-type medications are particularly susceptible. The natural course for a bruise is spontaneous healing over a period of days to weeks. As the blood beneath the surface breaks down chemically and is absorbed, the skin will change from red to black to green to yellow before there is complete resolution. *Contusion* is a fancy medical term for an injury to the soft tissues beneath the skin—in other words, a bump!

The primary herbal treatment here is external application of arnica as soon as possible. This should be accompanied by ingestion of internal remedies containing flavone constituents, which strengthen the walls of the traumatized small blood vessels. Examples are ginkgo and hawthorn. Aromatherapists suggest the use of rosemary oil once the distinctive colors have developed, to stimulate local circulation and so speed drainage. As rosemary may be irritating to sensitive skin, it should be diluted with a bland oil such as almond oil. (Formulations are given on pages 246–47.) It is advisable to supplement vitamin C with bioflavonoids.

Itching

Of course the cause of the itching—which may be just about anything from allergies, jaundice, or eczema to scratchy clothes or lice—must be identified and dealt with. Temporary relief can be easily obtained by applying distilled witch hazel to the irritated area. This convenient herbal preparation is still carried by drugstores and even supermarkets. Chickweed in any form can be applied or used in a bath and will often produce even more gratifying results. Formulations are given in the section on medicine making.

Scar Formation

Scar tissue is formed by the natural healing processes of the body. Certain remedies will help ensure a minimum of scar tissue buildup and a maximum of wound healing. Such treatment may be appropriate following surgery or in the case of wounds. The application of vitamin E oil is often enough but may be augmented by comfrey, calendula, or St. John's wort ointments.

Sunburn

About 5 percent of the sunlight that reaches the earth is made up of invisible ultraviolet (UV) light rays, UVA and UVB. The long wavelength ultraviolet (UVA) causes tanning by increasing the production of the natural skin pigment, melanin. The middle wavelength ultraviolet (UVB) is the major cause of sunburn. The sunlight between the hours of 10:00 a.m. and 3:00 p.m. is most direct, has the highest amount of UVA and UVB, and presents the greatest risk of sunburn. Whether one burns depends on a number of factors: skin color, the time of day, the duration of sun exposure, clouds, smog, altitude, the amount of reflected light, medications, and the presence—or lack—of protective clothing and sunscreen.

Aloe vera gel applied liberally to sunburned areas can have dramatic effects. St. John's wort oil, fresh cucumber juice, or an infusion of calendula are also helpful.

The Hair

Hair is actually a modified type of skin, growing everywhere on the body except the palms of the hands, soles of the feet, eyelids, and lips. Hair plays a number of essential protective functions. For example it reduces the loss of heat from the body. The hair in the nose, ears, and around the eyes protects these sensitive areas of the body from dust and other small particles. Eyebrows and eyelashes protect the eyes by decreasing the amount of light and particles that go into them.

Hair is damaged by modern lifestyles. A partial list of contributing factors would include blow dryers, chemical products, overzealous brushing, damaging hairstyles, and hair spray. Poor nutrition and illness will also lead to damage, and of course it is affected by the aging process.

- *Hair dries out.* The oil glands that lubricate the hair (and the skin) become increasingly inactive as we age. Lack of lubrication leaves it brittle, vulnerable to breaking, splitting, and further harm from the environment.
- *Hair gets finer.* The thickness of each hair shaft decreases as the protein-making machinery of the body slows down. At age forty, the hair shaft is 5 percent thinner than it was at twenty.
- *Hair loses its color.* In fact there is no such thing as gray hair: "gray" is the mix between normally pigmented hair and aging hair that has lost its pigment. (The way light bounces off it makes it appear white.)
- *Hair falls out.* Some shedding is part of the hair's normal growth cycle and not age-related. But as we get older, stress, diet, and drugs (especially hormones) can cause hair to fall out and not be replaced in kind.
- *Hair grows where it is not wanted.*

The herbal contribution to hair care most often falls under the umbrella of cosmetics, and many excellent suggestions can be found in herbal cosmetic guides. Some formulations are given in the section on medicine making (pages 251–52).

10  The Immune System

The immune system has become an increasingly crucial issue in all branches of medicine in recent years, especially because of the AIDS epidemic and the statistical explosion of a wide range of autoimmune diseases. To consider the possibilities of holistic approaches, it is important to have a grasp of the biological basis of immunity, but at least as important is a comprehension of the role the immune system plays in human life. The new—though still incomplete—understanding that immunology grants us illuminates much on the physical level, but much more is involved, and herbal medicine is as limited as allopathic medicine if it is used only in terms of blood chemistry without the benefit of a broader holistic context.

The immune system is one of the first body systems to experience a functional decline with age, and this reduction in efficiency may trigger several problems. For example, the degenerative diseases associated with aging usually develop only after the immune system begins to show signs of aging. One major function of this system is the cleansing of dead or defective cells from the body, and as its efficiency diminishes the subsequent buildup of what might be called "cellular garbage," in turn, contributes to the aging process in other body tissues. Infections and potentially fatal complications are more common in people as they age than in younger adults. Advancing age is accompanied by a gradual decline in the ability of the body to synthesize antibodies in response to antigens and to manifest cellular immunity.

Some important insights emerge when immune system functioning is placed in an ecological perspective and not simply a biochemical/medical one. It becomes clear that human immunity is a vital component of the interface between the individual and the world. Human activity is not simply resistance to a dangerous environment; it is a complex, beautiful dance flowing to and fro within the world.

The whole complex of human immunity has certain characteristics. Seen within the context of ecology, both human and environmental, immunity is about harmony, not simply resistance. It is a dynamic dance with the environment and not merely a series of barriers to it. This viewpoint leads to some insights that suggest exciting possibilities for the whole field of health care.

- Human immunity is ecology in action. In other words, there is a relationship. Both sides of the relationship, and the nature of the relationship itself, must be identified and understood. This can prove extremely challenging, as it will be in dynamic flux at all times.
- Immunity is an ecological interface between inner and outer environments. Such interfaces—between desert and savanna, rain forest and mountains, woodland and grassland, agriculture and wilderness—appear to be critical to the health and well-being of the planet herself. These transition zones facilitate the integration and fine-tuning of ecosystems and the health of the biosphere. Similarly, in human/nonhuman ecology, the immune system is a complex of procedures and processes that allow in and out, resistance and embrace, at the same time. To focus on only one side of this profound yin/yang is to miss the point and compromise the whole complex.
- Immunity is an expression of homeostasis. "Homeostasis" describes the body's wonderful integration of physiological processes that maintains a stable internal environment—body temperature, blood pressure, and glucose level, for example. This inner homeostasis is a reflection of the planetary homeostasis that characterizes Gaia. It was the recognition of these planetwide processes that originally led James Lovelock to propose the Gaia hypothesis, the concept that the planet as a whole can be seen as a single organism.
- Immunity is an expression of relationship. Implicit in everything said so far is the pivotal role that *relationship* plays in immune system well-being. Our relationship with the world is as important as our immunochemistry. This must be seen on many levels, from the food we eat and the people we love or hate to the way we relate to nature.

This ecological approach emphasizes that—as with all aspects of holistic healing—the approach to whole body immunity must address the following aspects of human life:

- *Bodily health and wholeness.* The physical body must have the correct nutrition and appropriate healing support for any ills it may be experiencing.
- *Emotional well-being.* A nurturing feeling life, encompassing both joy and pain, is needed for balance.
- *Mental vision and perspective.* One needs to create a mind-set within which to find one's place, to make choices from the center rather than from the stance of the victim.
- *Spiritual openness and vitality.* These can be encouraged in whatever form is appropriate for the individual.

Herbal Actions

The diverse herbal traditions of the world, with their unique cultural roots and expressions, have valuable insights into the many ways to use herbs to enhance immunological vitality. In fact, the field of herbal immune system support provides a good example of the confirmation of traditional knowledge by modern pharmacology. A growing number of remedies are now being shown in laboratory and clinical studies to have marked immunological effects. Some are stimulants to immunity, but most can best be described as "modulators"—that is, they enable the body's natural responses to be more flexible in the face of disease. But rather than focus on the plant, here again we shall look at the whole treatment process.

In the following sections, I shall present ideas that bridge a traditional European American approach and various insights offered by both oriental medicine and pharmacological research. Naturally, it is too soon in the process of cross-cultural synergy to say that the theories presented here are "the way it is," but the therapeutic suggestions are based upon clinical experience and historical precedence.

The Californian medical herbalist Christopher Hobbs has identified three levels of herbal activity. He describes these levels as deep immune activation, surface immune activation, and "adaptogenic" or hormonal modulation.

Deep Immune Activation

Increasing interest is being shown in plants that impact the immunological process within the tissue that mediates its work, termed *deep immune activation*. Pharmacology points to plant constituents such as saponins and complex polysaccharides as key components in the immunological role of herbs, but always remember that herbs act as biological wholes, not simply as vehicles for "active ingredients." Important immunomodulators now being introduced into Western herbal practice from China and Japan include *Astragalus membranaceous (huang-qi), Ligustrum lucidum* (Chinese privet), *Schizandra chinensis (wu-wei-zi), Ganoderma lucidum* (from the reishi mushroom), and *Codonopsis tangshen (dang shen)*.

In addition to specific remedies that directly impact immunochemistry, herbal support of general well-being will help homeostasis and so the immune system. Herbal actions and processes to take into account include the use of *bitter tonics* and *alteratives*. It is important to note that deep immune work involves support of the normal body functions of elimination and detoxification, discussed on page 218.

BITTER TONICS

It is becoming increasingly apparent that the bitter remedies have a major role to play in holistic herbal treatment and especially in preventive medicine. Because of their wide effect on the body's physiology, they help in treatment of the body as an integrated whole.

Bitters apparently work by triggering a sensory response in the mouth. The sensation of bitterness, probably along with many subtleties of which we are still unaware, is directed by the nerves to the central nervous system, setting off other responses in turn:

- The appetite is stimulated—a useful effect during convalescence and in conditions involving loss of appetite.
- There is a general stimulation of the flow of digestive juices from the pancreas, duodenum, and liver.
- Bitters also aid the liver in its detoxification work and increase the flow of bile. Possibilities for healing here are great, as many health problems have their roots in an overworked liver.
- There is a regulatory effect upon the secretion by the pancreas of the hormones that regulate blood sugar, insulin, and glucagon.

- Bitters help the gut wall repair damage through stimulation of self-repair mechanisms.

Bitters also affect the activity of heart and circulation in general. There can be a marked antidepressive action in some cases as well as a tonic effect with remedies such as mugwort and gentian. Moreover, as digestion and assimilation of food are fundamental to health, bitter stimulation can often fundamentally influence a medical picture that has nothing pathologically to do with the digestive process.

ALTERATIVES

They have not attracted the attention of researchers as the oriental remedies have, yet the herbs we know as alteratives bring about changes in the body that suggest they may work on the deep immune level. Important gentle alteratives include:

burdock	nettle	yellow dock
cleavers	sarsaparilla	

Surface Immune Activation

Surface immune activation is facilitated by herbs that promote the immune response to microbial infection. These are the many plants known as antimicrobials. These herbs, discussed in more depth below in the section on infection, include:

calendula	myrrh	western hemlock
echinacea	old man's beard	wild indigo
garlic	onion	

Hormonal Modulation

Remedies in this group work through some hormonal modulation of immune response. The feelings, thoughts, and dreams we have in response to daily life affect us in many ways, one of which is an immunological response. Most people, for example, have experienced getting a cold when work pressure is too great. Using adaptogens can help the body deal with such stress-related immunological problems. Please refer to the section on stress, where Siberian ginseng and ginseng are discussed (pages 118–21). Other endocrinological issues can be addressed herbally, as discussed below.

Detoxification

Helping the body to deal with removal of pollutants and potentially toxic metabolic waste produced internally is at the core of support for the immune system. One herbal approach to detoxification springs from the premise that the human body is a self-healing and homeostatic organism, and that the therapist simply has to support normal processes. The body has wonderfully effective mechanisms for ridding itself of waste and poisons, and this can be supported by using simple and safe herbs as long as the eliminative processes are addressed as a whole. This means that whenever such a program is undertaken, all the organs of elimination are supported at the same time. In addition, tonic help is given to the specific area of the body that has been most under toxic pressure. Examples would be the lungs in a tobacco smoker or the liver in a patient with alcohol-related problems. At the same time, symptomatic discomfort can be alleviated.

The key to detoxification is support of all the pathways with gentle herbs, not an attack with herbal Drano! The first step is to identify the appropriate herbs by considering what actions will gently support elimination in each pathway. If overly active plants are used, the effect may be unpleasant and uncomfortable and of no added therapeutic benefit. The herbal remedies listed below are effective, yet safe and mild.

Target System	Herbal Action	Remedy
Kidneys and urinary system	Diuretic	Dandelion leaf
Liver and blood	Hepatic, alterative	Dandelion root, milk thistle
Lymphatic system	Alterative, lymphatic tonic	Nettles, cleavers
Skin	Diaphoretic, alterative	Yarrow
Respiratory system	Expectorant, pulmonary, anticatarrhal	Mullein, coltsfoot
Systemic support	Tonic	Choose a remedy with relevant system affinity
	Adaptogen	Siberian ginseng
	Antimicrobial	Garlic

Immunological Actions

The range of information now available concerning the immune system and herbal approaches to treatments can be truly daunting! Since the approach I use throughout this book does not focus on isolated plant research but rather is *people*-based, the therapeutic suggestions that follow are based upon my own training and clinical experience in Wales.

As pharmacology has begun to newly explore the possibilities offered by the plant kingdom, new words have been coined to describe how the plants work:

- *Immunostimulants or immunopotentiators* provide general stimulation of the immunological defense system. Since their efficacy fades comparatively quickly, they have to be administered either in regular intervals or continuously. The immunity created by immunostimulants is brought about quickly and has been termed "paramunity."
- *Immunomodulators.* These herbs may stimulate T-suppressor cells and thereby reduce immune resistance. Here the terms immunomodulators or immunoregulators (in reference to their effect on immune responsiveness) have been proposed.
- *Immunoadjuvants* are substances that enhance the production of antibodies without acting as antigens themselves.

From the allopathic perspective, a number of therapeutic possibilities may be recognized, hinting at the changes in perspective that are underway within orthodox medicine today.

- Immunostimulation potentially provides an alternative to conventional chemotherapy for infections, especially in patients exhibiting an impaired immune response. Such herbal therapy promotes the body's own immune mechanisms and thereby may help to prevent opportunistic infections in patients at risk.
- Much that is being seen in work with immunostimulants can be utilized in the therapy of malignant diseases. It is well known, for example, that tumor growth can be inhibited by stimulating specific components of the immune system, such as macrophages or T-killer cells.

- Plant-based immune stimulation may also contribute new insights into the therapy of autoimmune disease.

As more research is done, the range of plant species and constituents that seem to be involved grows. There is still far too little research to make generalizations, but the excellent studies being undertaken by Chinese and Japanese scientists on their traditional remedies is revealing much of importance to immunology. However, the same attention is rarely given to traditional European or North American herbs. This is because of a lack of research grants, not because of an inherent lack of value in the plants. (Perhaps if nettle were given the same quality of attention that the East Asian remedy *Astragalus* has received, we might soon have the immunological "proof" of its profound effects!)

Immune System Problems

A number of immune system conditions may readily be addressed herbally. Immunological problems are grouped into the following categories:

Immunodeficiency diseases: Associated with some deficiency or malfunction of one or more of the major aspects of the immune response, such diseases are usually divided into two groups:
- Primary immune deficiency disease, hereditary or acquired, in which the immune deficiency is the cause of a disease.
- Secondary immune deficiency disease, in which the immune deficiency is a result of other diseases. An extreme example would be AIDS.

Hypersensitivity reactions: These are normal immunity processes that become damaging rather than protective. The pathological processes result from specific interactions between an antigen and components of the immune system.

Autoimmune disease: A condition in which lymphocytes produce antibodies that attack the body's own cells and tissues as if they were the foreign substances, thus causing pathological damage. Any organ or tissue may be involved.

Tumors and "cancer": There is a direct immunological relationship between the body and tumors. This fact highlights the possibilities of prevention and treatment through working with immunity.

Transplant problems: Transplant rejection is immunologically based.

When considering the possibilities offered by herbal therapy in this area, please remember that appropriate remedies for immune system problems must be selected based upon individual need, which can only be identified by careful diagnosis; thus the practitioner must be aware of the complexities of the process in play. Stimulating immunological activity may be inappropriate in some conditions and vital in others. In an attempt to clarify this for myself, I have established provisional guidelines for distinguishing between therapeutic situations calling for immunostimulation, and those where it may be contraindicated.

As a generalization, it seems safe to say that in conditions involving inappropriate activity of some aspect of the whole immunological complex, immunostimulant plants should be avoided. Thus, immunostimulants are probably contraindicated in autoimmune conditions, hypersensitivity reactions, and transplantation problems.

Conversely, in conditions involving inadequate or compromised activity of immunity, immunostimulant plants are fundamentally important in herbal treatment. In other words, immunostimulants are probably indicated in cases of infections, cancer, or immunodeficiency disease.

Why have I used the term *probably?* The experienced herbalist, who is completely at home with the multifactorial effects of plants, as well as the diversity of human beings, will never see a plant simply as "an immunostimulant." For example, a remedy may have specific value in the treatment of rheumatoid arthritis and may also be found to have immunostimulating activity. The long-standing experience of generations of practitioners and patients will have more value than the theoretical insights raised by in vitro or animal studies.

Infection

The risk of infection seems to be a natural consequence of life in the earth's biosphere. Humanity lives in constant ecological dialogue with vast numbers of bacteria, viruses, and fungi, yet our immune systems have evolved in such a way that this interaction only occasionally gives rise to health problems. In fact, our well-being is dependent on our healthy and positive relationships with a range of organisms that live within and on our body: two examples are the bacterial flora of the intestines and the microorganisms on the skin.

Infection occurs when the body is exposed either to pathogens or to organisms that are usually nonpathogenic but for some reason become a threat. If the immune response is compromised in some way, the ecological balance between host and microbe will change, allowing the microbe to thrive. Whichever the type of organism, an herbal treatment must focus on supporting immunity.

The herbal traditions of the world abound in plants reputed for their antimicrobial activities, but it must be borne in mind that they do not always achieve the results desired. Antibiotics are life-saving medicines when used appropriately. They have largely removed the scourge of epidemic infectious disease from the Western world. Thanks to systematic vaccination programs, smallpox is extinct. These are truly miraculous achievements. Herbalism cannot always deal adequately or quickly enough with severe acute infection, especially in patients with a weakened immune response. Such infections (meningitis, for example) necessitate the use of antibiotic therapy. As a dedicated herbalist who recognizes the limitations of my chosen therapy, I celebrate the existence of these medicines, for the role of the healer is the alleviation of suffering, not the promotion of a belief system. Still, much can be contributed by herbal treatment, including the following effects:

- boosting the immune response and thereby helping the body rid itself of the pathogen
- toning and strengthening tissue, organs, or whole systems that are the focus of the infection
- facilitating recuperation from the infection and also from the use of antibiotics

Antimicrobials widely used in British and American herbal therapy include:

aniseed	eucalyptus	rosemary
bearberry	garlic	St. John's wort
caraway	gentian	sage
calendula	goldenseal	thyme
cayenne	juniper	wild indigo
clove	marjoram	yarrow
coriander	myrrh	wormwood
echinacea	peppermint	
elecampane	rue	

All herbs rich in aromatic essential oils are antimicrobial. At one time, indeed, various essential oils were used in orthodox medicine to combat infection, particularly those of the bronchial and urinary tracts, and in preventing infection of burns and wounds. Some of these oils still find extensive use as disinfectants, as their antiseptic activity often exceeds that of phenol. Much clinical work is now under way with these oils in France, but, unfortunately, little has been translated into English thus far.

AN HERBALIST'S APPROACH TO INFECTION

Because of the similarity in the immune system's involvement in bodily response to one infection or another, it is possible to make certain generalizations regarding herbal treatment of infection. Of course, the details will vary according to the nature of the disease, the specific individual, and any medication the patient may be taking. Thus, the guidelines given here are only general suggestions.

First, select the appropriate antimicrobial remedy. Choice is based upon the most suitable herbs for:

- The particular site of infection. For example, use bearberry for bladder infections, elecampane for lung infections, and myrrh topically for the skin.
- The age and constitution of the person involved. For example, use gender herbs for the young, old, or debilitated.
- Use specific remedies for the particular pathogen involved wherever possible.

Always use antimicrobials along with tonic remedies. These may be selected based upon the following criteria:

- *The site of infection.* For example, use mullein in lung infections and cleavers for lymphatic tissue infections.
- *Specific prevention issues in the individual.* For example, use hawthorn if there is any concern about cardiovascular issues and ginkgo.
- *Any insights from the individual's medical or family history.*

Support the body by dealing with any fever that may accompany the infection. Also, alleviate symptomatic discomfort as necessary.

HERBAL SUPPORT OF ANTIBIOTIC THERAPY

There is no reason why the benefits of herbalism should not be utilized even when antibiotic treatment is under way. Here the herbal focus must be on tonics, helping the body cope with the intense biochemical battle raging within it. Selection of the tonic can be based upon these criteria:

- the site of infection
- support of the digestive system and liver, as intestinal side effects are common
- specific prevention issues pertaining to the individual patient
- any insights from the patient's medical or family history

Immune support is appropriate, but don't try to duplicate the work of the antibiotics by using excessive amounts of echinacea. Provide symptomatic support if appropriate.

RECUPERATION FOLLOWING ANTIBIOTIC THERAPY

Once a course of antibiotics has been completed, herbs may be used to speed convalescence, to help avoid any recurrence of infection, and to prevent secondary problems that might arise because of the temporarily weakened immune response.

Focus on general nutrition as well as herbal tonics:

- bitters to safely stimulate normal metabolism
- gentle diuretics and hepatics to support elimination
- specific tonics for the site of infection and/or the site of greatest symptomatic discomfort

Immune support is important. This may be both deep and surface work. Focus on deep immune support with the immunostimulant herbs if:

- the problem is a chronic or recurring one
- the patient is elderly or very debilitated following the infection
- the patient is under much psychological, social, or environmental stress and thus potentially immunocompromised

Cancer: A Holistic Approach

Herbs have a long and honorable history in the treatment of cancer, and it may surprise many readers to lean that herbs are still at the core of modern medicine's response to this disease.

Cancer is a term applied to a range of malignant diseases that may affect many different parts of the body. All are characterized by a rapid and uncontrolled formation of abnormal cells that may either mass together to form a growth (tumor) or proliferate throughout the body, initiating abnormal growth at other sites. If the process is not arrested, it may progress until it causes the death of the organism. Cancer is encountered in all higher animals, and plants also develop growths that resemble cancer.

The search among Western research scientists for a chemical anticancer "magic bullet" or a specific cytotoxic plant is predicated upon a rationale that is inherently flawed. To be sure, Western medicine has made great strides for a suffering humanity. Our pharmacology has furnished medicine with powerful tools for the treatment of life-threatening acute diseases and the alleviation of much suffering through speedy and effective amelioration of symptoms. Yet the major cause of death in the Western world is no longer acute infection but rather degenerative disease. On one hand, this change is a reflection of the successes of the allopathic approach: smallpox has been eradicated, polio no longer occurs in epidemic proportion, and tuberculosis is no longer the scourge it once was. On the other hand, these very successes serve to highlight the inadequacy of our approach to the degenerative diseases.

To use the unfortunately militaristic imagery of allopathic advocacy groups, acute infection has been "conquered," yet our investment of vast sums and resources into "conquering" cancer has not produced the results expected. The lobbyists of the "cancer industry" might conclude from this the need for more research funds—or the dearth of dramatic "breakthroughs" might suggest that the allopathic perspective has not perceived and addressed the complexity of factors at play. Multifactorial interactions are the strong suit of holistic medicine. This statement says nothing about specific techniques but emphasizes the need for a context that embraces far more than oncogenes, tumor pathology, and carcinogens.

From the perspective of holistic medicine, any approach to cancer must take into account the whole of a person's life; it is not simply a matter of destroying a tumor. A deep process of healing and reevaluation is essential, perhaps involving all of the following elements:

- *Some medical approach to destroying the tumor.* Therapy may focus on remedies that aim to improve the body's own immune response to cancer cells (herbal immunostimulants). Allopathic approaches might utilize cyto-toxic plants, chemotherapy, surgery, and/or radiation.
- *Therapeutics geared to the body as a whole,* taking into account the patient's noncancer-related concerns. Therapy might involve support for normal body processes such as elimination and general homeostatic integration, as well as tonics and other factors.
- *Nutritional reevaluation.* Therapy will not simply identify those foods that are "anticancerous" or carcinogenic but will ensure that the body is receiving appropriate nourishment.
- *Bodywork as appropriate for the individual.* For example, massage does not "cure" cancer, but it may be a vital part of a patient's stress management program and thus integrally belong to holistic cancer treatment.
- *Attention must be given to emotional and mental issues.* A complex and formidable proposition! Stress management is essential, but so is depth counseling of some sort. Within the context of transpersonal psychology, it is possible to see illness as a gift that offers many insights and directions for growth and transformation. This approach, as a component of a broad treatment of cancer, can facilitate major emotional, mental, and spiritual healing even in the face of terminal bodily disease.

HERBAL CANCER THERAPY

We all would like to find the magical herb to cure every possible disease, including cancer. But the term *anticancer herb*, promising as it sounds, is therapeutically meaningless. The National Cancer Institute has provided the following clear and useful definitions:

Anticancer is a term that is reserved for materials that are toxic to tumor cells in clinical trials with humans.

Antitumor activity occurs if this toxicity affects tumor cells in living animals.

A *cytotoxic* agent is a substance that is toxic to tumors in laboratory cultures.

Various cytotoxic herbs, such as American mandrake, are known, but just because we know about powerful poisons, powerful narcotics, and powerful purgatives does not mean that we use them. The selection of remedies in any therapeutic regimen is dictated by the practitioner's interpretation of need, which in turn will be an expression of the therapeutic philosophy that he or she espouses. The holistic practitioner's use of such powerful remedies would only be considered in the context of a treatment program that works in the broad way I have discussed earlier.

In fact, holistically orientated herbalists tend to minimize the role of cytotoxic plants in their approach to cancer because of the problems inherent in such remedies. For one thing, a common argument put forward by pharmacologists against the use of herbal medicines—that the variable amounts of active constituents in natural plants prevents accurate prescribing of standardized dosages—becomes relevant when considering cancer therapy. In most cases the herbal approach is based upon the use of normalizers, or, at most, effectors that do not contain potent constituents; but in the case of cytotoxic plants, the inherent variability of plant constituent levels makes the establishment of appropriate dosage extremely problematic. Thus, after experienced consideration of this therapeutic dilemma, I have been led to conclude that *chemotherapy may in fact well be safer than therapy based on the use of cytotoxic plants.* This may offend natural medicine purists, but the needs of my patients always outweigh any philosophical dogma I may be attached to. I believe that a holistic perspective combined with an approach based on immunostimulation and immunomodulation can provide a context of treatment that does not depend on the use of potentially poisonous plants. If extreme measures are needed, I do not hesitate to turn to the experts on poison—the allopaths.

Why are no prescriptions or treatment protocols suggested in this section? First, simply because each individual must be treated as just that: a unique individual, not a site for a tumor. As this approach proposes the avoidance of cytotoxic remedies, the factors to address will be fundamentally the same as those for general immune support, with possibly greater emphasis on the use of alteratives and lymphatics.

Another reason is a personal one. The herbal literature is replete with treatments and "cures" that sound wonderful but have no basis in reality. My own clinical experience in the treatment of cancer is not extensive enough for me to draw widely applicable conclusions beyond the following broad supportive guidelines:

- *Actions.* There is no "anticancer" herbal action. Theory suggests the relevance of alteratives, lymphatics, and general tonics. Other actions would be indicated by the symptom picture and issues unique to the kind of tumor involved.

- *System tonics.* Tonic support for the site of the tumor is essential, as is an address of other factors that may arise from a review of the patient's medical and family history.

- *Systemic support.* This involves immune system support with an emphasis on deep immune stimulation, eliminative support, and stress management.

- *Specific remedies.* Many plants around the world are reputed to be "anticancer" herbs. Unfortunately, they rarely work as claimed! The herbs in question are largely alterative, lymphatic, hepatic, or diuretic remedies that have much to contribute to the holistic approach I suggest but do not replace that broader approach. Common examples from Europe and North America are:

blue flag	mistletoe (European)	sweet violet
calendula	poke	western hemlock
chapparal	queen's delight	yellow dock
cleavers	red clover	

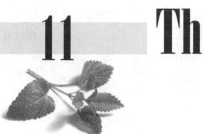

11 The Endocrine System

The herbal tradition suffers from a dearth of suggestions for treating the endocrine glands. In fact, our understanding of the functions of the endocrine system is very recent. Some contribution can be made by the use of herbs in the context of appropriate holistic therapy, but it is not always possible to achieve results that would adequately replace drug treatment. A comprehensive review of herbal medicine for the endocrine glands has yet to be written, and what follows is based on my own limited clinical experience in this field. Specifically, we will discuss the adrenal glands, the thyroid gland, and the pancreas.

The Adrenal Glands

Alternative medicine abounds in ideas about the adrenal glands and remedies for their ills. Unfortunately, such ideas often show lack of knowledge about the adrenals. The ideas couched in these terms are often valid and helpful, but the invocation of an "adrenal tonic" effect must be based upon actual physiology and not pseudoscience.

The two adrenals sit astride the kidneys, deep in the back of the abdomen. Each of these glands has two parts, a cortex or outer part, and a medulla or central portion. These have markedly different functions. When therapy is directed towards these glands, it must be appropriate to the specific adrenal function that needs to be addressed.

The adrenal medulla secretes the hormones epinephrine and norepinephrine, which are responsible for the rapid increases in nervous system and metabolic activity involved in the stress response. The adrenal cortex is responsible for production of hormones called glucocorticoids, including cortisone and hydrocortisone. They have a regulatory effect on metabolism, the immune system, certain aspects of behavior, and many other processes. The cortex also secretes aldosterone, which is fundamental to the homeostatic control of sodium and potassium secretion by the kidney.

Herbs for the Adrenal Cortex

Herbal medicines can impact the adrenal cortex in a variety of ways. Most important is the direct effect of plants that are rich in a specific variety of saponin. One such plant, licorice, is proving to be a controversial remedy because of its effects upon the adrenal cortex. Aldosterone, the substance secreted by the cortex, is part of a hormonal homeostatic complex that regulates electrolyte balance in the blood as well as the volume of urine passed. When licorice is eaten or taken in great excess, it has a direct impact upon aldosterone leading to potassium depletion. This is a very rare occurrence, but pharmacology books have pointed to it insistently to demonstrate the dangers of herbal medicine. Yet, on the other hand, British patients with Addison's disease have benefited greatly from this herb. However, to be completely safe, licorice should be avoided in overactivity; it is indicated in underactivity.

Herbs for the Adrenal Medulla

For a discussion of the contribution that can be made by herbs in support of the adrenal medulla when under stress, please refer to the section "Stress and the Adaptogens" (page 118–21). Adaptogens are the core of adrenal medulla support, with saponins such as the eleutherosides directly impacting the medulla. Nervine tonic support of some kind is usually indicated as well, although this does not directly impact the medulla. The contribution from such nervines is a more generalized systemic support that eases the impact of tension and anxiety. Bitter tonics can be helpful as well. Examples might include the following:

- *Adaptogens:* ginseng and Siberian ginseng
- *Nervine tonics:* skullcap, St. John's wort, and oats

The Pancreas

Two types of tissue are contained in the pancreas: the acini, responsible for the creation of digestive enzymes; and the islets, which produce hormones. The digestive enzymes are secreted by the pancreas into the duodenum, while the hormones are secreted (by the pancreas) into the bloodstream. The hormone insulin, which is released by the pancreas, controls how much sugar is in the blood; it enables the movement of sugar from the blood into the cells. When the body does not produce enough insulin for this to happen, an imbalance is created; this imbalance produces the symptoms and complications of diabetes, a multifaceted disease that potentially affects every organ in the body.

Diabetes

The regulation of blood sugar, a complex homeostatic process is, as noted above, dependent upon insulin, a hormone produced in the islets of Langerhans in the pancreas. After the insulin is produced by the pancreas, it is absorbed into the bloodstream and thereby carried to the rest of the body. Insulin has several functions: it causes glucose to leave the blood and enter the cells of the various body organs, facilitates metabolic processes that promote the storage of energy into fat and other substances, and prevents the release of such stores into the blood.

Insufficient insulin will cause the level of glucose in the blood to rise, especially after a meal. Without insulin, body organs are unable to extract glucose from the blood and begin to rely on alternate sources of energy, especially some fats. The fats' metabolites, called ketones, begin to accumulate in the blood. Metabolic changes in diabetes alters the way in which the body handles fats (including cholesterol), leading to their accumulation in the small arteries of the body, often those of the eyes, the kidney, the heart, and the brain, so that diabetes patients show increased incidence of blindness, kidney failure, heart attack, and stroke. Most cases of diabetes fall into one of two types:

- *Type I* (Insulin-dependent) is generally acquired in childhood, involving a near-total lack of insulin production. Such patients require ongoing insulin administration to sustain life.
- *Type II* (Non-insulin-dependent) is generally acquired in adulthood. As some degree of hormone production occurs, Type II may be treated with appropriate dietary measures; only a small minority of patients require

insulin. These people retain the ability to produce some insulin, but such activity (i.e., following a meal) is long delayed and often inadequate.

Symptoms of diabetes include fatigue, increased appetite if enough blood sugar is lost to the urine, and increased urination as the kidneys are forced to produce higher volumes to dissolve the excess load of sugar. Thirst is increased to replenish the lost body fluid. As levels of blood sugar rise and ketosis occurs, body fluids become excessively acid. One of the defenses against acidity is to decrease the carbon dioxide in the blood, leading to an increase in the rate and depth of respiration. Complications due to arterial blockage are common, including vision loss, heart problems, kidney damage, and peripheral neuropathy. Such problems usually require many years to develop.

How can herbal therapy help in diabetes? The plant kingdom includes many hypoglycemic plants (those acting to lower the blood sugar), which can contribute much to a comprehensive management program of non-insulin-dependant diabetes. Insulin-dependent patients will rarely respond well to hypoglycemics, however, as the islets of Langerhans are largely incapable of working. Herbs will not replace necessary insulin therapy. Laboratory screenings, similar to those for cytotoxic plants, have demonstrated the reality of plant hypoglycemics. Examples from Europe include:

bilberry	goat's rue	olive leaves
garlic	mulberry leaves	

Interestingly, goat's rue is also an effective galactagogue, an herb that increases the production of breast milk, a fact that suggests a possible pituitary or hypothalamus activity. Remember that gentle endocrine stimulation is one of the properties of the bitters, and in some people they can be dramatically effective in lowering blood sugar.

Many other plants have been shown to have experimental hypoglycemic effects to a greater or lesser degree, though the mechanisms are not always clear. The following examples are cited in *Medical Botany* by Walter H. Lewis and Memory P. F. Elvin-Lewis:

black cohosh	dandelion	oats
burdock	fenugreek	peyote
cashew	ginseng	pill-bearing spurge
cayenne	goldenseal	spinach
celery	gravel root	

The challenge for the practitioner in cases of diabetes is the appropriate application of the hypoglycemics. Such remedies can sometimes have a rapid impact on blood sugar levels, but one that varies from patient to patient. Their safe use can only be ensured within a comprehensive diabetes management program that is made for the particular individual. Very close observation must be kept on urine and blood signs, necessitating training of the patient by a skilled practitioner.

Herbal preventive work to avoid the various long-term complications of diabetes may be undertaken quite safely, even if no attempt is made to deal with insulin levels. Attention should be given to the cardiovascular system in particular; heart and vascular tonics are appropriate for long-term use, especially hawthorn, ginkgo, and bilberry.

The Thyroid Gland

The thyroid gland is a butterfly-shaped organ located at the base of the neck, just above the collarbone. The main function of this gland is to produce the iodine-containing hormone thyroxine. Thyroxine acts to control the rate and intensity of most physiologic functions of the body. Heart rate, sweating, digestive action, body temperature, calorie consumption, and many other activities depend in part on this hormone for regulation. The thyroid itself depends on the pituitary gland at the base of the front of the brain for control. Thyroid-stimulating hormone (TSH) from the pituitary is necessary for the thyroid gland to produce thyroxine. Pituitary TSR production is, in turn, dependent upon thyrotropin releasing hormone from the hypothalamus, higher in the brain, for its production. Thus, a complex set of delicate interactions oversees the thyroid's function; many physical and emotional factors can play a role as well.

Hypothyroidism

Hypothyroidism is an underactivity of the thyroid resulting in too little production of thyroid hormone. Although it may be caused by a variety of diseases that affect the hypothalamus and pituitary gland, this condition is due primarily to disorders of the thyroid gland itself. Inadequate secretion of thyroid hormone leads to a general slowing of all physical and mental processes. There is a general depression of most cellular enzyme systems and oxidative processes; metabolic activity of all cells of the body decreases, reducing oxygen consumption, decreasing oxidation of nutrients for energy, and producing less body heat.

The signs and symptoms, all resulting from the slowing of metabolism, range from nonspecific complaints to severe symptoms that may be life threatening if unrecognized and untreated. Fatigue, lack of energy, intolerance of cold temperatures, severe constipation, heavy menstrual periods, and weight gain despite a diminishing appetite may go unnoticed or may be attributed to other conditions such as stress, depression, or overwork. Symptoms worsen and become more obvious with time—the pulse slows; the skin becomes cool, dry, and coarse; muscles ache; there is puffiness around the eyes; hair falls out; the voice becomes hoarse; and the reflexes are sluggish. Changes in mood and personality simulating psychiatric illness may occur. The thyroid gland may enlarge, producing a goiter in the neck.

Orthodox therapy is based upon taking thyroid hormone daily to replace what is not there. Often this must remain the basis of therapy, in which case therapy will aim at helping the body deal with the repercussions of the condition. The use of bitters in mild cases is sometimes enough and in any event is sure to be beneficial. Kelp has been used in the past; although it has much to offer, it is only truly specific where iodine deficiency is present.

A number of important contributions can be made by herbs to support hormone replacement therapy. Hypothyroidism accelerates the onset of atherosclerosis; thus coronary artery disease may occur because of deposits of mucopolysaccharides in the heart muscle. This damage may be lessened through the use of cardiovascular tonics such as hawthorn, ginkgo, and garlic. Problems reflecting functional and structural changes in the skin can be eased, and while this may represent only symptomatic relief, it is essential. Emollients and circulatory stimulants can all find a role, but the specific remedies will depend upon the individual's experience. (Moisturizing is especially important as the skin is usually dry and scaly.)

Relieving some aspects of the symptomatic distress may be achieved herbally. Chronic constipation may be alleviated with laxatives. Hepatic laxatives are the best, as they support liver function; examples include yellow dock and butternut. In extreme cases, strong purgatives (e.g., cascara sagrada or senna) may be called for.

Nervine tonics and other varieties of nervine may be indicated, but avoid the stronger relaxing remedies such as hops and valerian. Antidepressant plants such as St. John's wort and mugwort can be helpful.

Hyperthyroidism

Overactivity of the thyroid gland may be caused by a functioning growth or tumor, such as a benign nodule or cancer, a self-limited inflammation of the gland from a probable viral infection, or Graves' disease (the commonest form). Graves' disease, which appears to be autoimmune in nature, is caused by the production of thyroid antibodies that have a stimulating effect on the gland and give rise to deposits of a thick substance within the skin, behind the eyes, and elsewhere.

Clinical manifestations of hyperthyroidism are the result of an increased metabolic rate, especially excessive body heat, increased neuromuscular and cardiovascular activity, and hyperactivity. For example:

- nervousness, emotional hyperexcitability, irritability, apprehension, sleeplessness
- difficulty in sitting quietly
- rapid pulse at rest as well as on exertion (ranges between 90 and 160); palpitations
- low heat tolerance; profuse perspiration; flushed skin (e.g., hands are warm and moist)
- fine tremor of hands; change in bowel habits (constipation or diarrhea)
- increased appetite and progressive weight loss
- muscle fatigability and weakness; amenorrhea
- bulging eyes (exophthalmos), producing a startled expression

This condition is served by one of the best examples of a specific remedy, bugleweed. It is a useful relaxing nervine but in addition has a sometimes dramatic effect in reducing the symptom picture associated with hyperthyroid conditions. I have seen no figures on thyroxin serum levels in patients using bugleweed and thus cannot say that improvement is due to the herb directly impacting the hormone, but something is definitely going on. The following approach is often effective:

Remedy for Symptoms of Hyperthyroidism

- bugleweed   4 parts
- motherwort   2 parts
- skullcap   2 parts
- hawthorn   1 part

As tincture: take 1 tsp (5 ml) of this mixture three times a day.

As dried herb: infuse 1–2 tsp to a cup and drink three times a day.

For Associated Insomnia

- valerian
- passionflower

Equal parts of tinctures.

Take 1–3 tsp (5–15 ml) thirty minutes before retiring.

12 Herbal Medicine Making

Cowritten with Diana DeLuca

There is nothing mysterious or even particularly clever or skillful about making healing formulations from plants. Intimidated by the pharmaceutical elite, we think that to be of any use a medicine must be made by a Ph.D. wearing a white lab coat, and then packaged with half an acre of rain forest material. Not so! If you can make a cup of tea or cook a simple meal that your family and friends are willing to eat, you are qualified. If this is not the case or if you have lost friends that way, then perhaps start with a simple cookbook.

Various ways of using plants to release and activate their healing properties have developed over the centuries. No doubt, our distant ancestors first used herbs by simply eating the fresh plant. Since then many other methods of preparation have been developed. With our modern knowledge of pharmacology, we can make conscious choices as to which process we use to release the biochemical constituents needed for healing without insulting the integrity of the plant by isolating fractions of the whole. Many excellent herb books now available contain detailed guides to making herbal preparations. (Please see the bibliography for titles we especially recommend.)

The most effective way of using herbs is to take them internally, since it is from within that healing takes place. The ways of preparing internal remedies are numerous, but in all cases it is essential to take care with the process to ensure the desired result. Three kinds of preparations are used for internal consumption: water-based extracts (teas), tinctures, and fresh or dried herbs in pill or capsule form.

Herbal Tea

Water-based extracts are decoctions and infusions. Certain basic rules of thumb may be used to select the method for a particular herb.

Decoction

If the herbs to be used are hard and woody, it is better to make a decoction to ensure that the soluble contents of the herbs actually reach the water. Roots, rhizomes, wood, bark, nuts, and some seeds are hard with very strong cell walls; to ensure that the constituents are transferred to the water, more heat is needed than for infusions, and the herb has to be boiled in the water.

- Place one teaspoonful of dried herb, or three teaspoons of fresh material, for each cup of water into a pot or saucepan. If large quantities are made, use one ounce of dried herb for each one pint of water. The container should be glass, ceramic, or earthenware. (If metal is used, it should be enameled.)
- Add the appropriate amount of water to the herbs.
- Bring to a boil and simmer for the time given for the mixture or specific herb, usually ten to fifteen minutes. If the herb contains volatile oils, put a lid on.
- Strain the tea while still hot.

If preparing a mixture containing soft and woody herbs, prepare an infusion and a decoction separately to insure that the more sensitive herbs are treated accordingly. For a woody herb that is volatile oil rich, it is best to powder finely and then make an infusion, thus ensuring that the oils do not boil away.

Decoctions are necessary if the herb contains any hard or woody material (e.g., roots, bark, or nuts). The denser the plant or the individual cell walls, the more energy will be needed to extract cell content into the tea; this explains the value of decocting. Infusions are most appropriate for nonwoody material such as leaves, flowers, and certain stems.

As with all generalizations, of course, there are exceptions! For example, in the case of a root rich in a volatile oil such as valerian root, the woodiness would suggest decocting, but if the roots are simmered, the therapeutically important volatile oil will boil off.

Infusion

If you know how to make tea, you know how to make an infusion, the simplest method of utilizing both fresh or dried herbs. In recipes that prescribe one part of dried herb, it can be replaced with three parts of the fresh herb, the difference being due to the higher water content of the fresh plant.

- In a china or glass teapot that has been warmed, place about one teaspoonful of the dried herb or herb mixture for each cup of tea.
- For each teaspoonful of herb in the pot, add a cup of boiling water and then put the lid on. Leave to steep for ten to fifteen minutes. Infusions may be drunk hot (normally best for a medicinal herbal tea) or cold. They may be sweetened to taste.

Tea bags can be made by filling little muslin bags with herbal mixtures, taking care to remember how many teaspoonfuls have been put into each bag. These can be used in the same way as ordinary teabags.

Larger quantities can be made in the proportion of one ounce of herb to one pint of water. An infusion is so full of life force that any microorganism entering the brew will multiply and thrive in it. If there is any sign of fermentation or spoilage, the infusion should be discarded. Whenever possible, infusions should be prepared fresh; if an infusion must be kept for any time at all, hold it in a thermos for a few hours or store it, tightly covered, in the refrigerator.

Infusions are best for nonwoody parts of the plant such as leaves, flowers, or green stems, where the substances wanted are easily accessible. If an infusion must be made of bark, root, seeds, or resin, it is best to powder such parts first to break down some of the cell walls and thus make them more accessible to water. Seeds such as fennel and aniseed should be slightly bruised before infusing to release the volatile oils from the cells. Any aromatic herb should be infused in a well-sealed pot to ensure that only a minimum of the volatile oil is lost through evaporation.

If the herbs are sensitive to heat, either because they contain highly volatile oils or because their constituents break down at high temperature, make a cold infusion. The proportion of herb to water is the same, but in this case the infusion should be left for six to twelve hours in a well-sealed pot. When ready, strain and use it.

Many herbs are not only medicines or alternatives to coffee, but in their own right make excellent beverages. Every individual will have his or her favorite herbs, but the following small list of herbs that may be used either singly or in combination offers a selection of popular choices. Selection can be based upon both taste and medicinal properties.

Flowers: chamomile, elder flower, hibiscus, linden blossom, and red clover
Leaves: peppermint, spearmint, lemon balm, rosemary, and lemon verbena
Berries: hawthorn and rose hips
Seeds: aniseed, caraway, celery, dill, and fennel
Roots: licorice

Tincture

Alcohol is a better solvent than water for most plant constituents. Mixtures of alcohol and water dissolve nearly all the ingredients, and the alcohol acts as a preservative. Alcohol preparations are called tinctures (an expression that is occasionally also used for preparations based on glycerin). The method given here is a basic approach; when tinctures are prepared professionally according to descriptions in a pharmacopoeia, specific water/alcohol proportions are used for each herb, but for the herbs described in this book such details are unnecessary.

- Place four ounces of finely chopped or ground dried herb into a container that can be tightly closed. If fresh herbs are used, twice the amount should be taken.
- Pour one pint of 60 proof vodka over the herbs and close tightly.
- Keep the container in a warm but dark place for two weeks and shake it once a day.
- After decanting the bulk of the liquid, pour the residue into a muslin cloth suspended in a bowl.
- Wring out all the liquid. (The residue makes excellent compost!)
- Pour the tincture into a dark bottle. It should be kept well stoppered.

As tinctures are much stronger, volume for volume, than infusions or decoctions, the dosage to be taken is much smaller, depending on the herb to be taken. Tinctures may be used in a variety of ways. They can be taken straight, mixed with water, or they can be added to a cup of hot water. If the latter course is followed, the alcohol will largely evaporate, leaving most of the extract in the water and possibly making the water cloudy, as resins and other constituents not soluble in water will precipitate. A few drops of tincture can be added to a bath or footbath, used in a compress, or mixed with oil and fat to make an ointment. Suppositories and lozenges can also be made using tincture.

Another way of making a kind of alcohol infusion is to infuse herbs in wine. Even though these wine-based preparations do not have the shelf life of tinctures and are not as concentrated, they can be both pleasant to take and effective.

Tinctures based on glycerin have the advantage of being milder on the digestive tract and do not involve the problems associated with alcohol. However, they have the disadvantage of not dissolving resinous or oily materials well. As a solvent, glycerin is generally better than water but not as good as alcohol. To make a glycerin tincture, make up one pint of a mixture consisting of one part glycerin and one part water, add four ounces of the dried ground herb and leave it in a well-stoppered container for two weeks, shaking it daily. After two weeks, strain and press or wring the residue as with alcoholic tinctures. For fresh herbs, which have a greater water content, put eight ounces into a mixture of 75 percent glycerin/25 percent water.

Dry Herb Preparations

There are two advantages to taking herbs in a dry form. Here the taste of the herb can be avoided, and the whole herb (including the woody material) can be taken. Unfortunately, a number of drawbacks are involved as well.

- Dry herbs are unprocessed, and their constituents are not always readily available for easy absorption. During infusion, heat and water help to break down the walls of the plant cells and dissolve the constituents, which is not always guaranteed during the digestive process.
- When the constituents are already dissolved in liquid form, they are available a lot faster and begin their action sooner.
- A subtler drawback lies in the very fact that you do not taste the herb when it is taken in capsule form. For reasons discussed elsewhere (see pages 16 and 216–17) the bitter herbs work best when tasted, as their effects result

from a neurological reflex. When bitters are put into a capsule or a pill, their action may well be lost or diminished.

Taking all these considerations into account, if herbs are to be used in dry form they should be powdered as finely as possible. This step guarantees that the cell walls are largely broken down, which will promote easier digestion and absorption of the herb.

Capsules

A convenient way to use powdered herbs is in gelatin capsules. The size needed depends on the amount of herbs prescribed per dose, the density of the plant, and the volume of the material. A capsule size 00 holds about $\frac{1}{6}$ ounce of finely powdered herb. Filling a capsule is easy:

- Place the powdered herbs in a flat dish and separate the halves of the capsule.
- Move the halves of the capsules through the powder, filling them in the process.
- Push the halves together.

Pills

There are several ways to make pills, depending on your degree of technical skill. The simplest way to take an unpleasant remedy is to roll the powder into a small pill using fresh bread, a method that works most effectively with herbs such as goldenseal or cayenne.

Formulations for the Skin

Absorption of herbal compounds can occur through the skin, and a range of methods have been developed that take advantage of this fact.

The Bath

The most pleasant way of absorbing herbal compounds through the skin is by taking a full bath with one pint of infusion or decoction added to the water. Alternatively, you can also take a foot or hand bath, in which case you would use the preparations in undiluted form. Any herb that can be taken internally can also be used in a bath. Herbs can, of course, also be used to give the bath an excellent fragrance. To give some idea of herbs that are particularly good to use for a bath that is relaxing and at the same time exquisitely scented, infusions can be made of:

elder flower	lemon balm
lavender flowers	rosemary leaves

For a bath that will bring about a restful and healing sleep, add an infusion of one of the following to the bath water. Bear in mind that although hops and valerian are very effective, they have strong aromas that may not be appealing.

cowslip	hops	valerian
cramp bark	linden blossom	

In feverish conditions or to help the circulation, stimulating and diaphoretic herbs can be used, including:

cayenne	mustard	yarrow
ginger	rosemary	

Try other possibilities for yourself. Ideas can be found in books about aromatherapy, a healing system based on the external application of herbs in the form of essential oils. These oils can also be used in baths by putting a few drops of oil into the bath water.

Instead of preparing an infusion of the herb beforehand, a handful of it can also be placed in a muslin bag, which is suspended from the hot water tap so that the water flows through it as the bath is filling. In this way, a very fresh infusion can be made.

An Invigorating Bath Mixture

- sage
- bay
- ginger
- eucalyptus
- peppermint
- rosemary

Equal parts of dried herbs.

A Relaxing Bath Mixture

- lavender
- roses
- chamomile
- hops

Equal parts of dried herbs.

The above blends may be infused in vegetable oil (almond, canola, etc.) for 1 week, or essential oils may be used, diluted as directed below. Use caution with the following essential oils, which can burn and irritate the skin: mints, basil, citrus, lemongrass, cinnamon, thyme.

Bath Oils

- 2 oz vegetable oil
- 2–10 drops of an appropriate essential oil

Mix well and add 1–2 tsp per tub.

Bath salts add trace minerals to the bath, soften the water, and gently cleanse the skin.

Bath Salts I

- 1 cup borax (sodium borate)
- 1 cup epsom salts (magnesium sulfate)
- 1/2 cup sea salt (sodium chloride)
- essential oil (lavender, rose geranium, and blue chamomile are soothing, relaxing, and balancing as are sandalwood, ylang ylang, and clary sage; rosemary and bergamot are more stimulating.)

Bath Salts II

borax	2 cups
sea salt	2 tbsp
white clay	2 tbsp
essential oils (see Bath Salts I, above)	

Compress

This is an excellent and simple way to apply a remedy to the skin. Compresses are used to treat insect bites, sprains, bruises, and swellings.

- Soak a clean linen or cotton cloth in hot herbal tea and apply to the affected part; use as hot as can be tolerated.
- Cover with a towel to hold in the heat.
- When cool, replace with another towel.
- For a cold compress, use the same method but with cool tea.

The Herbal Douche

Another method of using herbs externally is a douche, the application of herbs in water to the vagina; this method is particularly indicated for local infections.

- Prepare a new infusion or decoction for each douche.
- Allow the tea to cool to a temperature that will be comfortable internally.
- Pour into the container of a douche bag and insert applicator.
- Allow the liquid to rinse the inside of the vagina.

Note that the liquid will run out of the vagina, thus it is easiest to douche sitting on the toilet. It is not necessary to actively hold in the liquid. In most conditions that indicate a need for douching, it is advisable to use the tea undiluted three times daily for a number of days. If a three- to seven-day course of douching (as well as taking the appropriate internal herbal remedies) has not noticeably improved a vaginal infection, see a qualified practitioner for a diagnosis.

Liniments

Liniments are used in massages that aim at the stimulation of muscles and ligaments. They must only be used externally, never internally. To carry the herbal components to the muscles and ligaments, liniments are usually made of a mixture of herbs with alcohol or occasionally with apple cider vinegar, sometimes with the addition of herbal oils. The common ingredient of such a liniment is cayenne, which may be combined with lobelia or other remedies. A representative selection is given in the musculoskeletal section (pages 177–81). The following liniment is described by Jethro Kloss in his classic work *Back to Eden*.

Kloss Liniment

- 2 oz powdered myrrh
- 1 oz powdered goldenseal (optional)
- $^1/_2$ oz cayenne pepper
- 1 qt rubbing alcohol (70 percent)

Mix together and let stand 7 days. Shake well every day, decant off, and bottle in corked bottles.

Oils

Herbal oils can be used topically for massage, in a bath, or to moisturize the skin. They can be used in two forms, depending on the degree of sophistication of the extraction technique.

- Pure essential oils are extracted from the herb by a complex and careful process of distillation. These oils are best obtained from specialist suppliers who distill them for aromatherapy and take care that they are as pure as possible.
- A much simpler method resembles cold infusions. Instead of infusing the herb in water, it is put into an oil, thus obtaining a solution of the plant's essential oil in the oil base. The best oils for this purpose are vegetable oils such as olive, sunflower, or almond oil.

A Simple Herbal Oil

Chop about 1 oz of herb finely, cover with oil, and place in a clear glass container. Place in the sun or leave in a warm place for 2 to 3 weeks, shaking the container daily.

After that time, filter the liquid into a dark glass container and store the extracted oil.

St. John's Wort Oil

Pick about 1 oz of flowers when they are just opened and crush in a teaspoon of olive oil.

Cover with more oil, mix well, and put in a glass container in the sun or a warm place for 3 to 6 weeks, at the end of which the oil will be bright red. Press the mixture through a cloth to filter all the oil and let this stand. The water in the liquid will settle on the bottom, so decant oil from the top.

Store the oil in a well-sealed dark container.

Ointments

Ointments are semisolid preparations that can be applied to the skin. Depending on the purpose for which they are designed, ointments can vary in texture from very greasy ones to those made into a thick paste, depending on what base is used and what compounds are mixed together. Any herb can be used for making ointments, but particularly valuable for use in external healing mixtures are the following:

arnica	elder flower	plantain
calendula	eucalyptus	slippery elm bark
chickweed	goldenseal	thyme
comfrey	lady's mantle	woundwort
cucumber	marshmallow	yarrow

A simple way to prepare an ointment is by using petroleum jelly as a base. Although this has the disadvantage of being an inorganic base, it is easy to handle so a simple ointment can be made very quickly. For vegetable-based alternatives, try beeswax and olive oil. The basic method for such an ointment is to simmer two tablespoonfuls of herb in seven ounces of petroleum jelly for about ten minutes. A single herb, a mixture, fresh or dried herbs, roots, leaves, or flowers can be used.

A Simple Calendula Ointment

- 7 oz petroleum jelly
- 2 oz (a handful) freshly picked calendula flowers

Melt petroleum jelly over low heat. Add calendula. Bring the mixture to a boil and simmer very gently for about 10 minutes, stirring well. Sift it through fine gauze and press out all the liquid from the flowers. Pour the liquid into a container and seal after it has cooled.

Poultice

This more active topical method uses fresh or dried plants rather than a liquid form. A poultice is used on skin eruptions, boils, abscesses, cuts, and cysts.

- Mash or crush fresh plant material and mix with a small amount of boiling water to form a paste, or crush dried herb to powder and mix with hot water to form a paste.
- Apply directly to the skin as hot as possible and hold it in place with gauze.
- If using stimulating herbs such as mustard, apply between two layers of cloth to protect the skin from excessive irritation.

Suppositories

Suppositories are designed to facilitate the insertion of remedies into the orifices of the body. They can be shaped to be used in the nose or ears but are most commonly used for rectal or vaginal problems. They act as carriers for any herb that is appropriate to use; there are three general categories of such herbs:

1. herbs that act to soothe the mucous membranes, reduce inflammation, and aid the healing process, such as the root and leaf of comfrey, the root of marshmallow and goldenseal, and the bark of slippery elm

2. astringent herbs that can help in the reduction of discharge or in the treatment of hemorrhoids, such as periwinkle, pilewort, plantain, witch hazel, and yellow dock

3. remedies to stimulate intestinal peristalsis and so overcome chronic constipation (the laxatives)

It will often be appropriate in any of these three categories to include one of the antimicrobial herbs.

A number of different bases may be used, keeping in mind that the suppository has to be firm enough to be inserted into the orifice, yet be able to melt at body temperature once inserted to liberate the herbs it contains. The herbs should be distributed uniformly in the base—a point that is particularly important when using a powdered herb. The simplest form of preparing suppositories this way calls for gelatin and glycerin and either an infusion, a decoction, or a tincture, in the following proportions:

> ■ gelatin   10 parts
> ■ water (or infusion,
>   decoction, tincture)   40 parts
> ■ glycerin   15 parts
>
> Soak the gelatin in the liquid and gently heat to dissolve.
> Add the glycerin and heat the mixture over a water bath
> (double boiler) to evaporate the water, as the final consistency
> desired depends on how much water is removed. If it is
> removed completely, a very firm consistency will be achieved.

A mold to shape the suppository can be made very simply by shaping aluminium foil into the dimensions desired. The best shape is a torpedo-like, one-inch-long suppository. Pour the molten base into the mold and allow to cool. Store the suppositories in their molds in a refrigerator. It is best to make them as needed.

Facial Care

The following blend can be used as a tea for washing the face or for a facial steam. Herbal facial steam soothes muscles, increases circulation and color, softens the skin, and opens pores.

Facial Steam

- chamomile   1 part
- roses   1 part
- lavender   1 part
- comfrey   1 part
- lemon verbena   1 part
- calendula   1 part

Pour 2 cups of boiling water over a heaping tablespoon of herbs, cover, and steep for 3 to 5 minutes. After washing or scrubbing your face, tie hair back and put a bath towel over your head. Uncover the bowl, close your eyes, place your face over the bowl, and tuck the towel in like a tent. Steam for 5 minutes. You can take breaths by opening the towel.

Facial Scrub

- $1/3$ cup almonds
- 1 cup oats
- 1 cup clay
- 2 tbsp each ground roses and lavender
- optional: calendula, peppermint, comfrey leaf, chamomile

Grind almonds, oats, and herbs in a coffee grinder and add clay. This scrub can be stored dry in a container and mixed as needed with rosewater, tap water, and/or honey; massage on face and rinse. The face is now ready for a facial steam.

Lip Balm

- $1/2$ cup oil (almond, apricot, canola)
- 3 tbsp grated beeswax
- $1/2$ tsp vitamin E oil
- 1 tbsp honey
- natural flavoring: try a few drops of orange oil, spearmint oil, or anise oil

Melt beeswax and almond oil gently over low heat until wax is just melted.

Cool slightly; add vitamin E oil, honey, and flavor (optional). The balm will harden as it cools. To make an excellent ointment, steep herbs in the oil first and strain off before following recipe. (Add a little extra beeswax.)

Moisturizing Cream

- 1 tbsp grated beeswax, packed
- 2 tbsp coconut oil
- $^{1}/_{4}$ cup almond oil (or calendula oil)

Melt the oils gently over very low heat, just until wax melts. Cool in refrigerator until edges begin to congeal. Meanwhile, have ready in a blender $^{1}/_{2}$ cup rosewater or orange flower water, 2 tbsp aloe vera juice or gel, $^{1}/_{4}$ tsp vitamin E oil, 10 drops or so essential oil (lavender, geranium, or lemon is nice; a drop or so of peppermint makes a wonderful, refreshing foot cream!). When the oils have cooled, set blender on high and add the oils slowly in a steady stream (as if you were making mayonnaise). Scrape out all of the oil/wax mixture with a spatula. Store in a cool place.

Hair Care

Herbs provide delightful ingredients for easy-to-make hair care products that not only have cosmetic value but also provide gentle medicinal actions.

An Herbal Shampoo

- 4 oz unscented shampoo
- $^{1}/_{2}$ cup herbal mixture, according to shade of hair (see below)
- $^{1}/_{2}$ tsp rosemary oil
- $^{1}/_{2}$ tsp lavender oil

Shake ingredients together well in a plastic bottle.

Herbal Hair Rinse

Place herbal mixture (see below) in large glass jar and cover with apple cider vinegar.

Put lid on and let sit in a warm place for two weeks, then strain.

Place $^{1}/_{4}$ cup of this solution in 1 qt warm water and use as a last rinse after shampooing followed by plain water.

The following preparations will accentuate the natural colors of your hair.

Herbal Mixture for Dark Hair

- sage
- nettle
- rosemary
- cloves
- comfrey

Equal parts of dried herbs.

Infuse as tea and allow to cool.

Herbal Mixture for Light Hair

■ chamomile	2 parts
■ calendula	1 part
■ comfrey	1 part
■ safflower	1 part
■ yarrow	1 part

Infuse as tea and allow to cool.

13 Materia Medica

The potential materia medica available to us is the whole wonderful flora of our planet. The plants described on the following pages are relatively few in number, but they have been chosen as a representative core of herbs suitable for treating ailments relating to an older population. More extensive information about these herbs (and many others) can be found in the books listed in the bibliography.

The herbs listed here are all described according to a basic outline:

Common Name

Botanical (Latin) Name

Part Used: The part or parts of the herb used medicinally.

Actions: A listing of the physiological actions demonstrated by the herb. (These are explained in the opening chapter; see pages 15–18.)

Indications: A brief overview of the clinical indications of the herb, reflecting the training and experience of the writer. As there is so much variability among both people and plants, the indications given in herbals can rarely be all-encompassing. If there is material that you disagree with, please use that as an area for further research and personal insight. Always question authority!

Preparation and Dosage: The dosage range appropriate for older adults is listed. The older or frailer the person, the lower the dosage to be used.

Agrimony

Agrimonia eupatoria

Part Used: Dried aerial parts.

Actions: Astringent, bitter tonic, diuretic, vulnerary, antispasmodic, diaphoretic, carminative, hepatic, cholagogue.

Indications: Agrimony is a gently stimulating digestive system tonic. The combination of astringency and bitter tonic properties makes agrimony a valuable remedy, especially when astringency is needed in the digestive system, as it will also act as a tonic due to the bitter stimulation of digestive and liver secretions. It has a role in the treatment of colitis and other inflammatory conditions of the intestines. Used in cases of indigestion, it has a long tradition as a spring tonic. It may also be used to treat urinary incontinence and cystitis. As a gargle, it relieves sore throats and laryngitis. As an ointment, it will speed the healing of wounds and bruises.

Preparation and Dosage: An infusion is made from 1–2 teaspoonfuls of the dried herb and drunk three times a day. Tincture dosage is 1–2 milliliters three times a day.

Angelica

Angelica archangelica

Part Used: Roots and leaves are used medicinally, while the stems and seeds are used in confectionery.

Actions: Astringent, tonic, diuretic, vulnerary, cholagogue, anti-inflammatory.

Indications: This herb is a gentle expectorant for coughs, bronchitis, and pleurisy, especially when they are accompanied by fever, colds, or influenza. Angelica contains carminative essential oil, which explains its effectiveness in easing colic and flatulence. As a digestive agent, it stimulates appetite and may be used in the treatment of anorexia nervosa. It has been shown to help ease rheumatic inflammations. In cystitis it acts as a urinary antiseptic. Angelica is used frequently as a flavoring in liqueurs (e.g., chartreuse and benedictine) and in gin and vermouth; the leaves are used as a garnish or in salads; the candied stalks in cakes and puddings.

Preparation and Dosage: A decoction is made from 1 teaspoonful of the dried herb and drunk three times a day. Tincture dosage is 1–2 milliliters three times a day.

Aniseed

Pimpinella anisum

Part Used: Dried fruit.

Actions: Expectorant antispasmodic, carminative, antimicrobial, aromatic, galactogogue.

Indications: The aromatic oil in aniseed is the basis for its internal use to ease intestinal colic and flatulence. It also has an expectorant and antispasmodic action and may be used in cases of bronchitis whenever there is a persistent irritable cough as well as for whooping cough. The oil may be used externally in an ointment base for the treatment of scabies. By itself, the oil will help in the control of lice. It has been used in folk medicine to increase milk secretion, facilitate birth, and increase libido.

Preparation and Dosage: The seeds should be gently crushed just before use to release the volatile oils. An infusion is made from 1 teaspoonful of the seeds and drunk three times daily. To treat flatulence, the tea should be drunk slowly before meals.

Arnica

Arnica montana

Part Used: Flower heads.

Actions: Anti-inflammatory, vulnerary.

Indications: Although this herb should not be taken internally, as it is potentially toxic, it provides us with one of the best remedies for external local healing and may be considered a specific remedy when it comes to the treatment of bruises and sprains. The *homeopathic* preparation is entirely safe to take internally, especially when taken according to homeopathic directions. Used externally, the herb relieves muscular rheumatic pain and the pain and inflammation of phlebitis. It may be used wherever there is pain or inflammation on the skin, as long as the skin is not broken.

Preparation and Dosage: Arnica can be applied to unbroken skin as needed. You can prepare your own tincture of this herb as follows: pour 1 pint of 70 percent alcohol over 2 ounces freshly picked flowers. Seal tightly in a clear glass container and let stand for at least one week in the sun or in a warm place. Once filtered, it is ready for use. Store in a sealed container and protect from direct sunlight.

Astragalus

Astragalus membranaceus

Part Used: Root.

Action: Immunomodulator.

Indications: Used since ancient times in traditional Chinese medicine, astragalus has become an important remedy in the West ever since its effects upon the immune system came to light. As immunological research has focused on medicinal herbs, a whole new array of effects are being discovered. The polysaccharides contained in astragalus have been shown to intensify the activity of certain white blood cells, stimulate pituitary-adrenal cortical activity, and restore depleted red blood cell formation in bone marrow. Astragalus is also one of the herbs known to stimulate the body's natural production of interferon. The conclusion drawn by many Western herbalists is that astragalus is an ideal remedy for any one who might be immunocompromised in any way, from someone who easily catches cold to someone with cancer.

Preparation and Dosage: A decoction is made from 1–2 teaspoonfuls of the root and drunk three times a day. Tincture dosage is 2 milliliters three times a day.

Balm (Lemon Balm)

Melissa officinalis

Part Used: Dried aerial parts, or fresh in season.

Actions: Carminative, nervine, antispasmodic, antidepressive, diaphoretic, antimicrobial, hepatic.

Indications: Balm is an excellent carminative herb that relieves spasms in the digestive tract and is used in flatulent dyspepsia. Because of its mild antidepressive properties, it is primarily indicated where there is dyspepsia associated with anxiety or depression, as the gently sedative oils relieve tension and stress reactions, thus acting to lighten depression. The volatile oil appears to act on the interface between the digestive tract and nervous system. It has been described by some herbalists as being restorative to the nervous system, similar in some ways to oats. It may be used in migraine associated with tension; neuralgia; anxiety-induced palpitations; and insomnia. Balm has a tonic effect on the heart and circulatory system, causing mild vasodilation of the peripheral vessels and thus acting to lower blood pressure. It can be used in feverish conditions such as influenza. Hot-water extracts have antiviral properties, possibly due in part to the presence of rosmarinic acid and other polyphenolics. A lotion-based extract may be used for skin lesions of herpes simplex, its antiviral activity having been confirmed in both laboratory and clinical trials.

Preparation and Dosage: An infusion is made from 2–3 teaspoonfuls of the dried herb or 4 or 5 leaves of the fresh. A cup of this tea should be taken in the morning and the evening, or when needed. Tincture dosage is 2–4 milliliters three times a day.

Balmony

Chelone glabra

Part Used: Dried aerial parts.

Actions: Cholagogue, hepatic, antiemetic, stimulant, laxative.

Indications: Balmony is an excellent agent for liver problems. It acts as a tonic on the whole digestive and absorptive system. It has a stimulating effect on the secretion of digestive juices, and in this most natural way its laxative properties are produced. Balmony is used in cases of gallstones, inflammation of the gallbladder, and jaundice. It stimulates the appetite, eases colic, dyspepsia, and biliousness, and is helpful in debility. Externally it has been used on inflamed breasts, painful ulcers, and piles. It is considered a specific remedy in gallstones that lead to congestive jaundice. Suitable for both children and the elderly, especially for gastrointestinal disturbances after prolonged illness.

Preparation and Dosage: An infusion is made from 1–2 teaspoonfuls of the dried herb and drunk three times a day. Tincture dosage is 1–2 milliliters three times a day.

Bayberry

Myrica cerifera

Part Used: Bark of root.

Actions: Astringent, circulatory stimulant, diaphoretic.

Indications: As a circulatory stimulant, bayberry plays a role in many conditions when they are approached in a holistic way. Due to its specific actions, it is a valuable astringent in diarrhea and dysentery. It is indicated in mucous colitis. As a gargle it helps sore throats, it may be applied locally to bleeding gums, and used as a douche it can help in leukorrhea. It may be used in the treatment of colds and feverish conditions.

Preparation and Dosage: A decoction is made from 1 teaspoonful of the bark and drunk three times a day. Tincture dosage is 1–2 milliliters three times a day.

Bearberry *(Uva-Ursi)*

Arctostaphylos uva-ursi

Part Used: Leaves.

Actions: Diuretic, astringent, antimicrobial, demulcent.

Indications: Uva-ursi has a specific antiseptic and astringent effect upon the membranes of the urinary system, and it will generally soothe, tone, and strengthen them. It is specifically used where there is gravel or ulceration in the kidney or bladder. It may also be used in the treatment of infections such as pyelitis and cystitis or as part of a holistic approach to more chronic kidney problems. It has a useful role to play in the treatment of gravel or calculus in the kidney. Because of its high astringency, it is used in some bed-wetting remedies. Prepared as a douche, it may be helpful in vaginal ulceration and infection.

Preparation and Dosage: An infusion is made from 1–2 teaspoonfuls of the dried herb and drunk three times a day. Tincture dosage is 1–2 milliliters three times a day.

Birch

Betula alba

Part Used: Leaves and bark.

Actions: Diuretic, anti-inflammatory, antiseptic, tonic.

Indications: Birch leaves act as an effective remedy for cystitis and other infections of the urinary system as well as removing excess water from the body. Perhaps because of this cleansing diuretic activity, the plant has been used for gout, rheumatism, and mild arthritic pain. The bark will ease muscle pain if it is applied externally, with the fresh, wet internal side of the bark placed against the skin.

Preparation and Dosage: An infusion is made from 1–2 teaspoonfuls of the dried herb and drunk three times a day. Tincture dosage is 1–2 milliliters three times a day.

Black Catechu

Acacia catechu

Part Used: Extract from leaves and young shoots.

Actions: Astringent.

Indications: The powerful astringent may be used in chronic diarrhea, dysentery, and chronic catarrh. Useful for arresting excessive mucous discharges and checking hemorrhages, it is also recommended as a local application for sore mouths and gums. In practice, however, there are many other effective hypotensives that do not have the potential problem of constipation.

Preparation and Dosage: An infusion is made from 0.3–2.0 grams of the dried herb and drunk twice a day. The tincture is 1:5 in 45 percent alcohol at a dose of between 2.5 and 5 milliliters and is drunk twice a day.

Black Cohosh

Cimicifuga racemosa

Part Used: Root and rhizome; dried, not fresh.

Actions: Emmenagogue, antispasmodic, alterative, nervine, hypotensive.

Indications: Black cohosh is a most valuable herb with a powerful action as a relaxant and a normalizer of the female reproductive system. It may be used beneficially in cases of painful or delayed menstruation. Ovarian cramps or cramping pain in the womb will be relieved by black cohosh. It is very active in the treatment of rheumatic pains, but also in rheumatoid arthritis, osteoarthritis, and in muscular and neurological pain. It finds use also in the treatment of sciatica and neuralgia. It may be used in many situations where a relaxing nervine is needed, and it has been found beneficial in cases of tinnitus.

Preparation and Dosage: A decoction is made from ½–1 teaspoonful of the root and drunk three times a day. Tincture dosage is 1–2 milliliters three times a day.

Black Haw

Viburnum prunifolium

Part Used: Dried bark of root, stem, or trunk.

Actions: Antispasmodic, nervine, hypotensive, astringent.

Indications: Black haw has a very similar use to cramp bark, to which it is closely related. It is an effective relaxant of the uterus and is used for dysmenorrhea, false labor pains, and threatened miscarriage. Its relaxant and sedative actions explain its power in reducing blood pressure in hypertension, which happens through a relaxation of the peripheral blood vessels. It may be used as an antispasmodic in the treatment of asthma.

Preparation and Dosage: A decoction is made from 2–3 teaspoonfuls of the dried bark and drunk three times a day. Tincture dosage is 5 milliliters three times a day.

Black Root

Leptandra virginica

Part Used: Rhizome and root.

Actions: Cholagogue, hepatic, laxative, diaphoretic, antispasmodic.

Indications: Black root is used as a reliever of liver congestion and inflammation of the gallbladder. Chronic constipation can often be due to a liver dysfunction, in which case this herb is also ideal.

Preparation and Dosage: A decoction is made from 1–2 teaspoonfuls of the dried herb and drunk three times a day. Tincture dosage is 1–2 milliliters three times a day.

Bladderwrack

Fucus vesiculosus

Part Used: Whole plant.

Actions: Antihypothyroid, antirheumatic.

Indications: Bladderwrack has proved most useful in the treatment of underactive thyroid glands and goiter. Through the regulation of thyroid function, there is an improvement in all the associated symptoms. Where obesity is associated with thyroid trouble, this herb may be very helpful in promoting weight loss. It has a reputation in helping the relief of rheumatism and rheumatoid arthritis, both used internally and as an external application upon inflamed joints.

Preparation and Dosage: Bladderwrack may usefully be taken in tablet form as a dietary supplement or prepared as an infusion from 2–3 teaspoonfuls of the dried herb and drunk three times a day. (The tablets taste better!)

Bloodroot

Sanguinaria canadensis

Part Used: Dried rhizome.

Actions: Expectorant, antispasmodic, emetic, cathartic, nervine, cardioactive, topical irritant.

Indications: Bloodroot finds its main use in the treatment of bronchitis. While the stimulating properties show in its power as an emetic and expectorant, it demonstrates a relaxing action on the bronchial muscles and thus has a role in the treatment of asthma, croup, and also laryngitis. However, by far the most important contribution Sanguinaria has to make is in chronic congestive conditions of the lungs, including chronic bronchitis, emphysema, and bronchiectasis. It acts as a stimulant in cases of deficient peripheral circulation. It may be used as a snuff in the treatment of nasal polyps.

Preparation and Dosage: A decoction is made from 1 teaspoonful of the dried rhizome and drunk three times a day. Tincture dosage is 0.5–1 milliliter three times a day.

CAUTION: Do not exceed dosage because of potential toxicity.

Blue Cohosh

Caulophyllum thalictroides

Part Used: Root and rhizome.

Actions: Uterine tonic, emmenagogue, antispasmodic, antirheumatic, diuretic.

Indications: An excellent uterine tonic that may be used in any situation where there is a weakness or loss of tone. It may be used at any time during pregnancy if there is a threat of miscarriage. Similarly, because of its antispasmodic action, it will ease false labor pains and dysmenorrhea. However, when labor does ensue, the use of blue cohosh just before birth will help ensure an easy delivery. In all these cases, it is a safe herb to use. As an emmenagogue, it can be used to bring on delayed or suppressed menstruation while ensuring that any accompanying pain is relieved. Blue cohosh may be used in cases where an antispasmodic is needed, such as colic, asthma, or nervous coughs. It has a reputation for easing rheumatic pain.

Preparation and Dosage: A decoction is made from 1 teaspoonful of the dried root and drunk three times a day. Tincture dosage is 1–2 milliliters three times a day.

Bogbean (Buckbean)

Menyanthes trifoliata

Part Used: Leaves.

Actions: Bitter, diuretic, cholagogue, antirheumatic.

Indications: Bogbean is a most useful herb for the treatment of rheumatism, osteoarthritis, and rheumatoid arthritis. It has a stimulating effect upon the walls of the colon and thus acts as an aperient (laxative), so that it should not be used for rheumatism if colitis or diarrhea are present. It has a marked stimulating action on the digestive juices and on bile flow and so will aid in debilitated states that are due to sluggish digestion, indigestion, and problems of the liver and gallbladder.

Preparation and Dosage: An infusion is made from 1–2 teaspoonfuls of the dried herb and drunk three times a day. Tincture dosage is 1–2 milliliters three times a day.

Boldo

Peumus boldo

Part Used: Dried leaves.

Actions: Cholagogue, hepatic, diuretic.

Indications: Boldo is a specific remedy for gallbladder problems (stones or inflammations). It is also used when there is visceral pain due to other problems in the liver or gallbladder. Boldo has mild urinary demulcent and antiseptic properties and so could be used in cystitis.

Preparation and Dosage: An infusion is made from 1 teaspoonful of the dried herb and drunk three times a day. Tincture dosage is 1–2 milliliters three times a day.

Boneset

Eupatorium perfoliatum

Part Used: Dried aerial parts.

Actions: Diaphoretic, bitter, laxative, tonic, antispasmodic, carminative, astringent.

Indications: Boneset is one of the best remedies for the relief of the associated symptoms that accompany influenza. It will speedily relieve aches and pains as well as aid the body in dealing with fever. Boneset may also be used to help clear the upper respiratory tract of mucus. Its mild aperient activity will ease constipation. It may safely be used for any fever and also as a general cleansing agent. It may provide symptomatic aid in the treatment of muscular rheumatism.

Preparation and Dosage: An infusion is made from 1–2 teaspoonfuls of the dried herb and drunk three times a day. In cases of fever or flu, it should be drunk every half hour. Tincture dosage is 1–2 milliliters three times a day.

Buchu

Barosma betulina

Part Used: Leaves.

Actions: Diuretic, urinary antiseptic.

Indications: Buchu may be used in any infection of the genitourinary system, such as cystitis, urethritis, or prostatitis. Its healing and soothing properties are especially useful where dysuria is part of the symptom picture. The oil content may be too irritating for people with a history of serious kidney disease.

Preparation and Dosage: An infusion is made from 1–2 teaspoonfuls of the dried herb and drunk three times a day. Tincture dosage is 1–2 milliliters three times a day.

Bugleweed

Lycopus virginicus

Part Used: Aerial parts.

Actions: Diuretic, peripheral vasoconstrictor, astringent, nervine, antitussive.

Indications. Bugleweed is a specific remedy for overactive thyroid glands, especially where the symptoms include tightness of breathing, palpitations, and shaking. It may safely be used where palpitations of nervous origin occur. Bugleweed will aid the weak heart where there is an associated buildup of water in the body. As a sedative cough reliever, it eases irritating coughs, especially those of nervous origin.

Preparation and Dosage: An infusion is made from 1–2 teaspoonfuls of the dried herb and drunk three times a day. Tincture dosage is 1–2 milliliters three times a day.

Burdock

Arctium lappa

Part Used: Roots and rhizome.

Actions: Alterative, diuretic, bitter.

Indications: Burdock is a most valuable remedy for the treatment of skin conditions that result in dry and scaly skin. It may be most effective for psoriasis if used over a long period of time. It will be useful as part of a wider treatment for rheumatic complaints, especially those associated with psoriasis. Part of the action of this herb is through the bitter stimulation of the digestive juices and especially of bile secretion. Thus it will promote digestion and appetite. It has been used in anorexia nervosa and similar conditions, as well as to aid kidney function and to heal cystitis. In general, burdock will move the body to a state of integration and health, removing such indicators of systemic imbalance as skin problems and dandruff. Externally it may be used as a compress or poultice to speed up the healing of wounds and ulcers. Eczema and psoriasis may also be treated this way externally, but it must be remembered that such skin problems can only be healed from within and with the aid of internal remedies.

Preparation and Dosage: A decoction is made from 1 teaspoonful of the dried root and drunk three times a day. Tincture dosage is 1–2 milliliters three times a day.

Calendula

Calendula officinalis

Part Used: Petals, flower heads.

Actions: Anti-inflammatory, antispasmodic, lymphatic, astringent, vulnerary, emmenagogue, antimicrobial.

Indications: Calendula is one of the best herbs for treating local skin problems. It may be used safely for all cases of skin inflammation, whether due to infection or physical damage. It may be used for any external bleeding or wound, bruise, or strains. It will also be of benefit in slow-healing wounds and skin ulcers and is ideal for first-aid treatment of minor burns and scalds. Local treatments may be in lotion, poultice, or compress form, as appropriate. Internally it acts as a valuable herb for digestive inflammation and thus may be used in the treatment of gastric and duodenal ulcers. As a cholagogue, it will aid in the relief of gallbladder problems and through this process can also help many of the vague digestive complaints that go under the term *indigestion*. Calendula has marked antifungal activity and may be used both internally and externally to combat such infections. As an emmenagogue, it has a reputation of helping delayed menstruation and painful periods. It is in general a normalizer of the menstrual process.

Preparation and Dosage: An infusion is made from 1–2 teaspoonfuls of the dried herb and drunk three times a day. Tincture dosage is 1–2 milliliters three times a day. External use as a lotion or ointment for cuts, bruises, diaper rash, sore nipples, and burns.

California Poppy

Eschscholzia californica

Part Used: Dried aerial parts.

Actions: Nervine, hypnotic, antispasmodic, anodyne.

Indications: California poppy has the reputation of being a nonaddictive alternative to the opium poppy, though it is less powerful. It has been used as a sedative and hypnotic for children suffering from overexcitability and sleeplessness. It can be used wherever an antispasmodic remedy is required. The Native Americans used it for colic pains, and it may be useful in the treatment of gallbladder colic.

Preparation and Dosage: An infusion is made from 1–2 teaspoonfuls of the dried herb and drunk three times a day. A cup should be drunk at night to promote restful sleep. Tincture dosage is 1–4 milliliters three times a day.

Caraway

Carum carvi

Part Used: Seeds.

Actions: Carminative, antispasmodic, expectorant, emmenagogue, galactogogue, astringent, antimicrobial.

Indications: Caraway is used as a calming herb to ease flatulent dyspepsia and intestinal colic, especially in children. It will stimulate the appetite. Its astringency will help in the treatment of diarrhea, and it can be used in laryngitis as a gargle as well as in cases of bronchitis and bronchial asthma. Its antispasmodic actions help in the relief of menstrual pain. It has been used to increase milk flow in nursing mothers.

Preparation and Dosage: An infusion is made from 1 teaspoonful of the freshly crushed seeds and drunk three times a day. Tincture dosage is 1–2 milliliters three times a day.

Cascara Sagrada

Rhamnus purshiana

Part Used: Dried bark.

Actions: Laxative, hepatic, bitter.

Indications: Cascara sagrada may be used in chronic constipation. It encourages peristalsis and tones relaxed muscles of the digestive system.

Preparation and Dosage: A decoction is made from 1–2 teaspoonfuls of the bark and drunk at bedtime. Tincture dosage is 0.5–1 milliliter twice a day.

Cayenne

Capsicum frutescens

Part Used: Fruit.

Actions: Stimulant, carminative, anticatarrhal, sialagogue, rubefacient, antimicrobial.

Indications: Cayenne is the most useful of the systemic stimulants. It stimulates blood flow, strengthening the heart, arteries, capillaries, and nerves. A general tonic, it is also specific for both the circulatory system and the digestive system. It may be used in flatulent dyspepsia and colic. Cayenne may help if there is insufficient peripheral circulation, leading to cold hands and feet and possibly chilblains; it is also used for debility and for warding off colds. Externally it is used as a rubefacient in lumbago and rheumatic pains. As an ointment, it can help unbroken chilblains but must be used in moderation as it can cause a burning sensation to the skin! As a gargle for laryngitis, it combines well with myrrh. (This combination also makes a good antiseptic wash.)

Preparation and Dosage: An infusion is made from $\frac{1}{2}$–1 teaspoonful of cayenne. A tablespoonful of this infusion should be mixed with hot water and drunk when needed. Tincture dosage is 0.25–1 milliliter three times a day or when needed.

Celery Seed

Apium graveolens

Part Used: Dried ripe fruit.

Actions: Antirheumatic, anti-inflammatory, diuretic, carminative, antispasmodic, nervine.

Indications: Celery seeds are mainly used in the treatment of muscular rheumatism and arthritis. Their diuretic action is obviously involved in rheumatic conditions, but they are also used as a urinary antiseptic, largely because of the volatile oil apiol.

Preparation and Dosage: An infusion is made from 1–2 teaspoonfuls of the freshly crushed seeds and drunk three times a day. Tincture dosage is 1–2 milliliters three times a day.

Chamomile

Matricaria recutita

Part Used: Flowering tops.

Actions: Nervine, antispasmodic, carminative, anti-inflammatory, antimicrobial, bitter, vulnerary.

Indications: A comprehensive list of the medical uses of chamomile would include insomnia, anxiety, menopausal depression, loss of appetite, dyspepsia, diarrhea, colic, aches and pains of flu, migraine, neuralgia, teething, vertigo, motion sickness, conjunctivitis, inflamed skin, urticaria, and many other conditions. It is probably the most widely used relaxing nervine herb in the Western world. It relaxes and tones the nervous system and is especially valuable where anxiety and tension produce digestive symptoms such as gas, colic pains, or even ulcers. Safe in all types of stress and anxiety-related problems, it makes a wonderful late-night tea to ensure restful sleep. Used as an addition to the bath, it will help anxious children or teething infants. As an antispasmodic herb, it works on the peripheral nerves and muscles and so indirectly relaxes the whole body. When the physical body is at ease, ease in the mind and heart follows. It can prevent or ease cramps in the muscles (e.g., leg or abdomen). The essential oil acts on the digestive system, soothing muscle cramping in the intestinal walls, easing griping pains, and helping the removal of gas. A cup of hot chamomile tea is a simple, effective way to relieve indigestion, will help to calm inflammations such as gastritis, and helps prevent ulcer formation. Through use in steam inhalation, the essential oils can reach inflamed mucous membranes in the sinuses and lungs. As a mild antimicrobial, it helps the body destroy or resist pathogenic microorganisms. It also helps remove excess mucus in the sinus area, useful in colds and hayfever.

Preparation and Dosage: Used fresh or dried, the plant is best infused to make a tea. The tincture is an excellent way of ensuring that the plant's components are extracted and available for the body. The infusion is made from 2 teaspoonfuls of the dried herb and drunk three times a day. The tincture dosage is 1–4 milliliters three times a day.

Chasteberry

Vitex agnus-castus

Part Used: Fruit.

Actions: Uterine tonic.

Indications: Chasteberry may be called a balancing remedy, as it can produce apparently opposite effects though in truth it is simply normalizing. It has a reputation as both an aphrodisiac and an anaphrodisiac! It will usually enable what is appropriate to occur. The greatest use of chasteberry lies in normalizing the activity of the female sex hormones; it is used for menstrual cramping, premenstrual stress, and other disorders related to hormone function. It is especially beneficial during menopausal changes. In a similar way, it may be used to aid the body to regain a natural balance after the use of oral contraceptives. Scientists think that it regulates the pituitary gland, which detects increased estrogen levels and tells the ovaries to make less. Recent findings confirm that chasteberry helps restore a normal estrogen-to-progesterone balance. It can with time clear premenstrual syndrome, which has been linked to abnormally high levels of estrogen, especially if symptoms tend to disappear when menstruation begins. Chasteberry can also help in cases of fibroid cysts. Chasteberry can start to work on imbalances after about ten days, but it may take up to six months or longer.

Preparation and Dosage: An infusion is made from 1 teaspoonful of the dried berries and drunk three times a day. Tincture dosage is 1 milliliter three times a day.

Chickweed

Stellaria media

Part Used: Dried aerial parts.

Actions: Antirheumatic, vulnerary, emollient.

Indications: Chickweed is commonly used as an external remedy for cuts, wounds, and especially for itching and irritation. If eczema or psoriasis causes this sort of irritation, chickweed may be used with benefit. It also has a reputation as an internal remedy for rheumatism.

Preparation and Dosage: An infusion is made from 2 teaspoonfuls of the dried herb and drunk three times a day. To ease itching, a strong infusion of the fresh plant makes a useful addition to the bath water.

Cleavers

Galium aparine

Part Used: Dried aerial parts and freshly expressed juice.

Actions: Diuretic, alterative, anti-inflammatory, tonic, astringent.

Indications: Cleavers is a very valuable plant, being perhaps the best tonic available for the lymphatic system. As a lymphatic tonic with alterative and diuretic actions, it may be used safely in a wide range of problems where the lymphatic system is involved. These include swollen glands anywhere in the body, especially in tonsillitis and adenoid trouble. It is helpful in skin conditions, especially the dry kind such as psoriasis. It is helpful in the treatment of cystitis and other urinary conditions where there is pain and may be combined with urinary demulcents for this. There is a long tradition for the use of cleavers in the treatment of ulcers and tumors. This may have its basis in the plant's promotion of lymphatic drainage, which helps detoxify tissue. Cleavers also makes an excellent vegetable.

Preparation and Dosage: An infusion is made from 2 teaspoonfuls of the dried herb and drunk three times a day. Tincture dosage is 2–4 milliliters three times a day.

Coltsfoot

Tussilago farfara

Part Used: Dried flowers and leaves.

Actions: Expectorant, antitussive, antispasmodic, demulcent, anticatarrhal, diuretic.

Indications: Coltsfoot combines a soothing expectorant effect with an antispasmodic action. There are useful levels of zinc in the leaves, a mineral that has been shown to have marked anti-inflammatory effects. Coltsfoot may be used in chronic or acute bronchitis, irritating coughs, whooping coughs, and asthma. Its soothing expectorant action gives coltsfoot a role in most respiratory conditions, including the chronic states of emphysema. As a mild diuretic, it has been used in cystitis. The fresh bruised leaves can be applied to boils, abscesses, and suppurating ulcers.

Preparation and Dosage: An infusion is made from 1–2 teaspoonfuls of the dried flowers and drunk three times a day. Tincture dosage is 2–4 milliliters three times a day.

Comfrey

Symphytum officinale

Part Used: Root and rhizome, leaf.

Actions: Vulnerary, demulcent, anti-inflammatory, astringent, expectorant.

Indications: The impressive wound-healing properties of comfrey are partially due to the presence of allantoin, a chemical that stimulates cell proliferation and so augments wound healing both inside and out. The additional presence of much demulcent mucilage makes comfrey a powerful healing agent in gastric and duodenal ulcers, hiatus hernia, and ulcerative colitis. Its astringency will help hemorrhages wherever they occur. It has been used with benefit in cases of bronchitis and irritable cough, where it will soothe and reduce irritation as well as promote expectoration. Comfrey may be used externally to speed wound healing and guard against scar tissue developing incorrectly. Care should be taken with very deep wounds, however, as the external application of comfrey can lead to tissue forming over the wound before it is healed deeper down, possibly leading to abscesses. It may be used for any external ulcers, and for wounds and fractures as a compress or poultice. It is excellent in chronic varicose ulcers. It has a reputed anticancer action.

Preparation and Dosage: A decoction is made from 2 teaspoonfuls of the dried root and drunk three times a day. Tincture dosage is 2 milliliters three times a day.

Corn Silk

Zea mays

Part Used: Stigmas from the female flowers of maize. Fine soft threads 4 to 8 inches long.

Actions: Diuretic, demulcent, anti-inflammatory, tonic.

Indications: As a soothing diuretic, corn silk is helpful in any irritation of the urinary system. It is used for renal problems in children and as a urinary demulcent combined with other herbs in the treatment of cystitis, urethritis, prostatitis, and the like.

Preparation and Dosage: An infusion is made from 2 teaspoonfuls of the dried herb and drunk three times a day. Tincture dosage is 2 milliliters three times a day.

Couch Grass

Agropyron repens

Part Used: Rhizome.

Actions: Diuretic, demulcent, antimicrobial.

Indications: Couch grass may be used in urinary infections such as cystitis, urethritis, and prostatitis. Its demulcent properties soothe irritation and inflammation. It is of value in the treatment of enlarged prostate glands and may also be used in kidney stones and gravel. As a tonic diuretic, couch grass has been used with other herbs in the treatment of rheumatism.

Preparation and Dosage: A decoction is made from 2 teaspoonfuls of the rhizome and drunk three times a day. Tincture dosage is 2–4 milliliters three times a day.

Cramp Bark

Viburnum opulus

Part Used: Dried bark.

Actions: Antispasmodic, anti-inflammatory, nervine, hypotensive, astringent, emmenagogue.

Indications: Cramp bark shows by its name the richly deserved reputation it has as a relaxer of muscular tension and spasm. It has two main areas of use: First in muscular cramps and second in ovarian and uterine muscle problems. Cramp bark will relax the uterus and so relieve painful cramps associated with menstruation. It may similarly be used to protect from threatened miscarriage. Its astringent action gives it a role in the treatment of excessive blood loss in periods and especially bleeding associated with menopause.

Preparation and Dosage: A decoction is made from 2 teaspoonfuls of the dried bark and drunk three times a day. Tincture dosage is 2–4 milliliters three times a day.

Cranesbill

Geranium maculatum

Part Used: Rhizome.

Actions: Astringent, antihemorrhagic, anti-inflammatory, vulnerary.

Indications: Cranesbill is an effective astringent used in diarrhea, dysentery, and hemorrhoids. When bleeding accompanies duodenal or gastric ulceration, this remedy is used in combination with other relevant herbs. Where blood is lost in the feces, this herb will help, though careful diagnosis is vital. It may be used in cases of excessive blood loss during menstruation or a uterine hemorrhage. As a douche it can be used in leukorrhea.

Preparation and Dosage: A decoction is made from 1–2 teaspoonfuls of the rhizome and drunk three times a day. Tincture dosage is 2–4 milliliters three times a day.

Damiana

Turnera diffusa

Part Used: Dried leaves and stems.

Actions: Nerve tonic, antidepressant, urinary antiseptic, laxative.

Indications: Damiana is an excellent strengthening remedy for the nervous system. It has an ancient reputation as an aphrodisiac. While this may or may not be deserved, the herb has a definite tonic action on the central nervous system as well as the hormonal system. A useful antidepressant, damiana is considered to be a specific remedy in cases of anxiety and depression where there is a sexual factor. It may be used to strengthen the male sexual system.

Preparation and Dosage: An infusion is made from 1 teaspoonful of the dried herb and drunk three times a day. Tincture dosage is 1 milliliter three times a day.

Dandelion

Taraxacum officinale

Part Used: Root or leaf.

Actions: Diuretic, hepatic, cholagogue, antirheumatic, laxative, tonic, bitter.

Indications: Dandelion leaf is a safe but very powerful diuretic. The usual effect of a drug stimulating the kidney function is a loss of vital potassium from the body, which aggravates any cardiovascular problem present. In dandelion, however, we have one of the best natural sources of potassium. It thus makes an ideally balanced diuretic that may be used safely wherever such an action is needed, including in cases of water retention due to heart problems. As a hepatic, dandelion root may be used in inflammation and congestion of liver and gallbladder. It is specific for cases of congestive jaundice. As part of a wider treatment for muscular rheumatism, it can be most effective. This herb is a most valuable general tonic and perhaps the best widely applicable diuretic and liver tonic.

Preparation and Dosage: A decoction is made from 2–3 teaspoonfuls of the root and drunk three times a day. The leaves may be eaten raw in salads. Tincture dosage is 5 milliliters three times a day.

Devil's Claw

Harpagophytum procumbens

Part Used: Rhizome.

Actions: Anti-inflammatory, anodyne, hepatic.

Indications: This valuable plant has been found effective in the treatment of some cases of arthritis. This action appears to be due to the presence of a glycoside called harpagoside that reduces inflammation in the joints. Devil's claw is not always effective, but it is well worth considering in cases of arthritis where inflammation and pain are present. This plant also aids in liver and gallbladder complaints.

Preparation and Dosage: A decoction is made from 1 teaspoonful of the dried herb and drunk three times a day. Tincture dosage is 1–2 milliliters three times a day.

Dill

Anethum graveolens
Part Used: Seeds.
Actions: Carminative, aromatic, antispasmodic, anti-inflammatory, galactogogue.
Indications: Dill is an excellent remedy for flatulence and the colic that is sometimes associated with it. Chewing the seeds will help clear bad breath.
Preparation and Dosage: An infusion is made from 1–2 teaspoonfuls of the gently crushed seeds and drunk three times a day. Tincture dosage is 1–2 milliliters three times a day.

Echinacea

Echinacea spp.
Part Used: The root.
Actions: Antimicrobial, immunomodulator, anticatarrhal, alterative.
Indications: Echinacea is one of the best herbal remedies available to help the body rid itself of microbial infections. It is often effective against both bacterial and viral attacks. In conjunction with other herbs, it may be used for any infection in the body. For example, in combination with yarrow or bearberry, it will effectively stop cystitis. It is especially useful for infections of the upper respiratory tract such as laryngitis, tonsillitis, and for catarrhal conditions of the nose and sinus. In general it may be used widely and safely. The tincture or decoction may be used as a mouthwash in the treatment of pyorrhea and gingivitis. It may be used as an external lotion to help septic sores and cuts.
Preparation and Dosage: A decoction is made from 1–2 teaspoonfuls of the root and drunk three times a day. Tincture dosage is 1 to 4 milliliters three times a day. For the maintenance of a healthy immune system, echinacea is best used periodically—a few weeks on and a few weeks off, throughout the year.

Elder

Sambucus nigra

Part Used: Bark, flowers, berries, leaves.

Actions: Bark: purgative, emetic, diuretic. Leaves: externally as emollient and vulnerary; internally as purgative, expectorant, diuretic, and diaphoretic. Flowers: diaphoretic, anticatarrhal, antispasmodic. Berries: diaphoretic, diuretic, laxative.

Indications: The elder tree is a medicine chest by itself. The leaves are used for bruises, sprains, wounds, and chilblains. It has been reported that elder leaves may be useful in an ointment for tumors. Elder flower is ideal for the treatment of colds and influenza. They are indicated in any catarrhal inflammation of the upper respiratory tract, such as hayfever and sinusitis. Catarrhal deafness responds well to elder flower. Elderberries have similar properties to the flowers with the additional usefulness in rheumatism.

Preparation and Dosage: An infusion is made from 2 teaspoonfuls of the dried or fresh blossoms and drunk hot three times a day. Ointment is made from 3 parts of fresh elder leaves heated with 6 parts of melted petroleum jelly until the elder leaves are crisp. Strain and store this mixture; use as needed. Tincture dosage is 2–4 milliliters (made from the flowers) three times a day.

Elecampane

Inula helenium

Part Used: Rhizome.

Actions: Expectorant, antitussive, diaphoretic, hepatic, antimicrobial.

Indications: Elecampane is a specific remedy for irritating bronchial coughs, especially in children. It may be used wherever there is copious catarrh formed (e.g., in bronchitis or emphysema). This remedy shows the complex and integrated ways in which herbs work. The mucilage has a relaxing effect accompanied by the stimulation of the essential oils. Thus promotion of expectoration is accompanied by a soothing action, which in this herb combines with an antibacterial effect. Elecampane may be used in asthma and bronchitic asthma and has been used in the treatment of tuberculosis. The bitter principle makes it useful also to stimulate digestion and appetite.

Preparation and Dosage: An infusion is made from 1 teaspoonful of the shredded root and drunk three times a day. Tincture dosage is 1–2 milliliters three times a day.

Eyebright

Euphrasia officinalis

Part Used: Dried aerial parts.

Actions: Anticatarrhal, astringent, anti-inflammatory.

Indications: Eyebright is an excellent remedy for the problems of mucous membranes. The combination of anti-inflammatory and astringent properties makes it relevant in many conditions. Used internally it is a powerful anticatarrhal and thus may be used in nasal catarrh, sinusitis, and other congestive states. It is best known for its use in conditions of the eye, where it is helpful in acute or chronic inflammations, stinging and weeping eyes as well as oversensitivity to light. Used as a compress externally in conjunction with internal use, it is valuable in conjunctivitis and blepharitis.

Preparation and Dosage: An infusion is made from 1 teaspoonful of the dried herb and drunk three times a day. Tincture dosage is 1–2 milliliters three times a day. For a compress, place a teaspoonful of the dried herb in half a liter (1 pint) of water and boil for 10 minutes, let cool slightly. Moisten a compress in the lukewarm liquid, wring out slightly, and place over the eyes. Leave the compress in place for 15 minutes. Repeat several times a day.

False Unicorn Root

Chamaelirium luteum

Part Used: Dried rhizome and root.

Actions: Uterine tonic, diuretic, anthelmintic, anti-inflammatory, emmenagogue.

Indications: This herb, which comes to us via the North American Indians, is one of the best tonics and strengtheners of the reproductive system that we have. Though primarily used for the female system, it can be equally beneficial for men. It is known to contain precursors of the estrogens. However, it acts in an amphoteric way to normalize function. The body may use this herb to balance and tone and thus will aid in apparently opposite situations. While being of help in all uterine problems, it is specifically useful in delayed or absent menstruation. When ovarian pain occurs, false unicorn root may be safely used. It is also indicated to prevent threatened miscarriage and ease vomiting associated with pregnancy. However, large doses will cause nausea and vomiting.

Preparation and Dosage: A decoction is made from 1–2 teaspoonfuls of the dried herb and drunk three times a day. Tincture dosage is 2–4 milliliters three times a day.

Fennel

Foeniculum vulgare

Part Used: Seeds.

Actions: Carminative, aromatic, antispasmodic, anti-inflammatory, galactogogue, hepatic.

Indications: Fennel is an excellent stomach and intestinal remedy that relieves flatulence and colic while also stimulating the digestion and appetite. It is similar to aniseed in its calming effect on bronchitis and coughs. It may be used to flavor cough remedies. Externally the oil eases muscular and rheumatic pains. The infusion may be used to treat conjunctivitis and inflammation of the eyelids as a compress.

Preparation and Dosage: An infusion is made from 1–2 teaspoonfuls of slightly crushed seeds and drunk three times a day. To ease flatulence, take a cup half an hour before meals. Tincture dosage is 1–2 milliliters three times a day.

Fenugreek

Trigonella foenum-graecum

Part Used: Seeds.

Actions: Expectorant, demulcent, vulnerary, anti-inflammatory, antispasmodic, tonic, emmenagogue, galactogogue, hypotensive.

Indications: Fenugreek is an herb that has an ancient history. It was rarely used in Britain during the heyday of herbal medicine due to difficulties in obtaining the spice. Since becoming easily available, it has often been overlooked because herbal tradition rarely mentioned it. For a comprehensive discussion of fenugreek, one must refer to an herbal or materia medica of ancient Indian ayurvedic medicine. Its limited use in Britain demonstrates its value as a vulnerary, to heal and reduce inflammation in conditions such as wounds, boils, sores, fistulas, and tumors. It can be taken to help bronchitis and gargled to ease sore throats. Its bitterness explains its role in soothing disturbed digestion.

Preparation and Dosage: For external use, the seeds should be pulverized to make a poultice. A decoction is made from 1 teaspoonful of the seeds and drunk three times a day. Tincture dosage is 1–2 milliliters three times a day.

Feverfew

Tanacetum parthenium

Part Used: Leaves.

Actions: Anti-inflammatory, vasodilator, bitter, emmenagogue.

Indications: Feverfew has regained its deserved reputation as a primary remedy in the treatment of migraine headaches, especially those that are relieved by applying warmth to the head. It may also help arthritis in the painfully active inflammatory stage. Dizziness and tinnitus may be eased, especially if it is used in conjunction with other remedies. Painful periods and sluggish menstrual flow will be relieved by feverfew. It is the only herb used in European phytotherapy known to be specific for the treatment of migraine. It is also the best example of a remedy well known to medical herbalists that has recently been accepted and used by allopathic medicine. It has been used throughout recorded medical history as a bitter tonic and remedy for severe headaches.

Preparation and Dosage: It is best to use the equivalent of one fresh leaf one to three times a day. Preferably use fresh, but tincture or tablets are adequate. In this case, freeze-dried leaf preparations will be best (50–100 mg a day).

Figwort

Scrophularia nodosa

Part Used: Aerial parts.

Actions: Alterative, diuretic, laxative, heart stimulant.

Indications: Figwort finds most use in the treatment of skin problems. It acts in a broad way to help the body function well, bringing about a state of inner cleanliness. It may be used for eczema, psoriasis, and any skin condition where there is itching and irritation. Part of the cleansing occurs due to the purgative and diuretic actions. It may be used as a mild laxative in constipation. As a heart stimulant, figwort should be avoided where there is any abnormally rapid heartbeat.

Preparation and Dosage: An infusion is made from 1–2 teaspoonfuls of the dried herb and drunk three times a day. Tincture dosage is 2–4 milliliters three times a day.

Fringe Tree Bark

Chionanthus virginicus

Part Used: Root bark.

Actions: Hepatic, cholagogue, alterative, diuretic, tonic, antimetic, laxative.

Indications: This valuable herb may be safely used in all liver problems, especially when they have developed into jaundice. It is a specific remedy for the treatment of gallbladder inflammation and a valuable part of treating gallstones. It is a remedy that will aid the liver in general and as such is often used as part of a wider treatment for the whole body. Through its action of releasing bile, it acts as a gentle and effective laxative.

Preparation and Dosage: An infusion is made from 1–2 teaspoonfuls of the dried herb and drunk three times a day. Tincture dosage is 1–2 milliliters three times a day.

Garlic

Allium sativum

Part Used: Bulb.

Actions: Antimicrobial, diaphoretic, cholagogue, hypotensive, antispasmodic.

Indications: Garlic is among the few herbs that have a universal usage and recognition. Its daily usage aids and supports the body in ways that no other herb does. It is one of the most effective antimicrobial plants available, acting on bacteria, viruses, and alimentary parasites. The volatile oil is an effective agent, and as it is largely excreted via the lungs, it is used in infections of this system such as chronic bronchitis, respiratory catarrh, recurrent colds, and influenza. It may be helpful in the treatment of whooping cough and as part of a broader approach to bronchitic asthma. In general, garlic may be used as a preventive for most infectious conditions, digestive as well as respiratory. For the digestive tract, it has been found that garlic will support the development of the natural bacterial flora while killing pathogenic organisms. In addition to these amazing properties, garlic has an international reputation for lowering both blood pressure and blood cholesterol levels and generally improving the health of the cardiovascular system. A study was conducted on two groups: one consisted of twenty healthy volunteers who were fed garlic for six months and the other of sixty-two patients with coronary heart disease and raised serum cholesterol. Beneficial changes were found in all involved and reached a peak at the end of eight months. The improvement in cholesterol levels persisted throughout the two months of clinical follow-up. The clinicians concluded that the essential oil of garlic possessed a distinct fat-reducing action in both healthy people and patients with coronary heart disease. Garlic should be thought of as a basic food that will augment the body's health and protect it in general. It has been used externally for the treatment of ringworm and threadworm.

Preparation and Dosage: A clove should be eaten three times a day. If the smell becomes a problem, use garlic oil capsules; take 3 a day as a prophylactic or 3 capsules three times a day when an infection occurs.

Gentian

Gentiana lutea

Part Used: Dried rhizome and root.

Actions: Bitter, hepatic, antimicrobial, emmenagogue.

Indications: Gentian is an excellent bitter that (like all bitters) stimulates the appetite and digestion via a general stimulation of the digestive juices. Thus it promotes the production of saliva, gastric juices, and bile. It also accelerates the emptying of the stomach. It is indicated wherever there is a lack of appetite and sluggishness of the digestive system. It may thus be used where dyspepsia and flatulence, the symptoms of sluggish digestion, appear. Through the stimulation of the digestion it has a generally fortifying effect.

Preparation and Dosage: A decoction is made from ½ teaspoonful of the shredded root. This should be drunk warm about 15–30 minutes before meals, or at any time when acute stomach pains result from a feeling of fullness. Tincture dosage is 1–2 milliliters three times a day.

Ginger

Zingiber officinale

Part Used: Rootstock.

Actions: Stimulant, carminative, antispasmodic, rubefacient, diaphoretic, emmenagogue.

Indications: Ginger may be used as a stimulant of the peripheral circulation in cases of bad circulation, chilblains, and cramps. In feverish conditions it is a useful diaphoretic, promoting perspiration. As a gargle it may be effective in the relief of sore throats. Externally it is used in many muscle sprain treatments. Ginger has been used worldwide as an aromatic carminative and pungent appetite stimulant. In India, and in other countries with hot and humid climates, ginger is eaten daily and is a well-known remedy for digestion problems. Its widespread use is not only due to flavor, but to the antioxidant and antimicrobial effects, necessary for preservation of food in such climates.

Preparation and Dosage: An infusion is made from 1 teaspoonful of the fresh root and drunk whenever needed. A decoction is made from 1½ teaspoonfuls of the dried root in powdered or finely chopped form. This decoction can be drunk whenever needed. Ginger tincture comes in two forms: weak tincture, which should be taken in a dose of 1.5–3 milliliters three times a day, and the strong tincture, which should be taken in a dose of 0.25–0.5 milliliters three times a day.

Ginkgo

Ginkgo biloba

Part Used: Leaves. In oriental herbalism the seed kernel is used extensively.

Actions: Anti-inflammatory, vasodilatory, relaxant, digestive bitter, uterine stimulant.

Indications: While ginkgo is traditionally known as an antimicrobial and antitubercular agent, new research has shown a profound activity on cardiovascular circulation, brain function, and cerebral circulation. Clinically it is proving effective in a range of vascular disorders. To summarize, ginkgo has been suggested for the following conditions: vertigo; tinnitus; inner ear disturbances; impairment of memory and ability to concentrate; diminished intellectual capacity and alertness as a result of insufficient circulation; complications of stroke and skull injuries; diminished eyesight and hearing ability due to vascular insufficiency; intermittent claudication as a result of arterial obstruction; sensitivity to cold and pallor in the toes due to peripheral circulatory insufficiency; Raynaud's disease; cerebral vascular and nutritional insufficiency; arterial circulatory disturbances due to aging, diabetes, and nicotine abuse; arteriosclerotic, angiopathy of lower limbs; diabetic tissue damage with danger of gangrene; chronic arterial obliteration; and circulatory disorders of the skin.

Preparation and Dosage: Ginkgo is becoming available in a number of different forms. The clinically recommended dosage range is 40 milligrams of the dried herb in tablet form three times a day.

Ginseng

Panax spp.

Part Used: Root.

Actions: Adaptogen, tonic, stimulant, hypoglycemic.

Indications: Ginseng has an ancient history, and thus much has accumulated about its actions and uses. The genus name *Panax* derives from the Latin panacea meaning "cure all." Many of the claims that surround it are, unfortunately, exaggerated, but it is clear that this is an important remedy. A powerful adaptogen, it has a wide range of possible therapeutic uses. The best therapeutic application is with weak or elderly people, where the adaptogenic and stimulating properties can be profoundly useful. It should not be used indiscriminately, as its stimulating properties can be contraindicated in some pathologies; for example, Chinese herbalism warns about ginseng being used in acute inflammatory disease and bronchitis.

Preparation and Dosage: The root is often chewed, or a decoction may be made from ½ teaspoonful of the powdered root and drunk three times a day.

Goat's Rue

Galega officinalis

Part Used: Dried aerial parts.

Actions: Hypoglycemic, galactogogue, diuretic, diaphoretic.

Indications: Goat's rue is one of many herbal remedies with the action of reducing blood sugar levels. Its use is thus potentially indicated in the treatment of diabetes mellitus. This must not replace insulin therapy, however, and should be taken only under professional supervision. It is also an effective galactagogue, stimulating both the production and flow of milk, and has been shown to increase milk output by up to 50 percent in some cases. It may also stimulate the development of the mammary glands.

Preparation and Dosage: An infusion is made from 1 teaspoonful of the dried herb and drunk 3 times a day. Tincture dosage is 1–2 milliliters three times a day.

Goldenrod

Solidago virgaurea

Part Used: Dried aerial parts.

Actions: Anticatarrhal, anti-inflammatory, antimicrobial, astringent, diaphoretic, carminative, diuretic.

Indications: Goldenrod is perhaps the first plant to think of for acute or chronic upper respiratory catarrh. It may be used in combination with other herbs in the treatment of influenza. The carminative properties reveal its role in the treatment of flatulent dyspepsia. As an anti-inflammatory urinary antiseptic, goldenrod may be used in cystitis, urethritis, and the like. It can be used to promote the healing of wounds. As a gargle it can be used in laryngitis and pharyngitis.

Preparation and Dosage: An infusion is made from 2 teaspoonfuls of the dried herb and drunk three times a day. Tincture dosage is 2 milliliters three times a day.

Goldenseal

Hydrastis canadensis

Part Used: Rhizome and root.

Actions: Bitter, hepatic, alterative, anticatarrhal, antimicrobial, anti-inflammatory, astringent, laxative, expectorant, emmenagogue, oxytocic.

Indications: Goldenseal is one of our most useful remedies, owing much of its value to the tonic effects it has on the mucous membranes of the body. This is why it is of such help in all digestive problems, from peptic ulcers to colitis. Its bitter stimulation helps in loss of appetite, and the alkaloids it contains stimulate bile production and secretion. All catarrhal conditions improve with goldenseal, especially those involving the sinuses. The antimicrobial properties appear to be due to alkaloids present. As an example of research that has been done on plant constituents, we shall consider berberine. Berberine, found in a number of other herbs as well, has antibiotic, immunostimulatory, antispasmodic, sedative, hypotensive, uterotonic, cholerectic, and carminative activity. Traditionally goldenseal has been used during labor to help contractions, but it is for just this reason that it should be avoided during pregnancy. Applied externally it can be helpful in eczema, ringworm, itching, earache, and conjunctivitis.

Preparation and Dosage: An infusion is made from $1/2$–1 teaspoonful of the dried herb and drunk three times a day. Tincture dosage is 1 milliliter three times a day.

Gravel Root

Eupatorium purpureum

Part Used: Rhizome and root.

Actions: Diuretic, antilithic, antirheumatic.

Indications: Gravel root is used primarily for kidney stones or gravel. In urinary infections such as cystitis and urethritis, it may be used with benefit, while it can also play a useful role in a systemic treatment of rheumatism and gout.

Preparation and Dosage: A decoction is made from 1 teaspoonful of the dried herb and drunk three times a day. Tincture dosage is 1–2 milliliters three times a day.

Grindelia

Grindelia spp.

Part Used: Dried aerial parts.

Actions: Antispasmodic, expectorant, hypotensive.

Indications: Grindelia acts to relax smooth muscles and heart muscles. This helps to explain its use in the treatment of asthmatic and bronchial conditions, especially where these are associated with a rapid heartbeat and nervous response. It may be used in asthma, bronchitis, whooping cough, and upper respiratory catarrh. Because of the relaxing effect on the heart and pulse rate, there may be a reduction in blood pressure. Externally the lotion is used for the dermatitis caused by poison ivy.

Preparation and Dosage: An infusion is made from 1 teaspoonful of the dried herb and drunk three times a day. Tincture dosage is 1–2 milliliters three times a day.

Guaiac

Guaiacum officinale

Part Used: Heartwood.

Actions: Antirheumatic, anti-inflammatory, laxative, diaphoretic, diuretic.

Indications: Guaiac is a specific remedy for rheumatic complaints. It is especially useful where much inflammation and pain are present and is thus used in chronic rheumatism and rheumatoid arthritis. It will aid in the treatment of gout and may be used in the prevention of recurrence in this disease. Due to the high content of resins in this valuable herb, care must be taken with patients with gastritis or peptic ulceration.

Preparation and Dosage: A decoction is made from 1 teaspoonful of the dried herb and drunk three times a day. Tincture dosage is 1–2 milliliters three times a day.

Hawthorn

Crataegus oxyacantha, C. monogyna

Part Used: Berries and flowers.

Actions: Cardiotonic, diuretic, astringent, hypotensive.

Indications: Hawthorn can be considered a specific remedy in most cardiovascular disease; it is a tonic in the true sense. However, the therapeutic benefits are gained only when a whole-plant preparation is used. When the isolated constituents were tested separately in the laboratory, their individual effects were insignificant, whereas the whole plant has unique and valuable properties. Following a four-year study commissioned by the German Federal Ministry of Health, hawthorn has gained full recognition as a heart remedy in Europe. What is most important, no contraindications or side effects were noted. It brings about improvement in coronary circulation, dilating the coronary arteries and thus reducing the likelihood of angina attacks as well as relieving its symptoms. The herb thus directly affects the cells of the cardiac muscle, enhancing both activity and nutrition. It is quite different in activity to the cardiac glycoside-containing remedies. The latter impact the contractile fibers, while hawthorn is involved in the availability and utilization of energy. This facilitates a gentle but long-term, sustained effect on degenerative, age-related changes in the myocardium. It does not produce rapid results, but results are persistent once achieved. Hawthorn may be used in a range of cardiovascular degenerative conditions in which no disease state exists but a loss of function is experienced due to old age. No toxicity, accumulation, or habituation occurs; thus it may be used for long periods of time, achieving entirely safe results. Recovery from heart attacks is speeded by its use. Hypertension responds well to hawthorn when used in conjunction with other hypotensives. It will maintain the heart in a healthy condition, preventing the development of coronary disease.

Preparation and Dosage: An infusion is made from 2 teaspoonfuls of the dried herb and drunk three times a day. Tincture dosage is 1–2 milliliters three times a day.

Heartsease (Pansy)

Viola tricolor

Part Used: Herb.

Actions: Expectorant, diuretic, anti-inflammatory.

Indications: Traditionally used for bronchitis and rheumatism, heartsease is an especially valued remedy for treating skin disease. Used both internally and topically, it is good for eczema, psoriasis, and acne. The herb is employed in treating frequent and painful urination in conditions such as cystitis. Both the salicylates and the rutin contained in the plant are anti-inflammatory, a partial explanation of the traditional use herbalists have found for it in treating arthritis. The saponins in the plant account for its expectorant action, while its mucilage content soothes the chest. Heartsease is used to treat a range of respiratory disorders, including bronchitis and whooping cough. Due to the high concentration of rutin in the flowers, this herb may be employed to prevent bruising and broken capillaries, to check the buildup of fluid in the tissues, and to reduce atherosclerosis and thereby to help reduce blood pressure. It is mildly laxative.

Preparation and Dosage: An infusion is made from 1 teaspoonful of the dried herb and drunk three times a day. Tincture dosage is 1–2 milliliters three times a day.

Hops

Humulus lupulus

Part Used: Flower inflorescence.

Actions: Sedative, hypnotic, antimicrobial, antispasmodic, astringent.

Indications. Hops is a remedy with a marked relaxing effect upon the central nervous system. It is used extensively for the treatment of insomnia. It will ease tension and anxiety and may be used where this tension leads to restlessness, headache, and possibly indigestion. As an astringent with these relaxing properties, it can be used in conditions such as mucous colitis. Externally the antiseptic action is utilized for the treatment of ulcers.

Preparation and Dosage: An infusion is made from 1 teaspoonful of the dried herb and drunk three times a day. Tincture dosage is 1–2 milliliters three times a day.

CAUTION: Do not administer to patients suffering from extreme depression.

Horehound

Marrubium vulgare

Part Used: Dried leaves and flowering tops.

Actions: Expectorant, antispasmodic, bitter, vulnerary, emmenagogue.

Indications: Horehound is a valuable plant in the treatment of bronchitis where there is a nonproductive cough. It combines the action of relaxing the smooth muscles of the bronchus while promoting mucus production and thus expectoration. It is used with benefit in the treatment of whooping cough. The bitter action stimulates the flow and secretion of bile from the gallbladder, aiding digestion. Horehound is used externally to promote the healing of wounds.

Preparation and Dosage: An infusion is made from 1 teaspoonful of the dried herb and drunk three times a day. Tincture dosage is 1–2 milliliters three times a day.

Horse Chestnut

Aesculus hippocastanum

Part Used: Fruit (the horse chestnut itself).

Actions: Astringent, anti-inflammatory.

Indications: The unique action of horse chestnut is directed to the vessels of the circulatory system. It seems to increase the strength and tone of the veins in particular. It may be used internally to aid the body in the treatment of problems such as phlebitis, inflammation in the veins, varicosity, and hemorrhoids. Externally it may be used as a lotion for the same conditions as well as for leg ulcers.

Preparation and Dosage: An infusion is made from 1 to 2 teaspoonfuls of the dried herb and drunk three times a day or used topically. Tincture dosage is 1–2 milliliters three times a day.

Horsetail

Equisetum arvense

Part Used: Dried aerial stems.

Actions: Astringent, diuretic, vulnerary.

Indications: Horsetail grass is an excellent astringent for the genitourinary system, reducing hemorrhage and healing wounds thanks to its high silica content. While it acts as a mild diuretic, its toning and astringent actions make it invaluable in the treatment of incontinence and bed-wetting in children. It is considered a specific remedy in cases of inflammation or benign enlargement of the prostate gland. Externally it is a vulnerary. In some cases, it has been found to ease the pain of rheumatism and stimulate the healing of chilblains.

Preparation and Dosage: An infusion is made from 2 teaspoonfuls of the dried herb and drunk three times a day. Tincture dosage is 2 milliliters three times a day. A useful bath can be made to help in rheumatic pain and chilblains. Allow 3½ ounces of the herb to steep in hot water for an hour and add this to the bath.

Hydrangea

Hydrangea arborescens

Part Used: Dried roots and rhizome.

Actions: Diuretic, antilithic.

Indications: Hydrangea's greatest use is in the treatment of inflamed or enlarged prostate glands. It may also be used for urinary stones or gravel associated with infections such as cystitis.

Preparation and Dosage: A decoction is made from 2 teaspoonfuls of the dried herb and drunk three times a day. Tincture dosage is 2 milliliters three times a day.

Hyssop

Hyssopus officinalis

Part Used: Dried aerial parts.

Actions: Antispasmodic, expectorant, diaphoretic, nervine, anti-inflammatory, carminative, hepatic, emmenagogue.

Indications: Hyssop has an interesting range of uses that are largely attributable to the antispasmodic action of the volatile oil. It is used in coughs, bronchitis, and chronic catarrh. Its diaphoretic properties explain its use in the common cold. As a nervine, it may be used in anxiety states, hysteria, and petit mal.

Preparation and Dosage: An infusion is made from 1–2 teaspoonfuls of the dried herb and drunk three times a day. Tincture dosage is 1–2 milliliters three times a day.

Iceland Moss

Cetraria islandica

Part Used: Entire plant. It is a lichen.

Actions: Demulcent, anti-inflammatory, antiemetic, expectorant.

Indications: As a soothing demulcent with its high mucilage content, Iceland moss finds use in the treatment of gastritis, vomiting, and dyspepsia. It is often used in respiratory catarrh and bronchitis, soothing mucous membranes. Its nourishing qualities contribute to the treatment of cachexia, a state of malnourishment and debility.

Preparation and Dosage: A decoction is made from 1 teaspoonful of the shredded moss. A cup should be drunk in the morning and evening. Tincture dosage is 1–2 milliliters three times a day.

Irish Moss

Chondrus crispus

Part Used: Dried thallus. It is a seaweed.

Actions: Expectorant, demulcent, anti-inflammatory.

Indications: With modern attention on dramatically effective "miracle drugs," it is refreshing to remember the nourishing and strengthening food medicines such as Irish moss. Traditionally the main use of Irish moss is in respiratory illness; it is often the core of prescriptions to treat irritating coughs, bronchitis, and other lung problems. It may be freely used in digestive conditions where a demulcent is called for, such as gastritis and ulceration of the stomach and duodenum. The soothing activity is also seen in inflammations of the urinary system and was at one time used extensively, much as corn silk is used today. However, its primary role was in speeding recuperation from debilitating illness, especially tuberculosis and pneumonia. Irish moss and other tonic nutritive remedies can offer much in facilitating proper recovery of health. Indeed, in these times of degenerative disease, such perspectives cry out for attention.

Preparation and Dosage: To use fresh, wash it well and add one cup of Irish moss to three cups of milk or water and flavor to taste. Simmer slowly until most of the seaweed has dissolved. Remove any undissolved fragments and pour into a mold to set. The dried herb is best made into a decoction by steeping half an ounce of the dried herb in cold water for 15 minutes and then boiling it for 10–15 minutes in 3 pints of water (or milk). Strain and combine with licorice, lemon, ginger, or cinnamon. Sweeten to taste.

Jamaican Dogwood

Piscidia erythrina

Part Used: Stem bark.

Actions: Nervine, anodyne, antispasmodic.

Indications: Jamaican dogwood is a powerful sedative, used in its West Indian homeland as a fish poison. Although it is not poisonous to humans, the given dosage level should not be exceeded. It is a powerful remedy for the treatment of painful conditions such as neuralgia and migraine. It can also be used in the relief of ovarian and uterine pain. Its main use may be in insomnia due to nervous tension or pain.

Preparation and Dosage: A decoction is made from 1 teaspoonful of the root and drunk three times a day. Tincture dosage is 1–2 milliliters three times a day.

Juniper Berries

Juniperus communis

Part Used: Dried fruits.

Actions: Diuretic, antimicrobial, carminative, antirheumatic.

Indications: Juniper berries make an excellent antiseptic in conditions such as cystitis. The essential oil present is quite stimulating to the kidney nephrons; this herb should, therefore, be avoided in kidney disease. The bitter action aids digestion and eases flatulent colic. It is used in rheumatism and arthritis. Externally it eases pain in the joints or muscles.

Preparation and Dosage: An infusion is made from 1 teaspoonful of the dried herb and drunk three times a day. Tincture dosage is 1 milliliter three times a day.

CAUTION: Due to its action on the kidneys, juniper berries should be avoided in any kidney disease. They should also be avoided in pregnancy.

Kola

Cola vera

Part Used: Seed kernel.

Actions: Stimulant to central nervous system, antidepressive, astringent, diuretic.

Indications: Kola has stimulating effects on consciousness. It can be used wherever there is a need for direct stimulation, which is less often than is usually thought. As a short-term remedy, it may be used in nervous debility and in states of atony and weakness. It can act as a specific remedy in nervous diarrhea. It will aid in states of depression and may in some people give rise to euphoric states. In some varieties of migraine, it can help greatly. Through the stimulation it will be a valuable part of the treatment for anorexia. It can be viewed as a specific remedy in cases of depression associated with weakness and debility.

Preparation and Dosage: A decoction is made from 1 teaspoonful of the dried herb and drunk three times a day. Tincture dosage is 1–2 milliliters three times a day.

Lady's Mantle

Alchemilla vulgaris

Part Used: Leaves and flowering shoots.

Actions: Astringent, diuretic, anti-inflammatory, emmenagogue, vulnerary.

Indications: This and other species of alchemilla have been widely used in folk medicine throughout Europe. Lady's mantle will help reduce pains associated with periods as well as ameliorating excessive bleeding. It also has a role to play in easing the changes of menopause. As an emmenagogue, it stimulates the proper menstrual flow if there is any resistance. However, in the often apparently paradoxical way of herbal remedies, Lady's mantle is a useful uterine astringent, used in both menorrhagia and metrorrhagia. Its astringency provides a role in the treatment of diarrhea and as a mouthwash for sores and ulcers and as a gargle for laryngitis.

Preparation and Dosage: An infusion is made from 2 teaspoonfuls of the dried herb and drunk three times a day. To help diarrhea and as a mouthwash or lotion, a stronger dosage is made by boiling the herb for a few minutes to extract all the tannin. Tincture dosage is 1–2 milliliters three times a day.

Lavender

Lavandula officinalis

Part Used: Flowers.

Actions: Carminative, antispasmodic, antidepressant, rubefacient, emmenagogue, hypotensive.

Indications: This beautiful herb has many uses, culinary, cosmetic, and medicinal. It is an effective herb for headaches, especially when they are related to stress. Lavender can be quite effective in the clearing of depression, especially if used in conjunction with other remedies. As a gentle strengthening tonic of the nervous system, it may be used in states of nervous debility and exhaustion. It can be used to soothe and promote natural sleep. Externally the oil may be used as a stimulating liniment to help ease the aches and pains of rheumatism.

Preparation and Dosage: An infusion is made from 1 teaspoonful of the dried herb and drunk three times a day. The oil should not be taken internally but can be inhaled, rubbed on the skin, or used in baths.

Licorice

Glycyrrhiza glabra

Part Used: Dried root.

Actions: Expectorant, demulcent, anti-inflammatory, antihepatotoxic, antispasmodic, mild laxative.

Indications: Licorice is a traditional herbal remedy with an ancient history and worldwide usage. Modern research has shown it to have effects in particular upon the endocrine system and liver. The triterpenes of licorice are metabolized in the body to molecules that have a similar structure to the adrenal cortex hormones. (This may be the basis of the herb's anti-inflammatory action. As an antihepatotoxic, it can be effective in the treatment of chronic hepatitis and cirrhosis, for which it has been widely used in Japan. Much of the liver-oriented research has focused upon the triterpene glycyrrhizin, which inhibits hepatocyte injury caused by carbon tetrachloride, benzene hexachloride, and PCB. Antibody production is enhanced by glycyrrhizin, possibly through the production of interleukin. It has a wide range of uses in bronchial problems such as catarrh, bronchitis, and coughs in general. Licorice is used in allopathic medicine as a treatment for peptic ulceration, a similar use to its herbal use in gastritis and ulcers. It can be used in the relief of abdominal colic.

Preparation and Dosage: A decoction is made from $^{1}/_{2}$–1 teaspoonful of the dried herb and drunk three times a day. Tincture dosage is 1–3 milliliters three times a day.

CAUTION: There is a small possibility of affecting electrolyte balance with extended use of large doses of licorice. It has an ACTH-like effect, causing retention of sodium and thus raising the blood pressure. The whole herb has constituents that counter this, but it is best to avoid licorice if the patient suffers from hypertension or kidney disease or is pregnant.

Life Root

Senecio aureus

Part Used: Dried aerial parts. Never use the fresh plant.

Actions: Uterine tonic, diuretic, expectorant, anti-inflammatory, emmenagogue.

Indications: As a uterine tonic, life root may be used safely wherever strengthening and aid are called for. It is especially useful in cases of menopausal disturbances of any kind. Where there is delayed or suppressed menstruation, life root may be used. For leukorrhea it can be used as a douche. It also has a reputation as a general tonic for debilitated states and conditions such as tuberculosis.

Preparation and Dosage: An infusion is made from 1–2 teaspoonfuls of the dried herb and drunk three times a day. Tincture dosage is 1–2 milliliters three times a day.

Linden Blossom

Tilia europea

Part Used: Dried flowers.

Actions: Nervine, antispasmodic, hypotensive, diaphoretic, diuretic, anti-inflammatory, emmenagogue, astringent.

Indications: Linden is a relaxing remedy for use in nervous tension. It has a reputation as a prophylactic against the development of arteriosclerosis and hypertension. It is considered to be a specific remedy in the treatment of raised blood pressure associated with arteriosclerosis and nervous tension. Its relaxing action combined with a general effect upon the circulatory system give linden a role in the treatment of some forms of migraine. The sweating combined with the relaxation explain its value in feverish colds and flu.

Preparation and Dosage: An infusion is made from 1 teaspoonful of the blossoms and drunk three times a day. Tincture dosage is 1–2 milliliters three times a day.

Lobelia

Lobelia inflata

Part Used: Aerial parts.

Actions: Antiasthmatic, antispasmodic, expectorant, emetic, nervine.

Indications: Lobelia is one of the most useful systemic relaxants available to us. It has a general depressant action on the central and autonomic nervous system and on neuromuscular action. It may be used in many conditions in combination with other herbs to further their effectiveness if relaxation is needed. Its primary specific use is in bronchitic asthma and bronchitis. An analysis of the action of the alkaloids present reveals apparently paradoxical effects. Lobeline is a powerful respiratory stimulant, while isolobelanine is an emetic and respiratory relaxant; thus lobelia will stimulate catarrhal secretion and expectoration while relaxing the muscles of the respiratory system. The overall action is a truly holistic combination of stimulation and relaxation!

Preparation and Dosage: An infusion is made from $^{1}/_{4}$-$^{1}/_{2}$ teaspoonful of the dried leaves and drunk three times a day. Tincture dosage is $^{1}/_{2}$ milliliter three times a day.

Lungwort Herb

Pulmonaria officinalis

Part Used: Leaves.

Actions: Demulcent, expectorant, astringent, anti-inflammatory, vulnerary.

Indications: Lungwort has two broad areas of use. The one that provides its name is its use in the treatment of coughs and bronchitis, especially where associated with upper respiratory catarrh. The other broad area is that related to its astringency. This explains its use in the treating of diarrhea, especially in children, and in easing hemorrhoids. As with all plants, these two broad areas must be seen as part of the whole activity of the herb, acting as a unity. Externally, this plant may be used to heal cuts and wounds.

Preparation and Dosage: An infusion is made from 1–2 teaspoonfuls of the dried herb and drunk three times a day. Tincture dosage is 1–2 milliliters three times a day.

Ma Huang

Ephedra sinica

Part Used: Aerial stems.

Actions: Vasodilator, hypertensive, circulatory stimulant, antiallergic.

Indications: Ma huang has been used in China for at least five thousand years to treat a range of health problems, but especially those of the respiratory system. With the discovery of the alkaloids in ma huang, time-honored, traditional herbal wisdom has been verified, providing modern medicine with important healing tools. A range of therapeutically active alkaloids is found in *Ephedra,* sometimes amounting to up to 2.0 percent of the dried herb. Various species of Asian *Ephedra* are used as a source of the widely used alkaloids ephedrine and pseudoephedrine. Ma huang is an effective and safe treatment for nasal congestion and sinus pressure, whether due to the common cold, allergies, or sinusitis. The herb is used with great success in the treatment of asthma and associated conditions because of its power to relieve spasms in the bronchial tubes. It is thus used in bronchial asthma, bronchitis, and whooping cough. It also reduces allergic reactions, giving it a role in the treatment of hayfever and other allergies. It may be used in the treatment of low blood pressure and circulatory insufficiency.

Preparation and Dosage: A decoction is made from 1 teaspoonful of the dried herb and drunk three times a day. Tincture dosage is 1–2 milliliters three times a day.

CAUTION: Ma huang should not be used by people with cardiovascular conditions, thyroid disease, or diabetes, or by men experiencing difficulty urinating due to prostate enlargement, as the herb may aggravate (but not cause) such preexisting conditions.

Marshmallow

Althaea officinalis

Part Used: Root and leaf.

Actions: Demulcent, emmolient, diuretic, anti-inflammatory, expectorant.

Indications: Its abundance of mucilage makes marshmallow an excellent demulcent that is indicated wherever such an action is called for. The roots have been used more for the digestive system while the leaves are used primarily for the urinary system and lungs. All inflammatory conditions of the gastrointestinal tract will benefit from its use (inflammations of the mouth, gastritis, peptic ulceration, colitis, etc.). The leaves help in cystitis, urethritis, and urinary gravel as well as bronchitis, respiratory catarrh, and irritating coughs. Externally the herb is often used in drawing ointments for abscesses and boils or as an emollient for varicose veins and ulcers.

Preparation and Dosage: A cold infusion of the roots should be made with 2–4 grams to a cup of cold water and left to infuse overnight. Drink the infusion three times a day or as often as needed. Tincture dosage is 1–4 milliliters three times a day.

Meadowsweet

Filipendula ulmaria

Part Used: Aerial parts.

Actions: Antirheumatic, anti-inflammatory, carminative, antacid, antiemetic, astringent.

Indications: Meadowsweet is one of the best digestive remedies available and as such will be indicated in many conditions, if they are approached holistically. It acts to protect and soothe the mucous membranes of the digestive tract, reducing excess acidity and easing nausea. It is used in the treatment of heartburn, hyperacidity, gastritis, and peptic ulceration. Its gentle astringency is useful in treating diarrhea in children. The presence of aspirinlike chemicals explains meadowsweet's action in reducing fever and relieving the pain of rheumatism in muscles and joints.

Preparation and Dosage: An infusion is made from 1–2 teaspoonfuls of the dried herb and drunk three times a day. Tincture dosage is 1–2 milliliters three times a day.

Milk Thistle

Carduus marianus

Part Used: Seeds.

Actions: Hepatic, galactogogue, demulcent, cholagogue.

Indications: Milk thistle's traditional use as a liver tonic has been supported by research showing that it contains constituents that protect liver cells from chemical damage. Historically, this herb has been used in Europe as a liver tonic, and current phytotherapy indicates its use in a whole range of liver and gallbladder conditions, including hepatitis and cirrhosis. It may also have value in the treatment of chronic uterine problems. Much research being done in Germany is revealing exciting data about reversal of toxic liver damage as well as protection from potential hepatotoxic agents. A number of chemical components of the herb are now being shown to have this protective effect on liver cells. As its name implies, the herb promotes milk secretion and is perfectly safe to be used by all breast-feeding mothers.

Preparation and Dosage: An infusion is made from 1 teaspoonful of the ground seed and drunk three times a day. Tincture dosage is 1–2 milliliters three times a day.

Motherwort

Leonurus cardiaca

Part Used: Aerial parts.

Actions: Nervine, emmenagogue, antispasmodic, hepatic, cardiac tonic, hypotensive.

Indications: The names of this plant show its range of uses. Motherwort relates to its relevance to menstrual and uterine conditions, while the Latin *cardiaca* indicates its use in heart and circulation treatments. It is valuable in the stimulation of delayed or suppressed menstruation, especially where there is anxiety or tension involved. It is a useful relaxing tonic for aiding in menopausal changes. It may be used to ease false labor pains. It is an excellent tonic for the heart, strengthening without straining. It is considered to be a specific remedy in cases of heart palpitations, especially when brought on by anxiety or tension.

Preparation and Dosage: An infusion is made from 1–2 teaspoonfuls of the dried herb and drunk three times a day. Tincture dosage is 1–2 milliliters three times a day.

Mugwort

Artemisia vulgaris

Part Used: Leaves or root.

Actions: Bitter tonic, stimulant, nervine tonic, emmenagogue.

Indications: Mugwort can be used wherever a digestive stimulant is called for. It will aid the digestion through the bitter stimulation of the juices while also providing a carminative oil. Its mildly nervine action in aiding depression and easing tension appears to be due to the volatile oil, so it is essential that this oil not be lost in preparation. Mugwort may also be used as an emmenagogue to promote normal menstrual flow.

Preparation and Dosage: An infusion is made from 1–2 teaspoonfuls of the dried herb and drunk three times a day. Tincture dosage is 1–2 milliliters three times a day. Mugwort is used as a flavoring in a number of aperitif drinks—a pleasant way to take it!

Mullein

Verbascum thapsus

Part Used: Dried leaves and flowers.

Actions: Expectorant, demulcent, diuretic, anti-inflammatory, nervine, antispasmodic, vulnerary, alterative, astringent.

Indications: Mullein is a very beneficial respiratory remedy useful in most conditions that affect this vital system. It is an ideal remedy for toning the mucous membranes of the respiratory system, reducing inflammation while stimulating fluid production and thus facilitating expectoration. It is considered a specific remedy in bronchitis where there is a hard cough with pain. Its anti-inflammatory and demulcent properties indicate its use in inflammation of the trachea and associated conditions. Externally, an extract made in olive oil is excellent for soothing and healing any inflamed surface or easing ear problems.

Preparation and Dosage: An infusion is made from 1–2 teaspoonfuls of the dried herb and drunk three times a day. Tincture dosage is 1–2 milliliters three times a day.

Mustard

Brassica alba, B. nigra

Part Used: Seeds.

Actions: Rubefacient, irritant, stimulant, diuretic, emetic.

Indications: This well-known spice has its main use in medicine as a stimulating external application. The rubefacient action causes a mild irritation to the skin, stimulating circulation in that area and relieving muscular and skeletal pain. Its stimulating, diaphoretic action can be utilized much like cayenne and ginger. For feverishness, colds, and influenza, mustard may be taken as a tea or ground and sprinkled into a bath. The stimulation of circulation will aid chilblains as well as the conditions already mentioned. An infusion or poultice of mustard will aid in cases of bronchitis.

Preparation and Dosage: Mustard is most commonly used as a poultice, which can be made by mixing 100 grams (4 oz.) of freshly ground mustard seeds with warm water (at about 45°C) to form a thick paste. Spread the paste on a piece of cloth the size of the body area that is to be covered. To keep the paste from sticking to the skin, lay a piece of dampened gauze on the skin. Apply the cloth and remove after 1 minute. If the skin is reddened by this treatment, apply olive oil afterward. To make an infusion, pour a cup of boiling water over 1 teaspoonful of mustard flour and infuse for just 5 minutes to avoid bitterness. This may be drunk three times a day. To prepare a mustard footbath, make an infusion using 1 tablespoon of bruised seeds to 1 liter (2 pints) boiling water.

Nettle

Urtica dioica

Part Used: Aerial parts.

Actions: Astringent, diuretic, tonic, hypotensive.

Indications: One of the most widely applicable medicinal plants, nettle strengthens and supports the whole body. Throughout Europe they are used as a spring tonic and general detoxifying remedy. In some cases of rheumatism and arthritis, they can be astoundingly successful. They are very useful in cases of childhood eczema and beneficial in all the varieties of this condition, especially in nervous eczema. As an astringent, they may be used for nosebleeds or to relieve symptoms wherever hemorrhage occurs in the body (e.g., uterine hemorrhage).

Preparation and Dosage: An infusion is made from 1–2 teaspoonfuls of the dried herb and drunk three times a day. Tincture dosage is 1–2 milliliters three times a day.

Oats

Avena sativa

Part Used: Seeds and whole plant.

Actions: Nervine tonic, antidepressant, nutritive, demulcent, vulnerary.

Indications: Oats is one of the best remedies for "feeding" the nervous system, especially when under stress. It is considered a specific remedy in cases of nervous debility and exhaustion when associated with depression. It may be used with most of the other nervines, both relaxant and stimulatory, to strengthen the whole of the nervous system. It is also used in general debility. The high levels of silicic acid in the straw will explain its use as a remedy for skin conditions, especially in external applications.

Preparation and Dosage: An infusion is made from 1–3 teaspoonfuls of the dried straw and drunk three times a day. Tincture dosage is 3–5 milliliters three times a day. A soothing bath can also be made for use in neuralgia and irritated skin conditions from 1 pound of shredded straw boiled in 2 quarts of water for half an hour. The liquid is strained and added to the bath, or the cooked rolled oats may be placed into a muslin bag and so added to the bath water.

Oregon Grape

Berberis aquifolium

Part Used: Rhizome and root.

Actions: Alterative, cholagogue, laxative, antiemetic, anticatarrhal, tonic.

Indications: Oregon grape is similar in action to both goldenseal and barberry. It finds its main use in the treatment of chronic and scaly skin conditions such as psoriasis and eczema. As skin problems of this sort are due to systemic causes within the body, the tonic activity of Oregon grape on the liver and gallbladder may explain its potency. It can be used in stomach and gallbladder conditions, especially where there is associated nausea and vomiting. It may safely be used as a laxative to relieve constipation.

Preparation and Dosage: A decoction is made from 1 teaspoonful of the dried herb and drunk three times a day. Tincture dosage is 1 milliliter three times a day.

Parsley

Petroselinum crispum

Part Used: Tap root, leaves, and seeds.

Actions: Diuretic, expectorant, emmenagogue, carminative, antispasmodic, hypotensive.

Indications: The fresh herb, so widely used in cookery, is a rich source of vitamin C. Medicinally, parsley has three main areas of usage. First, it is an effective diuretic, helping the body get rid of excess water and so may be used wherever such an effect is desired. Remember, however, that the cause of the problem must be sought and treated; don't just treat symptoms. The second area of use is as an emmenagogue stimulating the menstrual process. It is advisable not to use parsley in medicinal dosage during pregnancy, as there may be excessive stimulation of the womb. The third use is as a carminative, easing flatulence and the colic pains that may accompany it.

Preparation and Dosage: An infusion is made from 1–2 teaspoonfuls of the dried herb and drunk three times a day. Tincture dosage is 1–2 milliliters three times a day.

Partridgeberry

Mitchella repens

Part Used: Aerial parts.

Actions: Parturient, emmenagogue, diuretic, astringent, tonic.

Indications: Partridgeberry is among the best remedies for preparing the uterus and whole body for childbirth. It may also be used for the relief of painful periods. As an astringent, it has been used in the treatment of colitis, especially if there is much mucus.

Preparation and Dosage: An infusion is made from 1 teaspoonful of the dried herb and drunk three times a day. Tincture dosage is 1–2 milliliters three times a day.

Pasqueflower

Anemone pulsatilla

Part Used: Aerial parts.

Actions: Nervine, antispasmodic, antibacterial.

Indications: Pasqueflower is an excellent relaxing nervine for use in problems relating to nervous tension and spasm in the reproductive system. It may be used with safety in the relief of painful periods, ovarian pain, and painful conditions of the testes. It may be used to reduce tension reactions and headaches associated with them. It will help insomnia and general overactivity. The antibacterial actions give this herb a role in treating infections that affect the skin, especially boils. It is similarly useful in the treatment of respiratory infections and asthma. The oil or tincture will ease earache.

Preparation and Dosage: An infusion is made from $1/2$–1 teaspoonful of the dried herb and drunk three times a day. Tincture dosage is 1 milliliter three times a day.

Passionflower

Passiflora incarnata

Part Used: Leaves and whole plant.

Actions: Nervine, hypnotic, antispasmodic, anodyne, hypotensive.

Indications: Passionflower has a sedating effect on central nervous system activity and is hypotensive; it is used to lower blood pressure, prevent tachycardia, and relieve insomnia. Its alkaloids and flavonoids have both been reported to have sedative activity in animals. Many of its flavonoids are well known for their antispasmodic and anti-inflammatory activities. Passionflower is the herb of choice for treating intransigent insomnia. It promotes restful sleep without any "narcotic hangover." It may be used wherever an antispasmodic is required, as in Parkinson's disease, seizures, and hysteria. It can be very effective in nerve pain such as neuralgia and the viral infection of nerves called shingles. It may be used in asthma where there is much spasmodic activity, especially when there is associated tension.

Preparation and Dosage: An infusion is made from 1 teaspoonful of the dried herb and drunk three times a day. Tincture dosage is 1–2 milliliters three times a day. Drink a cup in the evening for sleeplessness, or 1 cup twice a day for other conditions.

Peppermint

Mentha piperita

Part Used: Aerial parts.

Actions: Carminative, anti-inflammatory, antispasmodic, aromatic, diaphoretic, antiemetic, nervine, antimicrobial, analgesic.

Indications: Peppermint is an excellent carminative, having a relaxing effect on the muscles of the digestive system. It combats flatulence and stimulates bile and digestive juice flow. It is used to relieve intestinal colic, flatulent dyspepsia, and associated conditions. The volatile oil acts as a mild anesthetic to the stomach wall, allaying feelings of nausea (e.g., in pregnancy and travel sickness). Peppermint can play a role in the treatment of ulcerative conditions of the bowels. It is a traditional treatment of fevers, colds, and influenza. As an inhalant it is used as temporary relief for nasal catarrh. Where headaches are associated with digestion, peppermint may help. As a nervine it eases anxiety and tension. In painful periods it relieves the pain and eases associated tension. Externally it is used to relieve itching and inflammations.

Preparation and Dosage: An infusion is made from 1 teaspoonful of the dried herb and drunk three times a day. Tincture dosage is 1–2 milliliters three times a day.

Plantain

Plantago major

Part Used: Leaves or aerial parts.

Actions: Vulnerary, expectorant, demulcent, anti-inflammatory, astringent, diuretic, antimicrobial.

Indications: Both the greater plantain and its close relative ribwort plantain have valuable healing properties. It acts as a gentle expectorant while also soothing inflamed and sore membranes, making it ideal for coughs and mild bronchitis. Its astringency aids in diarrhea, hemorrhoids, and also in cystitis where there is bleeding.

Preparation and Dosage: An infusion is made from 2 teaspoonfuls of the dried herb and drunk three times a day. Tincture dosage is 1–2 milliliters three times a day.

Pleurisy Root

Asclepias tuberosa

Part Used: Rhizome.

Actions: Diaphoretic, expectorant, antispasmodic, carminative, anti-inflammatory.

Indications: Pleurisy root is effective against respiratory infections where it reduces inflammations and assists expectoration. It can be used in the treatment of bronchitis and other chest conditions. The addition of diaphoretic and anti-spasmodic powers will show why it is so highly valued in the treatment of pleurisy and pneumonia. It can be used in influenza.

Preparation and Dosage: An infusion is made from 1 teaspoonful of the dried herb and drunk three times a day. Tincture dosage is 1–2 milliliters three times a day.

Prickly Ash

Zanthoxylum americanum

Part Used: Bark and berries.

Actions: Stimulant (circulatory), tonic, alterative, carminative, diaphoretic, anti-rheumatic, hepatic.

Indications: Prickly ash may be used much like cayenne, although it is slower in action. It is used in many chronic problems such as rheumatism and skin disease. Any sign of poor circulation (e.g., chilblains, leg cramps, varicose veins, and varicose ulcers) calls for the use of this herb. Externally, it may be used as a stimulation liniment for rheumatism and fibrositis. Due to its stimulating effect upon the lymphatic system, circulation, and mucous membranes, it will have a role in the holistic treatment of many specific conditions.

Preparation and Dosage: An infusion is made from 1 teaspoonful of the dried herb and drunk three times a day. Tincture dosage is 1–2 milliliters three times a day.

Red Clover

Trifolium pratense

Part Used: Flower heads.

Actions: Alterative, expectorant, antispasmodic.

Indications. Red Clover, one of the most useful remedies for children with skin problems, can also be of value for adults. The expectorant and antispasmodic action give this remedy a role in the treatment of coughs and bronchitis, but especially in whooping cough. As an alterative it is indicated in a wide range of problems when approached in a holistic sense.

Preparation and Dosage: An infusion is made from 1–2 teaspoonfuls of the dried herb and drunk three times a day. Tincture dosage is 2 milliliters three times a day.

Red Sage

Salvia officinalis var. *rubia*

Part Used: Leaves.

Actions: Carminative, antispasmodic, antimicrobial, astringent, anti-inflammatory.

Indications: Red sage is the classic remedy for inflammations of the mouth, throat, and tonsils, its volatile oils soothing the mucous membranes. It may be used internally and as a mouthwash for inflamed and bleeding gums, inflamed tongue, or generalized mouth inflammation. It is an excellent remedy in mouth ulcers. As a gargle, it will aid in the treatment of laryngitis, pharyngitis, tonsillitis, and quinsy. It is a valuable carminative used in dyspepsia. It reduces sweating when taken internally. As a compress it promotes the healing of wounds.

Preparation and Dosage: An infusion is made from 1–2 teaspoonfuls of the leaves and drunk three times a day. For a mouthwash, put 2 teaspoonfuls of the leaves in ½ liter (1 pint) water, bring to a boil, and let stand covered for 15 minutes. Gargle deeply with the hot tea for 5–10 minutes several times a day. Tincture dosage is 2–4 milliliters three times a day.

Rhubarb Root

Rheum palmatum

Part Used: Rhizome of *Rheum palmatum* and other species, not the garden rhubarb.

Actions: Bitter, laxative, astringent.

Indications: Rhubarb root has a purgative action for use in the treatment of constipation but also has an astringent effect following this. It therefore has a truly cleansing action upon the gut, removing debris and then astringing with antiseptic properties as well. Note: rhubarb root may color the urine yellow or red.

Preparation and Dosage: A decoction is made from ½–1 teaspoonful of the ground root and drunk in the morning and evening. Tincture dosage is 1–2 milliliters three times a day.

Rosemary

Rosmarinus officinalis

Part Used: Leaves and twigs.

Actions: Carminative, antispasmodic, antidepressive, rubefacient, antimicrobial, emmenagogue.

Indications: Rosemary is a circulatory and nervine stimulant that has a toning and calming effect on digestion and is also used where psychological tension is present, as in cases of flatulent dyspepsia, headache, or depression associated with debility. Externally, it may be used to ease muscular pain, sciatica, and neuralgia. It acts as a stimulant to the hair follicles as well as to scalp circulation and thus may be helpful in cases of premature baldness. The oil is most effective here.

Preparation and Dosage: An infusion is made from 1–2 teaspoonfuls of the dried herb and drunk three times a day. Tincture dosage is 1–2 milliliters three times a day.

St. John's Wort

Hypericum perforatum

Part Used: Aerial parts.

Actions: Anti-inflammatory, astringent, vulnerary, nervine, antimicrobial.

Indications: Taken internally, St. John's wort has a sedative and pain-reducing effect, which gives it a place in the treatment of neuralgia, anxiety, tension, and similar problems. It is especially regarded as an herb to use where there are menopausal changes triggering irritability and anxiety. It is increasingly recommended in the treatment of depression. In addition to neuralgic pain, it will ease fibrositis, sciatica, and rheumatic pain. Externally, it is a valuable healing and anti-inflammatory remedy. As a lotion, it will speed the healing of wounds and bruises, varicose veins, and mild burns. The oil is especially useful for the healing of sunburn.

Preparation and Dosage: An infusion is made from 1–2 teaspoonfuls of the dried herb and drunk three times a day. Tincture dosage is 1–2 milliliters three times a day.

Sarsaparilla

Smilax officinalis

Part Used: Root and rhizome.

Actions: Alterative, antirheumatic, diuretic, diaphoretic.

Indications: Sarsaparilla is a widely applicable alterative. It may be used to aid proper functioning of the body as a whole and in the correction of such diffuse systemic problems as skin and rheumatic conditions. It is particularly useful in scaling skin conditions such as psoriasis, especially where there is much irritation. It should be considered as part of any wider treatment for chronic rheumatism and is especially useful for rheumatoid arthritis. It has been shown that sarsaparilla contains constituents with properties that aid testosterone activity in the body.

Preparation and Dosage: A decoction is made from 1–2 teaspoonfuls of the root and drunk three times a day. Tincture dosage is 1–2 milliliters three times a day.

Saw Palmetto

Serenoa serrulata

Part Used: Berries.

Actions: Diuretic, urinary antiseptic, endocrine agent.

Indications: Saw palmetto is an herb that acts to tone and strengthen the male reproductive system. It may be used with safety where a boost to the male sex hormones is required. It is a specific remedy in cases of enlarged prostate glands. It will be of value in infections of the genitourinary tract.

Preparation and Dosage: A decoction is made from ½–1 teaspoonful of the berries and drunk three times a day. Tincture dosage is 1–2 milliliters three times a day.

Senna

Cassia angustifolia, C. senna

Part Used: Dried fruit pods and leaves.

Actions: Cathartic.

Indications: Senna is a powerful cathartic used in the treatment of constipation that works through a stimulation of intestinal peristalsis. It is vital to recognize, however, that constipation is a symptom of some causal condition and that this cause must be sought and dealt with specifically.

Preparation and Dosage: An infusion is made from the dried pods or leaves steeped in warm water for 6–12 hours. If they are Alexandrian senna pods *(C. senna),* use 3–6 in a cup of water; if they are Tinnevelly senna pods *(C. angustifolia),* use 4–12 in a cup of water. Tincture dosage is 1–2 milliliters to be taken before bedtime.

Shepherd's Purse

Capsella bursa-pastoris

Part Used: Aerial parts.

Actions: Astringent, diuretic, anti-inflammatory.

Indications: This herb is easily recognized by its characteristic seed pods that look like medieval purses. It may be used wherever a gentle diuretic is called for (e.g., in water retention due to kidney problems). As an astringent, it will prove effective in the treatment of diarrhea, wounds, nosebleeds, and other conditions. It is specific for stimulation of the menstrual process yet can also be used to reduce excess flow.

Preparation and Dosage: An infusion is made from 1–2 teaspoonfuls of the dried herb. If it is used for menstrual conditions, it should be drunk every 2–3 hours just before and during the period. Otherwise, drink it three times a day. Tincture dosage is 1–2 milliliters three times a day.

Skullcap

Scutellaria laterifolia

Part Used: Aerial parts.

Actions: Nervine tonic, antispasmodic, hypotensive.

Indications: Skullcap is perhaps the most widely relevant nervine available to us. It relaxes states of nervous tension while at the same time it renews and revives the central nervous system. It has specific use in the treatment of hysterical states as well as epilepsy and other conditions involving seizures. It may be used in all exhausted or depressed conditions, and it can be used with complete safety in the easing of premenstrual tension.

Preparation and Dosage: An infusion is made from 1–2 teaspoonfuls of the dried herb and drunk three times a day. Tincture dosage is 2–4 milliliters three times a day.

Slippery Elm

Ulmus fulva

Part Used: Inner bark.

Actions: Demulcent, emollient, nutrient, astringent, anti-inflammatory.

Indications: Slippery elm bark is a soothing nutritive demulcent that is perfectly suited for sensitive or inflamed mucous membrane linings in the digestive system. It may be used in gastritis, gastric or duodenal ulcer, enteritis, colitis, and the like. It is often used as a food during convalescence as it is gentle and easily assimilated. In cases of diarrhea it will soothe and astringe at the same time. Externally, it makes an excellent poultice for boils, abscesses, or ulcers.

Preparation and Dosage: A decoction is made by using 1 part of the powdered bark to 8 parts of water. Mix the powder in a little water initially to ensure it will mix. Bring to a boil and simmer gently for 10–15 minutes. Drink half a cup three times a day. For a poultice, mix the coarsely powdered bark with enough boiling water to make a paste.

Stone Root

Collinsonia canadensis

Part Used: Root and rhizome.

Actions: Antilithic, diuretic, diaphoretic.

Indications: As its name suggests, stone root finds its main use in the treatment and prevention of stone and gravel in the urinary system and the gallbladder.

It can be used as a prophylactic but is also excellent when the body is in need of help in passing stones or gravel. It is also a strong diuretic.

Preparation and Dosage: A decoction is made from 1–2 teaspoonfuls of the dried root and drunk three times a day. Tincture dosage is 1–2 milliliters three times a day.

Sweet Violet

Viola odorata

Part Used: Leaves and flowers.

Actions: Expectorant, alterative, anti-inflammatory, diuretic.

Indications: Sweet violet has a long history of use as a cough remedy and especially for the treatment of bronchitis. It may also be used to aid in the treatment of upper respiratory catarrh. With the combination of actions present, it has a use in skin conditions such as eczema and in a long-term approach to rheumatism. It may be used for urinary infections. Sweet violet has a reputation as an "anticancer" herb, and although this is a misnomer, the herb definitely has a role to play in any holistic treatment of cancer.

Preparation and Dosage: An infusion is made from 1 teaspoonful of the dried herb and drunk three times a day. Tincture dosage is 1–2 milliliters three times a day.

Thuja

Thuja occidentalis

Part Used: Young twigs.

Actions: Expectorant, antimicrobial, diuretic, astringent, alterative.

Indications: Thuja's main action is due to its stimulating and alterative volatile oil. In bronchial catarrh, thuja combines expectoration with a systemic stimulation beneficial if there is also heart weakness. It should be avoided where the cough is due to overstimulation, as in dry irritable coughs. Where ordinary incontinence occurs due to loss of muscle tone, thuja may be used. It has a role to play in the treatment of psoriasis and rheumatism and may be used externally to treat warts. It is reported to counter the ill effects of smallpox vaccination. A marked antifungal effect is found if it is used externally for ringworm and thrush.

Preparation and Dosage: An infusion is made from 1 teaspoonful of the dried herb and drunk three times a day. Tincture dosage is 1–2 milliliters three times a day

CAUTION: Avoid during pregnancy, as thuja has a specific reflex action on the uterus.

Thyme

Thymus vulgaris

Part Used: Leaves and flowering tops.

Actions: Carminative, antimicrobial, antispasmodic, expectorant, anthelmintic, astringent.

Indications: With its high content of volatile oil, thyme makes a good carminative for use in dyspepsia and sluggish digestion. This oil is also a strongly antiseptic substance, which explains many of thyme's uses. It can be used externally as a lotion for infected wounds, but also internally for respiratory and digestive infections, it may be used as a gargle in laryngitis and tonsillitis, easing sore throats and soothing irritable coughs. It is an excellent cough remedy, producing expectoration and reducing unnecessary spasm. It may be used in bronchitis, whooping cough, and asthma. As a gentle astringent, it has found use in childhood diarrhea and bed-wetting.

Preparation and Dosage: An infusion is made from 1–2 teaspoonfuls of the dried herb and drunk three times a day. Tincture dosage is 1–2 milliliters three times a day.

Tea Tree

Melaleuca alternifolia

Part Used: Essential oil.

Actions: Antimicrobial.

Indications: The essential oil of tea tree is an important antimicrobial that has recently become available in North America. An undoubtedly useful oil, it has become the object of an exaggerated promotion reminiscent of the old snake oil sales pitches! Claims are being made that have a kernel of truth but are exaggerated for promotional reasons. Never believe advertisements about herbs; question them instead. The claims may be true, but get the evidence and make up your own mind. The conditions that *Melaleuca* is claimed to heal include sinusitis, the common cold, sinus blockage, laryngitis, coughs, canker sores, boils, cuts, bites, sunburn, miliaria, parasites, head lice, herpes simplex, herpes progenitalis, impetigo, psoriasis, infected seborrheic dermatitis, ringworm of the scalp, ringworm, athlete's foot, fungal infections of the nails, thrush, and trichomoniasis.

Preparation and Dosage: The oil is for external use, and for those with sensitive skin, it should be diluted with a bland fixed oil such as almond oil. Many products currently on the market contain the oil, including toothpastes, soaps, shampoos, and deodorants.

Valerian

Valeriana officinalis

Part Used: Rhizome, stolons, and roots.

Actions: Nervine, hypnotic, antispasmodic, carminative, hypotensive, emmenagogue.

Indications: Valerian's main indications are anxiety, nervous sleeplessness, and the bodily symptoms of tension such as muscle cramping or indigestion. It may be used safely where tension and anxiety are present, whether the symptoms are purely psychological and behavioral or physical in nature. For some people valerian can be an effective mild pain reliever. As one of the best gentle herbal sleeping remedies, it promotes the natural process of slipping into sleep. For elders who do not need as much sleep as they once did, it also ensures that simply lying in bed becomes a restful and relaxing experience, one that can often be as revivifying as sleep itself. Valerian is a safe muscle relaxant and can be used in muscle cramping, uterine cramps, and intestinal colic. Valerian is used worldwide as a relaxing remedy in hypertension and stress-related heart problems. Its effect goes beyond simple nerve relaxation, as its constituents include mild hypotensives.

Preparation and Dosage: To be effective valerian has to be used in sufficiently high dosage. The tincture dosage is from 2.5–5 milliliters ($^1/_2$–1 tsp) to as much as 10 milliliters in some cases (2 tsp). For situations of extreme stress where a sedative or muscle relaxant effect is needed fast, the single dose of 1 teaspoonful may be repeated two or three times at short intervals. An infusion is used to ensure no loss of the volatile oils from 2 teaspoonfuls of the dried root for each cup of tea prepared. A cold infusion may be made from a glass of cold water poured over 2 teaspoonfuls of valerian root and left to stand for 8–10 hours. A nighttime dose should thus be set up in the morning, and the morning dose is prepared the night before.

Vervain

Verbena officinalis

Part Used: Aerial parts.

Actions: Nervine tonic, sedative, antispasmodic, diaphoretic, hypotensive, galactagogue, hepatic.

Indications: Vervain is an herb that will strengthen the nervous system while relaxing any tension and stress. It can be used to ease depression and melancholia, especially following an illness such as influenza. Vervain may be used to help in seizure and hysteria. As a diaphoretic, it can be used in the early stages of fevers. As a hepatic remedy, it will help in inflammation of the gallbladder and jaundice. It may be used as a mouthwash to prevent caries and gum disease.

Preparation and Dosage: An infusion is made from 1–2 teaspoonfuls of the dried herb and drunk three times a day. Tincture dosage is 1–2 milliliters three times a day.

Wahoo

Euonymus atropurpureus

Part Used: Root bark.

Actions: Cholagogue, hepatic, laxative, diuretic, circulatory stimulant.

Indications: Wahoo is one of the primary liver herbs. It acts to remove congestion from the liver, allowing the free flow of bile and so helping the digestive process. It may be used in the treatment of jaundice and gallbladder problems such as inflammation and pain or congestion due to stones. It will relieve any constipation related to liver or gallbladder problems. Through its normalizing action upon the liver, it may help in a range of skin problems where there is a possible involvement of the liver.

Preparation and Dosage: A decoction is made from ¹/₂–1 teaspoonful of the bark and drunk three times a day. Tincture dosage is 1–2 milliliters three times a day.

White Poplar

Populus tremuloides

Part Used: Bark.

Actions: Anti-inflammatory, astringent, antiseptic, anodyne, cholagogue, bitter tonic.

Indications: White poplar is an excellent remedy to use in the treatment of arthritis and rheumatism where there is much pain and swelling. In this area, its use is quite similar to willow; it is most effective when used as part of a broad therapeutic regimen. It is very helpful during flare-ups of rheumatoid arthritis. As a cholagogue, it can be used to stimulate digestion and especially stomach and liver function, particularly where there is loss of appetite. It may be considered for use in feverish colds and infections such as cystitis. As an astringent it can be used in the treatment of diarrhea.

Preparation and Dosage: A decoction is made from 1–2 teaspoonfuls of the dried herb and drunk three times a day. Tincture dosage is 1–2 milliliters three times a day.

Wild Carrot

Daucus carrota

Part Used: Dried aerial parts and seeds.

Actions: Diuretic, antilithic, carminative, antispasmodic.

Indications: The volatile oil that is present in wild carrot is an active urinary antiseptic, which helps explain its use in the treatment of such conditions as cystitis and prostatitis. It has long been considered a specific remedy in the treatment of kidney stones. In the treatment of gout and rheumatism, it is used in combination with other remedies to support its cleansing diuretic action. The seeds can be used as a settling carminative agent for the relief of flatulence and colic.

Preparation and Dosage: An infusion is made from 1 teaspoonful of the dried herb and drunk three times a day. Tincture dosage is 1–2 milliliters three times a day.

Wild Cherry Bark

Prunus serotina

Part Used: Dried bark.

Actions: Antitussive, expectorant, astringent, nervine, antispasmodic.

Indications: Because of its powerful sedative action on the cough reflex, wild cherry bark finds its main use in the treatment of irritating coughs and thus has a role in the treatment of bronchitis and whooping cough. It can be used together with other herbs to help control asthma. It must be remembered, however, that mere inhibition of a cough does not represent the healing of a chest infection, which will still need to be treated. It may also be used as a bitter where digestion is sluggish. The cold infusion of the bark may be helpful as a wash in cases of inflammation of the eyes.

Preparation and Dosage: An infusion is made from 1 teaspoonful of the dried herb and drunk three times a day. Tincture dosage is 1–2 milliliters three times a day.

Wild Indigo

Baptisia tinctoria

Part Used: Root.

Actions: Antimicrobial, anticatarrhal.

Indications. Wild indigo is an herb to be considered wherever there is a focused infection. It is especially useful in the treatment of infections and catarrh in the ear, nose, and throat. It may be used for laryngitis, tonsillitis, pharyngitis, and catarrhal infections of the nose and sinus. Taken both internally and as a mouthwash, it will heal mouth ulcers and gingivitis and help in the control of pyorrhea. As a systemic remedy, it may be helpful in the treatment of enlarged and inflamed lymph glands and may also help to reduce fever. Wild indigo ointment will help infected ulcers and ease sore nipples.

Preparation and Dosage: A decoction is made from ¹/₂–1 teaspoonful of the dried herb and drunk three times a day. Tincture dosage is 1–2 milliliters three times a day.

Wild Lettuce

Lactuca virosa

Part Used: Dried leaves.

Actions: Nervine, anodyne, hypnotic, antispasmodic.

Indications: The latex of the wild lettuce was at one time sold as "Lettuce Opium," naming the use of this herb quite well! It is a valuable remedy for use in insomnia, restlessness, excitability, and other manifestations of an overactive nervous system. As an antispasmodic, it can be used as part of a holistic treatment of whooping cough and dry irritated coughs in general. It will relieve colic pains in the intestines and uterus and so may be used in dysmennorhea. It will ease muscular pains related to rheumatism. It has been used as an anaphrodisiac.

Preparation and Dosage: An infusion is made from 1–2 teaspoonfuls of the dried herb and drunk three times a day. Tincture dosage is 1–2 milliliters three times a day.

Wild Yam

Dioscorea villosa

Part Used: Dried underground parts.

Actions: Antispasmodic, anti-inflammatory, antirheumatic, hepatic, cholagogue, diaphoretic.

Indications: This valuable herb was at one time the sole source of the chemicals that were used as the raw materials for contraceptive hormone manufacture. In herbal medicine, wild yam is a remedy that can be used to relieve intestinal colic, to soothe diverticulitis, and to ease dysmenorrhea and ovarian and uterine pains. It is of great use in the treatment of rheumatoid arthritis, especially in the acute phase of intense inflammation.

Preparation and Dosage: A decoction is made from 1–2 teaspoonfuls of the dried herb and drunk three times a day. Tincture dosage is 1–2 milliliters three times a day.

Willow

Salix spp.

Part Used: Bark.

Actions: Analgesic, anti-inflammatory, tonic.

Indications: Willow is an ancient remedy that has been used in various forms for rheumatism, gout, fevers, and aches and pains of all kinds. It is usually considered to be the natural form and origin of aspirin.

Preparation and Dosage: A decoction is made from 1–2 teaspoonfuls of the bark and drunk three times a day. Tincture dosage is 1–2 milliliters three times a day.

Witch Hazel

Hamamelis virginiana

Part Used: Bark or leaves.

Actions: Astringent, anti-inflammatory.

Indications: This herb can be found in most households in the form of distilled witch hazel. The most easily used astringent known, this herb may be used wherever there has been bleeding, both internally or externally. It is especially useful in the easing of hemorrhoids. It has a deserved reputation in the treatment of bruises, inflamed swellings, and also varicose veins. Witch hazel will control diarrhea and help to relieve dysentery.

Preparation and Dosage: An infusion is made from 1 teaspoonful of the dried herb and drunk three times a day. Tincture dosage is 1–2 milliliters three times a day.

Wood Betony

Betonica officinalis

Part Used: Dried aerial parts.

Actions: Nervine, bitter.

Indications: Betony gently tones and strengthens the nervous system and also has a relaxing action. It finds use in the treatment of nervous debility associated with anxiety and tension. It will ease headaches and neuralgias of nervous origin and especially those caused by hypertension.

Preparation and Dosage: An infusion is made from 1–2 teaspoonfuls of the dried herb and drunk three times a day. Tincture dosage is 1–2 milliliters three times a day.

Yarrow

Achillea millefolium

Part Used: Aerial parts.

Actions: Diaphoretic, hypotensive, astringent, anti-inflammatory, diuretic, antimicrobial, bitter, hepatic.

Indications: One of the best diaphoretic herbs known, yarrow is a standard remedy for aiding the body to deal with fevers. It lowers blood pressure due to a dilation of the peripheral vessels. It stimulates the digestion and tones the blood vessels. As a urinary antiseptic, it is indicated in infections such as cystitis. Used externally, it will aid in the healing of wounds. It is considered to be a specific remedy in thrombotic conditions associated with hypertension.

Preparation and Dosage: An infusion is made from 1–2 teaspoonfuls of the dried herb and drunk three times a day. Tincture dosage is 1–2 milliliters three times a day.

Yellow Dock

Rumex crispus

Part Used: Root.

Actions: Alterative, laxative, hepatic, tonic, cholagogue.

Indications: Yellow dock is used extensively in the treatment of chronic skin complaints such as psoriasis. The anthraquinones it contains have a markedly cathartic action on the bowel, but in this herb they act in a mild way, possibly tempered by the tannin content. Thus, it makes a valuable remedy for constipation, working as it does in a much wider way than simply stimulating the gut muscles. It promotes the flow of bile and has that somewhat obscure action of being a "blood cleanser." The action on the gallbladder gives it a role in the treatment of jaundice when due to congestion.

Preparation and Dosage: A decoction is made from 1 teaspoon of the dried root and drunk three times a day. Tincture dosage is 1–2 milliliters three times a day.

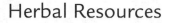

Useful Internet Addresses

Herbal Resources

There is a bewildering amount of information concerning herbs, their use and abuse on the internet. I'm afraid to say that the bulk of it is not very reliable. What follows are links to databases, treatment suggestions, or the writings of herbalists that are dependable.

Herbalists

David Winston
www.herbaltherapeutics.net

Jonathan Treasure's Herbal Bookworm
www.herbological.com

Medical Herbalism/Paul Bergner
www.medherb.com

Robyn Klein's Recommended Reading
www.rrreading.com

Rosemary Gladstar's Sage Mountain
www.sagemountain.com

Christopher Hobbs' Virtual Herbal
www.christopherhobbs.com

Herbal Databases

Herbal Medicine Center—HealthWorld Online

www.healthy.net/scr/center.asp?centerid=24

HealthWorld Online is the Internet's leading resource on alternative medicine, wellness, and mind/body health. It has a comprehensive herbal section.

HerbMed

www.herbmed.org

HerbMed an interactive, electronic herbal database—provides hyperlinked access to the scientific data underlying the use of herbs for health. It is an impartial, evidence-based information resource.

Finding Practitioners

American Herbalist Guild (AHG)

www.americanherbalistsguild.com

American Association of Naturopath Physicians

www.naturopathic.org

Alternative and Complementary Medicine

Healthy Aging Center—HealthWorld Online

www.healthy.net/scr/center.asp?centerid=3

Possibly the best online Alternative Medicine site, Health World provides a comprehensive package of resouces in their Healthy Aging Center. Apart from the numerous named conditions discussed, they cover nutrition, herbalism, naturopathic, and integral medicine. Their discussions of wellness, fitness, and sexuality in the aging process are worth exploring.

General Health Web Sites

Arthritis Foundation

www.arthritis.org

A voluntary health agency covering all arthritis-related conditions.

MEDLINEplus from the National Library of Medicine

www.nlm.nih.gov/medlineplus

MEDLINEplus information pages direct you to resources containing information that will help you research your health questions.

Healthfinder

www.healthfinder.gov

A government site that directs you to online publications, databases, Web sites, and support and self-help groups, as well as government agencies and not-for-profit organizations that produce reliable information for the public.

Hardin Meta Directory of Internet Health Sources

www.lib.uiowa.edu/hardin/md/index.html

Hardin MD points to the most complete and frequently cited lists for health subjects, a list of lists.

MayoClinic.com

www.mayoclinic.com

A wealth of easy-to-understand information on health and medical topics.

The Columbia University College of Physicians and Surgeons Complete Home Medical Guide

http://cpmcnet.columbia.edu/texts/guide

The online version of the Third Revised Edition of this standard consumer health text.

Women's Health Web Sites

Ask NOAH About: Women's Health

www.noah-health.org/english/wellness/healthyliving/womenshealth.html

The New York Online Access to Health (NOAH) is a bilingual health information site. Sponsors include the City University of New York, the New York Academy of Medicine, and the New York Public Library.

Feminist.com Health and Sexuality Links

www.feminist.com/resources/links/links_health.html

A comprehensive list of links to pages concerning breast cancer/cancer, reproductive health, reproductive rights, sexuality, women & AIDS, and general women's health provided by feminist.com, a grassroots community. Benefactors include the Gloria Steinem Fund.

National Women's Health Resource Center (NWHRC)

www.healthywomen.org

The National Women's Health Resource Center is a nonprofit, national clearing-house for women's health information.

WebMD Women's Health Center

http://women.webmd.com

WebMD has online information, research, educational services, and communities for consumers and physicians.

Men's Health Web Sites

American Academy of Family Physicians—Men's Health

www.aafp.org/patientinfo/health5.html

Information pamphlets on a range of health topics including prostate cancer screening, hypertension, diet, lowering cholesterol, and lifestyle.

American Cancer Society Man to Man

www.cancer.org/m2m/m2m.html

Prostate cancer education and support.

New York Times Men's Health

www.nytimes.com/library/national/science/menshealth/resources.html

Resources for specific health issues such as aging, AIDS, alcohol, arthritis, back pain, cholesterol, colorectal cancer, coronary artery disease, depression, diet and exercise, headache, prostate, smoking, sexually transmitted diseases, stress, and stroke.

Drug Information Resources

RxList—The Internet Drug Index

www.rxlist.com

A very useful drug index. Information on various disease categories is also provided as is Taber's Medical Encyclopedia.

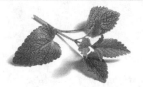

Bibliography

Herbal

Bremness, Lesley. *The Complete Book of Herbs*. New York: Viking Studio Books, 1994.

Fünfgeld, E. W. Rökan. *Ginkgo biloba*. Berlin: Springer-Verlag, 1988.

Green, James. *The Herbal Medicine Maker's Handbook*. Berkeley: Crossing Press, 2000.

———. *The Male Herbal*. Berkeley: Crossing Press, 2007.

Grieve, Mrs. M. *A Modern Herbal*. 2 vols. New York: Dover Publications, 1971.

Griggs, Barbara. *Green Pharmacy*. Rochester, Vt.: Healing Arts Press, 1997.

Hoffmann, David. *An Herbal Guide to Stress Relief*. Rochester, Vt.: Healing Arts Press, 1991.

———. *Medical Herbalism*. Rochester, Vt.: Healing Arts Press, 2003.

———. *The New Holistic Herbal*. Shaftsbury, U.K.: Element Books, 1991.

Lewis, Walter H., and Memory P. F. Elvin-Lewis. *Medical Botany*. 2nd ed. New York: John Wiley & Sons, 2003.

Mabey, Richard. *The New Age Herbalist*. New York: Collier Books, 1988.

Mowrey, Daniel. *Next Generation Herbal Medicine*. New Canaan, Ct.: Keats Publishing Co., 1990.

Pizzorno, Joseph E., and Michael T. Murray. *Textbook of Natural Medicine*. 3rd ed. New York: Churchill Livingstone, 2005.

Rose, Jeanne. *Herbal Body Book*. Berkeley: Frog Ltd., 2000.

Theiss, Barbara and Peter. *The Family Herbal*. Rochester, Vt.: Healing Arts Press, 1989.

General

American Medical Association. *AMA Handbook of First Aid and Emergency Care*. New York: Random House, 2000.

Dychtwald, Ken. *The Age Wave*. New York: Bantam, 1990.

Fries, James F. *Aging Well*. Reading, Pa.: Addison Wesley, 1989.

———. *Arthritis*. 5th ed. New York: Perseus Books, 1999.

Kübler-Ross, Elizabeth. *On Death and Dying*. New York: Scribner, 1997.

MacLean, Helene. *Caring for Your Parents: A Sourcebook of Options and Solutions for Both Generations*. Garden City, N.Y.: Doubleday and Co., 1987.

Martin, Raquel, and Judi Gerstung. *The Estrogen Alternative*. 4th ed. Rochester, Vt.: Healing Arts Press, 2004.

Murray, Michael, and Joseph Pizzorno. *Encyclopedia of Natural Medicine*. 2nd ed. New York: Three Rivers Press, 1997.

Pfeiffer, George J., and Louise Williams. *Taking Care of Today and Tomorrow*. Reston, Va.: The Center for Corporate Health, 1991.

Portnow, Jay, and Martha Houtmann. *Home Care for the Elderly: A Complete Guide*. New York: McGraw-Hill, 1987.

Ojeda, Linda. *Menopause Without Medicine*. 5th ed. Claremont, Calif.: Hunter House, 2003.

Simonton, Carl and Stephanie. *Getting Well Again*. New York: Bantam, 1992.

Weil, Andrew. *Natural Health, Natural Medicine*. Boston: Houghton Mifflin Co., 2004.

Wilson, Josleen. *Woman: Your Body, Your Health*. New York: Harcourt, Brace, Jovanovich, 1990.

Vickery, Donald, and James Fries. *Take Care of Yourself*. New York: Perseus Books, 2006.

Index

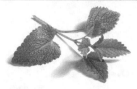

absorption, 22, 36
Acacia catechu. See black catechu
Achillea millefolium. See yarrow
actions. *See* herbal medicines
activities of daily living (ADL) devices, 188
adaptogens
    adrenal gland, 15, 229–30
    defined, 15, 126
    nervous system, 106, 118–21
adrenal. *See* glands
Aesculus hippocastanum.
        See horse chestnut
aging
    biology of (theories), 7
    cultural views on, 8
    health issues and, 13
    herbal medicine and, 7
    population and, 2
    psychology of, 104, 127
    sexuality and, 166
Agrimonia eupatoria. See agrimony
agrimony, 254
Agropyron repens. See couch grass
Alchemilla vulgaris. See lady's mantle
Allium sativum. See garlic

alteratives
    defined, 15
    immune system, 217
    musculoskeletal system, 173–74, 186, 190
    osteoarthritis, 186
    rheumatoid arthritis, 190
Althaea officinalis. See marshmallow
Alzheimer's disease, 121–28
American Cancer Society, 79, 80
American Lung Association, 80
Ammon, H. P., 58
analgesics
    nervous system, 131, 139
    osteoarthritis, 186
Anemone pulsatilla.
        See pasqueflower
Anethum graveolens. See dill
angelica, 254
Angelica archangelica. See angelica
angina pectoris, 64
    remedy for, 59
aniseed, 255
anticatarrhals
    defined, 15–16, 81
    respiratory system, 96, 100, 102

anticonvulsants, 195
antidepressant, 106, 160
anti-inflammatories
    defined, 16
    digestive system, 25, 31–32, 33, 34
    herbal, 174–76
    musculoskeletal system, 174–76, 186, 190
    skin, 202
    urinary system, 145, 151, 153, 154
antilithics
    gallstone, 55
    urinary system, 145
antimicrobials
    defined, 16
    digestive system, 31, 39, 43, 54
    respiratory system, 87, 91, 96, 102
    skin, 202
    urinary system, 145, 148, 154
antipruritics
    eczema and, 202
    for jaundice, 53
antirheumatics, 173–74
    rheumatism and, 183–84
antispasmodics
    cardiovascular system, 67, 72, 76
    defined, 16
    digestive system, 25
    musculoskeletal system, 174, 179, 183, 186, 190, 192
    nervous system, 106, 107, 113, 129
    reproductive system, 159, 161
    respiratory system, 81, 87, 91, 95
aphrodisiacs, 167
Apium graveolens. See celery seed
appendicitis, 28
applications, 177–81
Arctium lappa. See burdock
Arctostaphylos uva-ursi. See bearberry

arnica, 209, 255
    for bruises, 210
Arnica montana. See arnica
arrhythmias, 56, 59
Artemisia vulgaris.
        See mugwort
arteriosclerosis
    cholesterol and, 65
    remedy for, 66
    risk factors, 65–66
arthritis
    defined, 184
    psoriasis and, 205
    rubefacient herbs and, 18, 183
    rubs and poultices for, 209, 248
    See also osteoarthritis;
        rheumatoid arthritis
Arthritis Foundation, 188
Asclepias tuberosa.
        See pleurisy root
ashwaganda, 122–23
asthma
    action for, 83
    attack of, 84
    remedy for, 83
astragalus, 9, 256
    immune system, 216, 220
Astragalus membranaceous, 216.
        See also astragalus
astringents
    defined, 16
    digestive system, 25, 43, 48, 50
    reproductive system, 159, 168
    skin, 202
    urinary system, 145
atherosclerosis, 65–66
    cholesterol and, 61
    menopause and, 163
athlete's foot, 204–5
Avena sativa. See oats

Bach Flower Remedies, 86
balm (lemon balm), 256–57
balmony, 257
Baptisia tinctoria. See wild indigo
Barosma betulina. See buchu
baths, 242–44
bayberry, 257
bearberry *(Uva-Ursi),* 258
Berberis aquifolium. See oregon grape
beth root, 156
Betonica officinalis. See wood betony
Betula alba. See birch
birch, 258
bitters
    defined, 16
    digestive system, 25
    immune system, 216–17
black catechu, 258–59
black cohosh, 259
black haw, 259
black mustard, 177
black root, 260
bladderwrack, 260
blood
    loss in uterine, 159
    stools with, 48
bloodroot, 260–61
blue cohosh, 261
bogbean (buckbean), 261–62
boldo, 262
boneset, 262
Brassica alba, Brassica nigra. See mustard
Brazilian suma (Pfaffia paniculata), 7–8
Brekhman, L. L., 118
bronchitis
    acute, 87–90
    chronic, 83, 90–93
    steam inhalations, 88–90
bruises, 210–11
buchu, 262–63

bugleweed, 263
burdock, 263–64
burns, 210
bursitis, 191–92

calabar bean, 123
calendula, 264
    applications, 209
Calendula officinalis. See calendula
California poppy, 264–65
cancer
    digestive system, 28
    herbal therapy, 226–28
    holistic approach, 225–28
    immune system and, 220
canker sores, 30–31
Capsella bursa-pastoris. See shepherd's
        purse
Capsicum frutescens. See cayenne
caraway, 265
cardiovascular disease, 58–60
    cholesterol and, 61–63
    gallbladder and, 54–55
    stress and personality, 63–64
cardiovascular system, 56–78
    defined, 11
    hawthorn and, 59
    hemorrhoids and, 50
    maintenance of, 60
    remedies, 9
    respiratory system, 83
    surgery and, 113
    tonic herbs, 12–13
    See also heart
Carduus marianus. See milk thistle
carminatives
    defined, 16–17
    digestive system, 25
Carum carvi. See caraway
Cascara sagrada, 265

Cassia angustifolia. See senna
Cassia senna. See senna
catarrh
    action for, 15–16, 81
    pollen induced, 97
Caulophyllum thalictroides.
        See blue cohosh
cayenne, 265–66
    external application, 177–78
celery seed, 266
Cetraria islandica. See Iceland moss
Chamaelirium luteum, 156. *See also*
        false unicorn root
chamomile, 266–67
    reflux and, 33
chasteberry, 267–68
Chelone glabra. See balmony
chickweed, 268
    external application, 178
    recipe, 53
Chinese privet, 216
Chionanthus virginicus.
        See fringe tree bark
cholecystitis, 54
cholesterol
    defined, 61
    gallstones and, 55
    herbs for, 62–63
Chondrus crispus. See Irish moss
Cimicifuga racemosa. See black cohosh
circulatory system
    hypnotics for, 136
    inflammation, 176
    nervines for, 187
    stimulants for, 183, 187, 190
claudication, 75–76
cleavers, 268–69
climacteric, 157
    genital symptoms and, 162
Codonopsis tangshen, 216

coffee, 74
Cola vera. See kola
cold hands and feet, 66–67
colds, 96–99
colitis, 40
    inflammation, 48
    ulcerative (remedy), 48–49
Collinsonia canadensis.
        See stone root
coltsfoot, 269
comfrey, 209
    for wounds, 38
compress, 245
constipation
    causes of, 40–41
    remedy for, 41–42
corn silk, 270
couch grass, 270
coughs, 93–94
cramp bark, 271
cranesbill, 271
Crataegus oxyacantha, C. monogyna.
        See hawthorn
Culpeper, Nicholas, *134*
cuts, *209*
Cypripedium spp., 156
cystitis, 146–50
    remedies for, 148–49

dairy products
    age and, 24
    bowel and, 45
    bronchitis, 93
    catarrh and, 99
    eczema and, 203
    lactose intolerance, 27
    sinusitis and, 103
    ulcers and, 36–37
damiana, 271–72
dandelion, 272

dang shen, 216
Daucus carrota. See wild carrot
decoction technique, 238
dementia, 121–28
demulcents
    defined, 17
    digestive system, 25
    reproductive system, uterine, 160
    respiratory system, 100
    urinary system, 145
depression, 128–30
    menopause and, 163
dermatitis, 200–1
detoxification, 218
devil's claw, 272–73
diabetes, 231–33
    cystitis and, 147
diaphoretic, 17
diarrhea, 43–45
digestive system, 22–55
    aging and, 23–24
    herbal actions for, 24–26
    hypnotics and, 136
    maintenance of, 26–27
    medications and, 27
    NSAIDs and, 182
    process of, 23
    relaxants for, 136
    stimulants for, 109
    tonics for, 13
dill, 273
Dioscorea villosa. See wild yam
diuretics
    cardiovascular system, 57, 68,
        72
    defined, 17
    musculoskeletal system, 193
    urinary system, 145
diverticulitis, 47–48
douche, 245

echinacea, 9, 273
    gum disease and, 30–31
eczema, 200–3
effectors, 14
elder, 274
elecampane, 274
electrolyte loss, 44
Ellingwood, Finley, 58
emmenagogues
    defined, 17
    reproductive system, female, 158–59
emphysema, 94–95
endocrine system, 229–36
Ephedra sinica. See ma huang
Equisetum arvense. See horsetail
Eschscholzia california.
        See California poppy
esophagitis, 32–34
Euonymus atropurpureus. See wahoo
Eupatorium perfoliatum. See boneset
Euphrasia officinalis. See eyebright
expectorants
    defined, 17
    herbal, 82–83
    respiratory system, 81–82
eyebright, 275

facial care, 249–51
false unicorn root, 275
feet. *See* athlete's foot
fennel, 276
fenugreek, 276
feverfew, 277
fiber diets, 26
    digestive system and, 26, 47–48, 49
    diverticulitis and, 47, 48
    hemorrhoids, 51
figwort, 277
Filipendula ulmaria. See meadowsweet
flu. *See* influenza

Foeniculum vulgare. See fennel
fringe tree bark, 278
Fucus vesiculosus. See bladderwrack
Fünfgeld, E. W., 141

Gaia hypothesis, 214
galantamine, 123
Galanthus nevalis, 123
Galega officinalis. See goat's rue
Galium aparine. See cleavers
gallbladder, 53–54
    inflammation of, 54
gallstones
    gallbladder and, 54–55
    remedy for, 55
    symptoms of, 28
Ganoderma lucidum, 216
garlic, 9, 278–79
    fat-rich diets and, 62
gastritis, 34–35
gastroesophageal reflux, 32–34
gastrointestinal distress, 27
general adaptation syndrome (GAS),
    110, 120
gentian, 279
Gentiana lutea. See gentian
Geranium maculatum. See cranesbill
Gerard, John, 134
German Federal Ministry of Health, 58,
    284
ginger, 279–80
gingivitis, 31–32
ginkgo, 9, 280
    dementia, Alzheimer's and, 124–28
Ginkgo biloba. See ginkgo
ginseng and siberian ginseng, 9, 281
    studies on, 119–21
glands
    adrenal, 229–30
    thyroid, 233

Glycyrrhiza glabra. See licorice
goat's rue, 281
goldenrod, 281–82
goldenseal, 282
gout, 193–94
gravel root, 283
Green, James, 169, 171
grindelia, 283
guaiac, 283–84
Guaiacum officinale. See guaiac
guarana, 74
gum (application), 32

hair, 212
    care, 251–52
Hamamelis virginiana. See witch hazel
Handel, M., 58
Harpagophytum procumbens.
    See devil's claw
hawthorn, 9, 58–60, 284
headaches, 130–35
    migraine, 132–35
health care
    costs and constraints of, 3
    iatrogenic disease and, 20
    preventive, 3, 21
heart
    attack recovery, 69–70
    burn, 28, 33
    failure (congestive), 68–69
    stomach acid and, 33
heartsease (pansy), 285
hemorrhoids, 49–51
    inflammation of, 50
hepatics
    defined, 17
    digestive system, 26
herb impact assessment, 12–14
Herb Research Foundation, 8
herbal antirheumatics, 173–74

herbal medicine, 7–9
    actions, 15–18
    aesthetic criteria, 19
    antibiotic therapy and, 224
    choosing herbs for, 11–12
    dosage, 12
    economic criteria, 20
    efficacy of, 8, 10, 194
    elders and, 8–9, 90
    environmental criteria, 20
    holistic approach model for, 14–15
    preparation techniques, 237–52
    research of, 15
    surgery and, 4
    tonics in, 18
herbal tea, 238–40
    cough, 94
hiatal hernia
    reflux and, 33
    remedy for, 38
high blood pressure
    drugs and, 167
    herbs for lowering, 13, 62
Hildegard of Bingen, 2
Hobbs, Christopher, 215
holistic medicine, 3–7
    cancer and, 225–28
    herbs and, 11–12
    immune system and, 225–26
    nervous system and, 113
    vs. allopathic, 5
hops, 285
horehound, 286
hormonal
    modulation, 217
    normalizers, 159
horse chestnut, 286
horsetail, 286–87
hot flashes, 163
huang-qi, 216

Humulus lupulus. See hops
Huperzia serrata, 123. *See also Qing Ceng Ta*
hydrangea, 287
Hydrangea arborescens. See hydrangea
Hydrastis canadensis. See goldenseal
Hylands, D. M., 133
Hypericum perforatum. See St. John's wort
hypertension
    arteriosclerosis and, 65
    dietary factors, 74–75
    menopause and, 163
    patient statistics, 70
    remedies for, 71–73
    Siberian ginseng and, 71
hyperthyroidism, 235–36
hypnotics, 106
    herbal, 135–38
    osteoarthritis, 187
hypotensives
    cardiovascular system, 57
    defined, 17
hypothyroidism, 234–35
hyssop, 287
Hyssopus officinalis. See hyssop

Iceland moss, 287–88
immune system, 213–28
    aging and, 213
    ecology and, 214–15
    herbal actions for, 215–18
    illnesses in, 220
    immune activation, 219–20
    surgery and, 226
indigestion, 38–40
infections
    douche for, 147
    fungal skin, 204
    herbal approach, 223
    tonic herbs for, 14
    urinary tract and, 147–48

influenza, 99–100
  remedy, 99
  Siberian ginseng and, 119
infusion technique, 239–40
insomnia. *See* sleep
intermittent claudication, 75–76
intestinal blockage, 28
Inula helenium. See elecampane
Irish moss, 288
irritable bowel syndrome
  gallbladder and, 54
  remedy for, 45–46
  symptoms of, 27
itching, 211

Jamaican dogwood, 288–89
juniper berries, 289
Juniperus communis. See juniper berries

kidney
  age and, 147
  detoxification, 218
  maintenance of, 145–46
  problems, 28
  role of, 143
  stones, 28, 150–53
kola, 289–90
Krameria triandra. See rhatany
Kuhn, Maggie, 105

Lactuca virosa. See wild lettuce
lady's mantle, 290
lady's slipper, 156
laryngitis, 100–1
Lavandula officinalis. See lavender
lavender, 290–91
  external application, 179
laxatives
  avoidance of, 18, 25–26, 27
  defined, 18

digestive system, 25–26
  herbs as, 25–26
  types, 41–42
Leonurus cardiaca. See motherwort
Leptandra virginica. See black root
Lewis, Walter H., 232
licorice, 291
life root, 292
Ligustrum lucidum, 216
linden blossom, 292
liver, 51–52
  age and, 24, 51
  cholesterol and, 61
  cirrhosis, 51–52
  detoxification, 25, 218
  disease of, 8
  herbal actions, 15, 16, 17, 52
  jaundice, 53
  tonics for, 14
lobelia, 292–93
  external application, 179
Lobelia inflata. See lobelia
London Migraine Clinic, 133
Longevity (magazine), 7, 8
Lovelock, James, 214
lungwort herb, 293
Lycopus virginicus. See bugleweed

ma huang, 85, 293–94
malabsorption, 43
  syndrome, 44
Marrubium vulgare. See horehound
marshmallow, 294
  reflux and, 33
Matricaria recutita. See chamomile
McCaleb, Rob, 8, 9
meadowsweet, 295
medicine
  absorption, 22, 36
  dosage, 12

herbal. *See* herbal medicine
holistic (concept of), 3–7
iatrogenic, 3, 20
preventive, 21
Melaleuca alternifolia. See tea tree
Melissa officinalis. See balm
Ménière's disease, 140
menopause, 157–58
Mentha piperita. See peppermint
Menyanthes trifoliata. See bogbean
milk products. *See* dairy products
milk thistle, 9, 295
Mitchella repens. See partridgeberry
Monet, Claude, 105
Moses, Grandma, 105
motherwort, 296
mouthwash (recipe), 30
mucous colitis, 45
mugwort, 296
mullein, 297
    external application, 179
musculoskeletal system, 172–96
    actions for, 173
    external applications, 177–81
    herbal anti-inflammatories, 174–76
    herbal anitrheumatics, 173–74
    hypnotics and, 136
    relaxants for, 107
    remedies, 177
    stimulants for, 109
    tonics, 14
mustard, 177, 180, 297–98
myocardial problems, 59
Myrica cerifera. See bayberry
myrrh, 180

Narcissus, 123
National Headache Foundation
    (tips list), 131–32
National Kidney Foundation, 144

nervines
    cardiovascular system, 72
    defined, 18
    digestive system, 26
    heart failure, 68
    relaxant, 107–8
    reproductive system, 159
    respiratory system, 82
    stimulant, 109
    tonic, 108
nervous system, 104–42
    aging and, 104–5
    herbal remedies and, 105–7
    hypnotics for, 136
    inflammation in, 130
    relaxants for, 18, 107–8
    stimulants for, 18, 109
    surgery and, 120
    tonics, 14, 18
nettle, 298
neuritis, 138
normalizers, 13–14
NSAIDs (nonsteroidal anti-inflammatory
    drugs), 181–82
nutritional supplements
    asthma, 86
    cirrhosis, 52
    cold hands/feet, 67
    depression, 130
    eczema, 203
    osteoporosis, 196
    peptic ulcer, 37
    reproductive system, 169
    teeth and gums, 32
    ulcerative colitis, 49

oats, 298–99
Ojeda, Linda, 160
operations. *See* surgery
Oregon grape, 299

osteoarthritis
  actions for, 173
  herbal therapy, 186
  meadowsweet and, 186
  nutritional factors, 187–88
  predisposing factors, 185
  remedies, 173–74, 187
osteoporosis, 194–96
  menopause and, 164

Panax spp. *See* ginseng
pancreas, 231–33
  age and, 24
  inflamed, symptoms of, 28
Parkinson's disease, 40, 122, 124
parsley, 299
partridgeberry, 300
pasqueflower, 300
Passiflora incarnata.
    See passionflower
passionflower, 300–301
peppermint, 301
peptic ulcers
  remedy for, 36
  symptoms of, 28
perimenopause, 157
peripheral neuropathy, 138–39
Petroselinum crispum. See parsley
Peumus boldo. See boldo
Physostigma venenosurn.
    See calabar bean
Pimpinella anisum. See aniseed
Piper methysticum. See kava
Piscidia erythrina. See Jamaican dogwood
Plantago major. See plantain
Plantago ovata. See psyllium
plantain, 302
  for wounds, 209
pleurisy root, 302
Populus tremuloides. See white poplar

postmenopause, 157
prickly ash, 302–3
prostate
  enlargement, 169–70
  prostatitis, 170–71
Prunus serotina. See wild cherry bark
psoriasis, 205–8
psyllium, 26, 41, 48
Pulmonaria officinalis. See lungwort herb
pulmonary system.
    See respiratory system, lower
pyorrhea, 31

Qing Ceng Ta, 123

red clover, 303
red sage, 303–4
  canker sores and, 30
  gum disease and, 31–32
reflux, 28, 32–34
relaxants, nervine, 107–8
reproductive system, 156–71
  female herbal remedies, 158–60
  female sexuality, 157–58
  hypnotics and, 136
  inflammation and, 165
  male herbal remedies, 168–69
  male sexuality, 166–67
  relaxants for, 136
  stimulants for, 109
  tonics, 14
respiratory system, 79–103
  detoxification, 218
  expectorants, 17, 82–83
  hypnotics for, 136
  lower, 81–82, 96–103
  relaxants for, 82
  stimulants for, 109
  tonics, 14, 83
  upper, 79–95

Rhamnus purshiana. See Cascara sagrada
rhatany, 32
rheumatism, 182–84
    rubs and poultices for, 178–81, 248
rheumatoid arthritis
    remedies, 190
    symptoms, 189
Rheum palmatum. See rhubarb root
rhubarb root, 304
rosemary, 304
Rosmarinus officinalis. See rosemary
rubefacients
    defined, 18
    osteoarthritis, 187
    rheumatoid arthritis, 190
Rumex crispus. See yellow dock
Russell, Bertrand, 105

St. John's wort, 304–5
    for burns and wounds, 223
    oil, 211
sage, 123
Salix spp. *See* willow
salmonella, 48
Salvia officinalis. See sage
Salvia officinalis var. *rubia. See* red sage
Sambucus nigra. See elder
Sanguinaria canadensis. See bloodroot
sarsaparilla, 305
sassafras, 180
saw palmetto, 305–6
scar formation, 211
Schizandra chinensis, 216
Selye, Hans, 96
Scrophularia nodosa. See figwort
Scutellaria laterifolia. See skullcap
Senecio aureus. See life root
senna, 11, 306
Serenoa serrulata. See saw palmetto
Shaw, George Bernard, 105

shepherd's purse, 306
shigella, 48
shingles, 139–40
sinusitis, 101–3
skin, 197–211
    aging and, 198–99
    applications, 177–80
    detoxification, 218
    dry, 200
    eczema, 200–203
    first aid for, 208–10
    functions of, 197–98
    herbal actions for, 199–200
    hypnotics for, 136
    inflammation, 200–1
    relaxants for, 108
    stimulants for, 109
    surgery of, 211
    tonics, 14
skullcap, 307
sleep
    herbs for, 9
    insomnia, 135–38
    menopause and, 163
    pain and, 191
slippery elm, 307
Smilax officinalis. See sarsaparilla
Solidago virgaurea. See goldenrod
spastic colon, 45
Stellaria media. See chickweed
stimulants, 109
    nervine, 108
stomach
    acid, 32–33
    age and, 24
    flu, 28
    gas, 27
    gastritis, 34–35
    NSAIDs and, 181–82
    See also ulcers

stone root, 307–8
stress
    adaptogens and, 15, 118–21
    canker sores and, 30
    defined, 148
    digestion and, 27
    gastritis and, 34
    heart disease and, 63–64
    herbs for, 9, 15
    management of, 112–21
    physiological responses to, 111
    psychological responses to, 111–12
    from surgery, 120
sunburn, 211
suppositories, 248–49
surgery
    postoperative care, 120
    scar formation, 211
    symptomatic discomfort, 224
sweet violet, 308
Symphytum officinale. See comfrey

Tanacetum parthenium. See feverfew
Taraxacum officinale. See dandelion
teeth, 31–32
tendinitis, 191–92
therapeutic ecology, 4–5, 6, 10, 11
thuja, 308–9
Thuja occidentalis. See thuja
thyme, 309
Thymus vulgaris. See thyme
Tilia europea. See linden blossom
tinctures, 240–41
tinea, 204
tinnitus, 140–42
tea tree, 309–10
tonics
    affinity to body, 18
    bitter, 16, 216–17
    cardiac, 81

defined, 12–13, 18
    nervine, 108
    respiratory system, 83
    system, 13–14
    uterine, 160
Trifolium pratense. See red clover
Trigonella foenumgraecum. See fenugreek
Trillium spp., 156
tumors
    garlic and, 9
    immune system and, 220
Turnera diffusa. See damiana
Tussilago farfara. See coltsfoot

ulcers
    canker sores and, 30–31
    drugs and, 27
    herbs for, 18
    inflammation and, 189
    peptic, 28, 35–37
Ulmus fulva. See slippery elm
urinary system, 143–55
    age and, 143
    diuretics, 17, 144–45
    hypnotics and, 136
    inflammation in, 146
    maintenance of, 145–46
    relaxants for, 136
    stimulants for, 109
    tonics, 14
    urination, 153–54
uterine fibroids, 161–62
Urtica dioica. See nettle

vaginitis, 165
valerian, 9, 310–11
Valeriana officinalis. See valerian
Valium, 33
    reflux and, 33
varicose veins, 76–78

vascular tonics, 57

Verbascum thapsus. See mullein

Verbena officinalis. See vervain

vervain, 311

Viburnum opulus. See cramp bark

Viburnum prunifolium. See black haw

Viola odorata. See sweet violet

Viola tricolor. See heartsease (pansy)

Vitex agnus-castus. See chasteberry

vulneraries

   defined, 18

   digestive system, 36, 38, 48

   skin, 109

wahoo, 311

water retention, 154–55

   hypertension and, 72

Weiss, Dr., 44

white mustard, 180

white poplar, 312

wild carrot, 312

wild cherry bark, 312–13

wild indigo, 313

wild lettuce, 313–14

wild yam, 314

willow, 314

witch hazel, 315

Withania somonifera. See ashwaganda

wood betony, 315

World Health Organization, 3, 4

   cerebral aging and, 128

   electrolyte formula, 45

   holistic medicine views, 3–7

wu-wei-zi, 216

yarrow, 315–16

yellow dock, 316

Zanthoxylum americanum.

   See prickly ash

Zea mays. See corn silk

Zingiber officinale. See ginger

Books of Related Interest

Medical Herbalism
The Science and Practice of Herbal Medicine
by David Hoffmann

The Herbal Handbook
A User's Guide to Medical Herbalism
by David Hoffmann

An Herbal Guide to Stress Relief
Gentle Remedies and Techniques for Healing
and Calming the Nervous System
by David Hoffmann

The Estrogen Alternative
A Guide to Natural Hormonal Balance
by Raquel Martin and Judi Gerstung, D.C.

The Natural Testosterone Plan
For Sexual Health and Energy
by Stephen Harrod Buhner

Adaptogens
Herbs for Strength, Stamina, and Stress Relief
by David Winston and Steven Maimes

The Book of Ginseng
And Other Chinese Herbs for Vitality
by Stephen Fulder, Ph.D.

Natural Therapies for Emphysema and COPD
Relief and Healing for Chronic Pulmonary Disorders
by Robert J. Green Jr., ND

Inner Traditions • Bear & Company
P.O. Box 388
Rochester, VT 05767
1–800–246–8648
www.InnerTraditions.com

Or contact your local bookseller